D0603762

Food Porn Daily

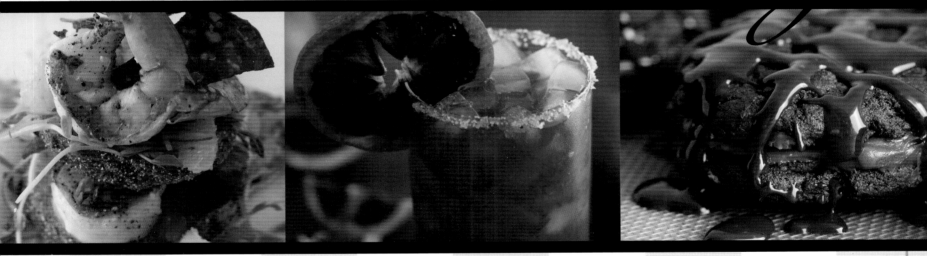

THE COOKBOOK

Food Porn Daily

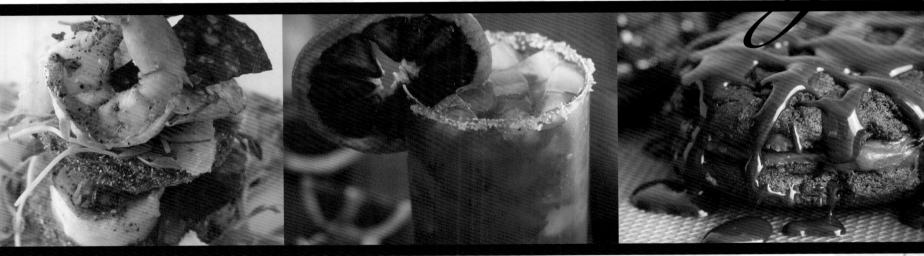

THE COOKBOOK

AMANDA SIMPSON

© 2010 Amanda Simpson

All rights reserved.

No part of this book may be reproduced in any form whatsoever, whether by graphic, visual, electronic, film, microfilm, tape recording, or any other means, without prior written permission of the publisher, except in the case of brief passages embodied in critical reviews and articles.

ISBN 13: 978-1-59955-399-3

Published by Sweetwater Books, an imprint of Cedar Fort, Inc., 2373 W. 700 S., Springville, UT 84663
Distributed by Cedar Fort, Inc., www.cedarfort.com

LIBRARY OF CONGRESS CATALOGING-IN-PUBLICATION DATA

Simpson, Amanda, 1980-
 Food porn daily / Amanda Simpson.
    p. cm.
 ISBN 978-1-59955-399-3
 1. Cookery. I. Title.

 TX714.S5854 2010
 641.5--dc22

2010020588

Cover and page design by Tanya Quinlan
Cover design © 2010 by Lyle Mortimer
Edited by Megan E. Welton

Printed in China

10 9 8 7 6 5 4 3 2 1

Printed on acid-free paper

For Tyler . . .

With your endless support, love, and humor, anything is possible.
I love you.

The Food Porn Definition

To some, food porn is defined as high-fat, artery-clogging food, dripping with grease. To others, it refers to the flirtatious presentation style or overt sexuality of a cooking show host. Neither of these are definitions that we at FoodPornDaily embrace. As Bill Buford notes in his article called "TV Dinners," which he wrote for *The New Yorker*, "The point [of Food Porn] is to get very close to what you are filming, so close that you can see an ingredient's 'pores' (you should believe the dish is in your living room), which then triggers some kind of Neanderthal reflex. If you're flicking from channel to channel and come upon food that has been shot in this way, you will be hardwired as a human being to stop, look, and bring it back to your cave."

Mr. Buford's statement most closely resembles our definition of food porn. To us, food porn is a high-resolution, close-up image of any food that gets your salivary glands flowing, whether a huge, juicy cheeseburger or a healthy-yet-flavorful piece of grilled fish. Calories play no role in our definition. On FoodPornDaily.com, our motto is "Click, Drool, Repeat." Perhaps for the book, we should change that to "Flip, Drool, Repeat," or even better, "Flip, Drool, Cook, Eat, Repeat."

About FoodPornDaily.com

After tinkering with the idea of starting a food porn site for almost a year, FoodPornDaily.com was released to the public in June 2008 with the goal of providing at least one delicious, high-resolution food photo a day. We've been astounded and amazed at the wonderful reception FPD has received since its release, garnering tens of millions of views in the first two years alone. Every day, we receive dozens of requests for the recipes of the food featured on the site. This cookbook is our response to those requests.

Contents

Introduction

The recipes that appear in this book are meant to be building blocks so that you can create your own dishes as well as replicate those that I have created. Use the recipes as a starting point. For example, if you taste a sauce and think it could use more acid, don't be afraid to add that extra squeeze of lemon juice or if you love the crust for the halibut, don't be afraid to try it on another type of protein. Recipes are simply guidelines. In my opinion, there is no definitive right or wrong way to create a dish so long as the outcome is a tasty, satisfying experience.

ON SEASONING:

The most fundamental element to good-tasting food is proper seasoning. Without enough salt, food that would otherwise be tasty seems dull and flavorless. On the other hand, food that has been over-salted is downright inedible. The best way to season food is to taste the dish first, add small amounts of salt (and frequently freshly cracked black pepper), stir, and then taste again. Continue tasting and adding small dashes of seasoning until your mouth tells you that the food is well-seasoned. Different people like different levels of seasoning, so what I may consider well-seasoned may be either over- or under-seasoned to someone else. For this reason, in most recipes I will recommend you season the dish "to taste." The best you can do is cook the food to your liking and hope that those around you have similar tastes!

When seasoning water for pasta, boiled potatoes, or blanched vegetables, I almost always add handfuls of salt to the water in order to properly season the ingredients that will be boiled. On the other hand, when simmering a sauce or soup that will cook for hours and reduce the amount of liquid, I always under-season in the beginning. As the liquid evaporates, the salt content in the dish will intensify. When making desserts and sweets, it's also important to add a small amount of salt. As a natural flavor enhancer, both sweet and savory dishes will benefit from the addition of salt.

ON PREHEATING:

A fatal error that novice cooks often make is throwing ingredients into a cold pan or oven and expecting good results. Preheating is an essential step to good caramelizing and for anything from searing meat to sautéing mushrooms. This is due to the Maillard reaction (also called the browning reaction), which is a chemical reaction that takes place between the amino acids and natural sugars present in foods, creating a "meaty" flavor and a caramel color—both of which enhance the taste of most foods. This reaction most frequently occurs between 300 and 500 degrees Fahrenheit, making it essential to start with a hot pan. If you put a steak into a cold pan, it will be overcooked on the inside by the time the caramelizing occurs on the outside.

Cooking bacon is my one exception to this rule. When cooking bacon, add it to a cold pan and cook it over medium to medium-low heat for best results. The fat will render out slowly and leave a flat, crisp, perfectly cooked piece of bacon rather than a curled-up, spottily cooked specimen.

Throughout these recipes, I direct the reader to heat the oil until it ripples. This refers to the point just before the oil will begin to smoke. The heat beneath the pan is high enough that it sends small waves through the oil. As soon as you can see the ripples, you can be certain the pan is hot enough to sear the food well.

ON FRYING:

Always be very cautious when frying. Once the oil reaches its smoke point (also known as flash point) combustion can occur, which means you could easily have an oil fire on your hands. The smoke point for canola oil (expeller pressed) is 464 degrees Fahrenheit, refined safflower oil is 450 degrees, and refined peanut oil is also 450 degrees. These are my three preferred types of oil for deep frying due to their high smoke points. It's worth mentioning—although you likely already know this—that adding water to an oil fire will worsen the fire; doing so causes the oil and fire to splash and sputter out of the pot and spread around the kitchen. When frying, always keep a watchful eye on the oil temperature and keep a fire extinguisher within reach (just in case).

When deep frying, never fill the pot more than halfway full. The oil will bubble profusely and expand when whatever you're frying is added. Also, use caution when placing items with high-water content into hot oil because these will also cause the oil to splatter viciously when first added.

Modern deep fryers virtually eliminate the dangers of frying on the stove top by self-regulating the temperature of the oil and by keeping the heating element on the inside of the device so that if oil spills over the edge of the deep-fryer, it will not touch the heating element and catch on fire. By using a device manufactured especially for deep frying or by keeping a watchful eye on the temperature of the oil when deep frying on the stove, there is no reason to be afraid of cooking in oil or enjoying the occasional deep-fried treat.

ON MEASURING FLOUR:

When cooking savory dishes, most of the time you don't need to be absolutely precise in your measurements. Actually, cooking using your senses generally produces the best results. When it comes to baking, though, precise measuring is much more important. When you measure flour for a recipe, always use a spoon to scoop the flour into the measuring cup, loosely mounding it over the rim and then swiping the flat back side of a knife over it to level the ingredients without compacting the flour. Flour scooped directly with the required measuring cup will contain a much denser amount than if you had spooned it into the cup. This is why professional bakers often weigh their ingredients rather than using measuring cups. I am not a professional baker, so all of the measurements in this book are listed by cups.

SPECIALIZED INGREDIENTS:

While I mainly try to use ingredients that are available to most people in the average grocery store, there are several specialty ingredients that appear throughout the book. For those ingredients, refer to the sources section at the back of the book. Ingredients that were once nearly impossible to find can now be delivered to your door via some of the amazing gourmet food sources on the Internet.

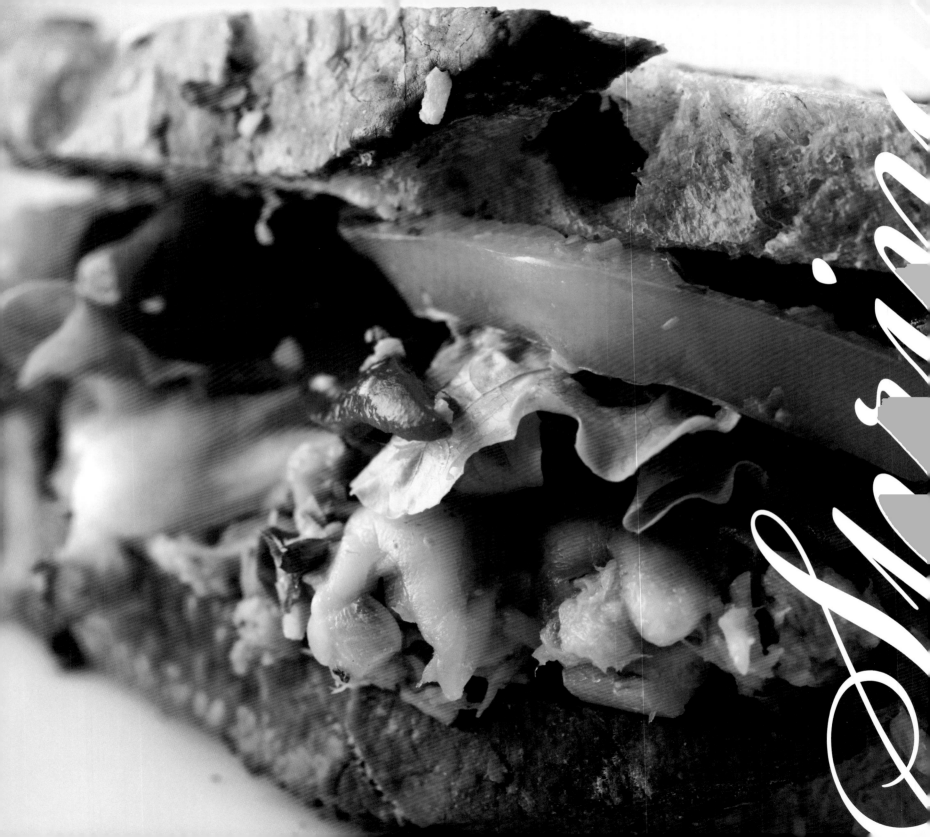

Chorizo Bistro Salad

with Caramelized Cremini Mushrooms,
Poached Egg and Sherry Vinaigrette

One of my all-time favorite salads is made with fresh frisee, lardons of bacon, and a poached egg with a basic vinaigrette. For this salad we've replaced the bacon with browned chorizo, added sautéed cremini mushrooms, and made the vinaigrette with sherry vinegar. If you can't find frisee, feel free to substitute your greens of choice.

Vinaigrette:

3 Tbsp.	sherry vinegar
1 Tbsp.	Dijon mustard
¼ tsp.	kosher salt, plus extra
¼ tsp.	freshly cracked black pepper, plus extra
6 Tbsp.	canola or safflower oil

1 tsp.	canola oil
½ lb.	fresh chorizo sausage
12	cremini mushrooms, quartered
6	cups frisee
	shaved Parmesan cheese

Poached Eggs:

1 Tbsp.	distilled white vinegar
4	eggs

SALAD & VINAIGRETTE

Prepare vinaigrette: Whisk together first 4 ingredients in a small mixing bowl. While whisking continuously, slowly drizzle oil into sherry-vinegar mixture for an emulsified vinaigrette. Set dressing aside and allow flavors to develop for at least 20 minutes.

Heat 1 teaspoon canola oil in a saucepan over medium-high heat for 2 to 3 minutes or until oil ripples with heat. Once pan is heated, brown chorizo and cook through. Remove from pan and drain on a paper towel.

Drain all but 1 tablespoon of fat from pan and return to heat. Reduce heat to medium and add cremini mushrooms. Sprinkle with kosher salt and freshly cracked black pepper. Sauté mushrooms over medium heat for about 10 minutes until caramelized and cooked through, stirring occasionally to ensure even cooking. (*Note: Do not stir constantly—the mushrooms will not be able to caramelize if they are continuously disturbed.*) Remove from heat and set aside.

Toss frisee with vinaigrette to coat. Adjust seasonings to taste to taste with kosher salt and freshly cracked black pepper.

Divide frisee among 4 plates or bowls. Sprinkle equal amounts of browned chorizo and sautéed mushrooms over each salad. Place one poached egg in the center of each salad and garnish with a few pieces of shaved Parmesan. Sprinkle with freshly cracked black pepper, if desired.

POACHED EGGS

In a large saucepan bring approximately 3 inches of water to a simmer over medium heat and add vinegar. Do not allow the water boil—adjust heat as necessary to maintain a simmer.

Crack 1 egg into a small cup or bowl. Gently slide egg from cup into simmering water. Repeat with remaining eggs. Cook for 2 to 3 minutes until egg whites have cooked through but yolks are still runny. Remove from water using a slotted spoon or spider. If using immediately, drain egg briefly on a paper towel.

Poached eggs can be made up to 1 day in advance and stored in ice-cold water in the refrigerator. To reheat, simply slip them into simmering water for about 30 seconds.

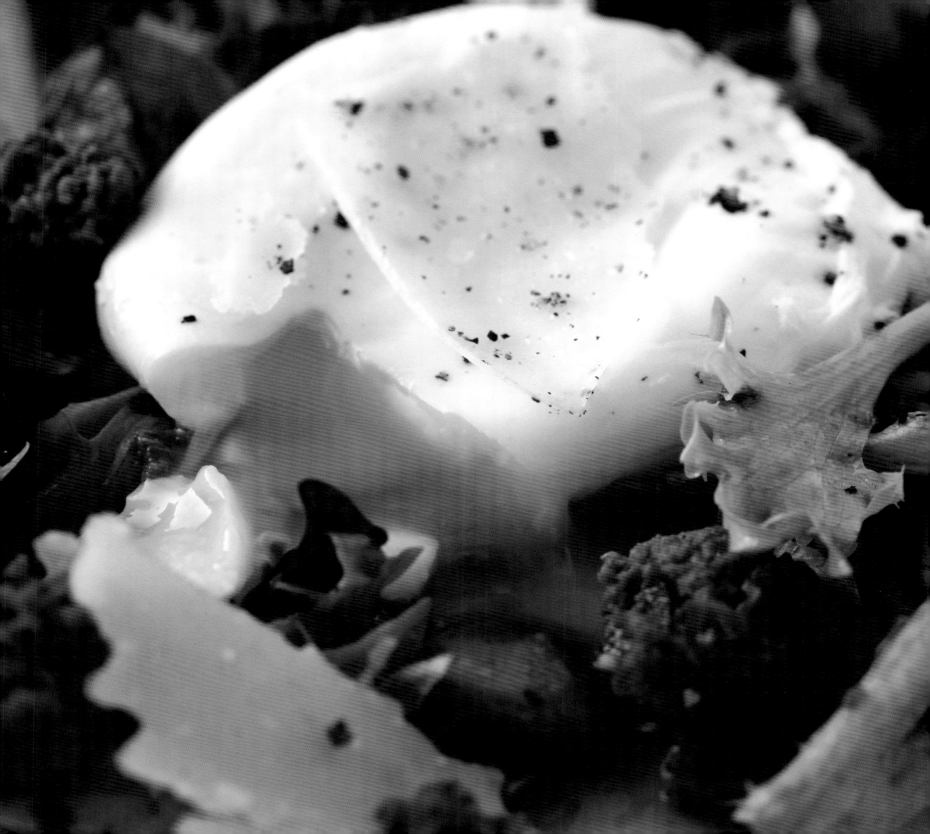

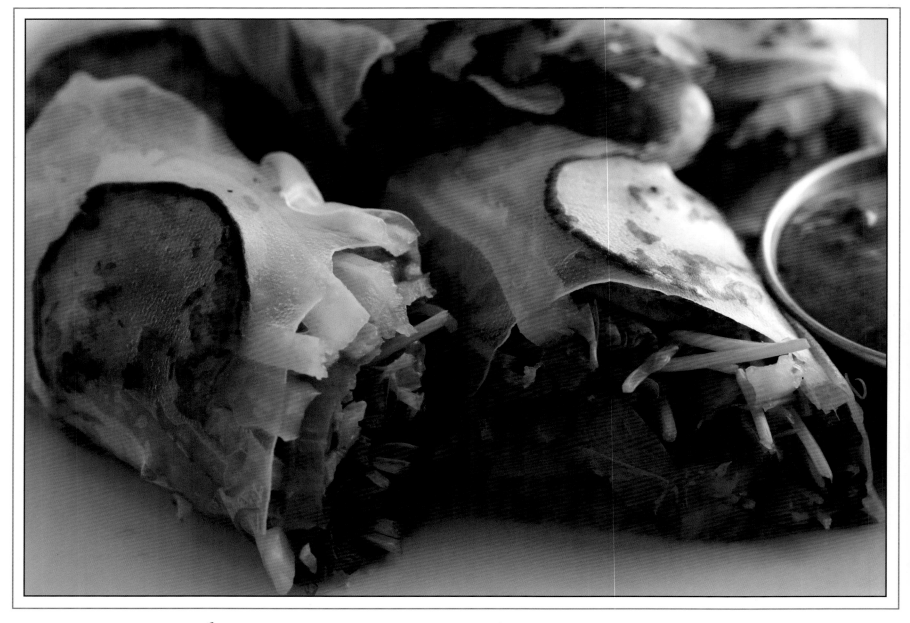

Shrimp Confit Fennel Spring Rolls

with Fig Vinaigrette Dipping Sauce

Preserved lemons have a very strong flavor. While two small strips of the lemon in each spring roll may not seem like much, the flavor will shine through in the finished product. Adding more of the preserved lemon will cover up the other flavors in the spring roll and overpower the dish.

Confit Fennel and Garlic

1 cup	extra virgin olive oil
1	large bulb fennel, cut in half and sliced ⅛-inch thick, reserving fronds
10	cloves raw garlic, peeled
1 tsp.	kosher salt
6	black peppercorns

Fig Vinaigrette

4	dried mission figs
¼ cup	white wine vinegar
¼ cup	extra virgin olive oil, from confit fennel and garlic
3 Tbsp.	water
¼ tsp.	kosher salt
¼ tsp.	freshly cracked black pepper
4	confit garlic cloves, can substitute roasted garlic
1 tsp.	minced preserved lemon, rinsed, peel only (see page 238)

Spring Rolls

6	jumbo shrimp, peeled and de-veined
	kosher salt
	freshly cracked black pepper
1 Tbsp.	butter
½ Tbsp.	canola oil
6	rice paper spring roll wrappers
½	preserved lemon, pulp removed, rinsed well, cut in a thin julienne
1	recipe confit fennel and garlic
3 cups	pea shoots or micro greens

Heat oil in small saucepan and heat over low heat until temperature reaches 150 degrees. Stir remaining ingredients into heated oil. Slowly confit the fennel and garlic until tender and fully cooked through—1 to 1½ hours—stirring occasionally. (*Note: Be sure to watch your temperature. You want to slowly and gently braise the fennel in oil; you don't want to fry it.*) Strain off oil using a fine mesh sieve. Allow fennel and garlic to strain in sieve for at least 30 minutes in order to drain off as much oil as possible. Reserve oil for future use by storing in an airtight container in the refrigerator for up to 1 week..

FIG VINAIGRETTE

Place all ingredients into a blender or food processor. Process until smooth. Adjust seasoning to taste with kosher salt and freshly cracked black pepper.

SPRING ROLLS

Preheat a sauté pan over medium-high heat. Season shrimp liberally with kosher salt and freshly cracked black pepper. Add butter and canola oil to preheated pan. Sear shrimp in melted butter over medium-high heat until just cooked through—about 2 minutes per side, 4 minutes total. Remove from heat. When cool enough to handle, slice shrimp down middle, where vein has been removed.

Fill a wide bowl or pot with 1 inch of water. The container should be wider than spring roll wrappers. Completely submerge 1 spring roll wrapper in water for 3 to 4 seconds. Remove from water and lay flat on a clean surface. Place two shrimp halves, seared-side facing down, in a row down center of spring roll wrapper, leaving about 1½ inches of space to both left and right of shrimp. Top shrimp with two thin strips of preserved lemon. Evenly spread ⅙ of the confit fennel mixture over shrimp and follow with about ½ cup of pea shoots.

Fold outer left and right edges in over filling. Gently lift the edge of the wrapper closest to you (at the bottom) and roll up tightly like a burrito. The spring roll wrapper will stick to itself, creating a seal without needing any assistance. Try to roll spring rolls as tightly as possible without tearing wrappers. Repeat this process with remaining filling and wrappers.

Cut spring rolls in half at a diagonal and serve with fig vinaigrette dipping sauce.

Grilled Artichokes
with Thai Red Curry Beurre Blanc

Thai red curry paste is made from lemongrass, galangal, lime leaves, garlic, bird's eye chiles, and coriander seeds as well as several other ingredients. Because this recipe doesn't require much of the paste, I suggest purchasing pre-made red curry paste, which is commonly available in the Asian section of most grocery stores or at Asian markets. We prefer the Maesri brand red or panang curry paste.

GRILLED ARTICHOKES

Grilled Artichokes:

kosher salt

4   medium globe artichokes

2   lemons, cut in halves

canola or extra virgin olive oil for brushing

Thai Red Curry Beurre Blanc

See Page 243

Garnish:

finely chopped cilantro

Bring a large pot of water to a boil over high heat. Add liberal amount of kosher salt—about a handful—and the juice of 1½ lemons to water.

When water is near boiling, prepare artichokes. Working with one artichoke at a time, snap off outermost leaves 3 or 4 layers deep. Using a sharpened chef's knife or a serrated blade, cut off the third of the artichoke opposite the stem. (*Note: The artichoke will oxidize rapidly once cut, so to prevent browning, rub the freshly cut parts of the artichoke with lemon half to coat in juice.*) Trim end of stem and then, using a vegetable peeler, peel off outer part of stem to remove stringy, fibrous layer. Coat entire stem in lemon juice. Set aside and repeat process with remaining artichokes.

Prepare a grill for medium-high heat.

Boil prepared artichokes until crisp-tender—15 to 20 minutes. Remove artichokes from water and let cool until able to handle. (*Note: Prepared artichokes may be stored in the refrigerator for up to 24 hours.*)

Cut artichokes in half lengthwise. Using a spoon, remove choke and any tough prickly or purple leaves from the middle of each half. Repeat this process with remaining artichokes. Once chokes have been removed, brush the artichokes on all sides with oil and sprinkle with kosher salt and freshly cracked black pepper.

Grill artichokes, cut-side down, for 4 to 5 minutes until grill marks have been charred into artichokes. Flip and grill another 4 to 5 minutes. Remove from grill.

Place artichokes onto a serving platter, cut-side up, and pour red curry beurre blanc evenly over artichokes. Serve immediately. (*Note: If not serving immediately DO NOT plate the beurre blanc. The sauce will separate as it cools.*)

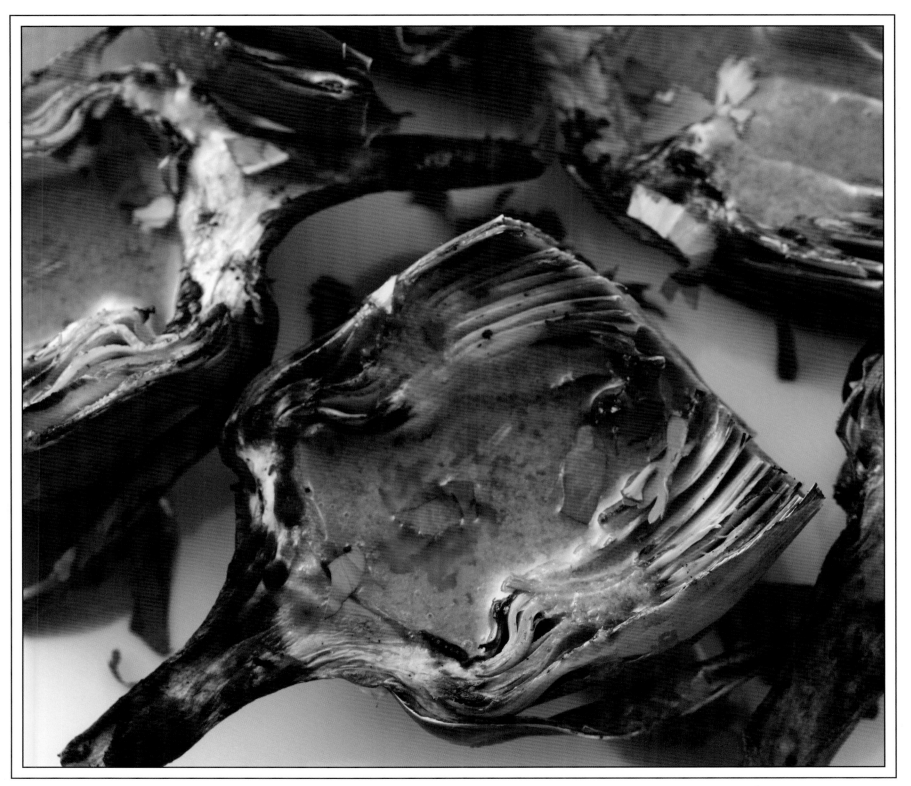

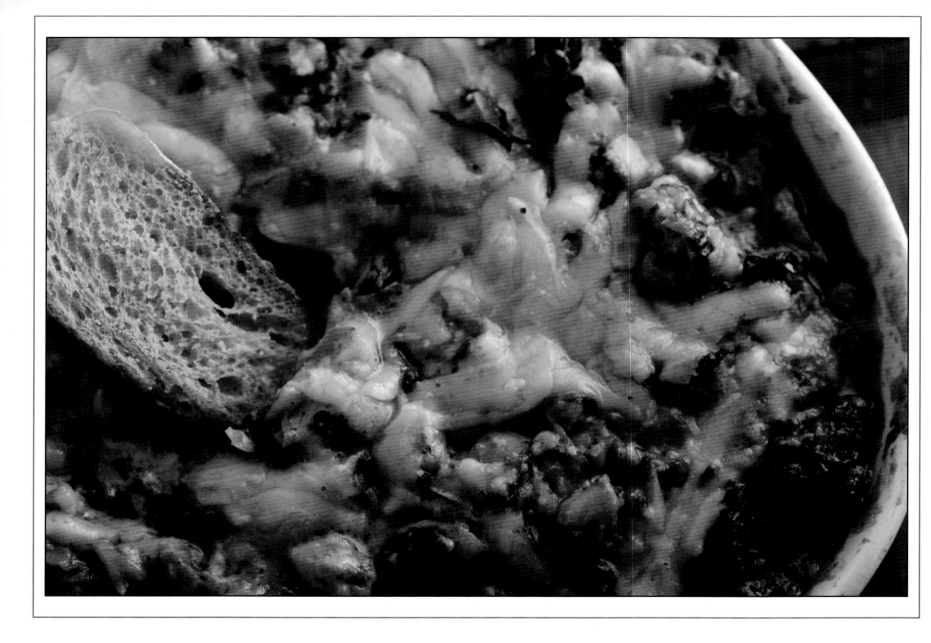

Artichoke Dip

with Crawfish, Mascarpone, and Arugula

Crawfish season begins in the early spring and runs through about June. If possible, purchase crawfish from the U.S. (mainly from Louisiana), and avoid those from China. U.S. crawfish farming is generally more environmentally-friendly.

½ Tbsp.	butter
1 (7-oz.)	bag pre-washed, trimmed arugula
6 oz.	frozen artichoke hearts
4	thick slices bacon, cooked and crumbled
	cloves from 1 bulb roasted garlic (see page 240)
8 oz.	mascarpone cheese, at room temperature
8 oz.	cooked crawfish tails, roughly chopped and toweled dry of any excess moisture
½ tsp.	granulated garlic
½ tsp.	onion powder
½ tsp.	freshly cracked black pepper, plus extra
½ tsp.	kosher salt, plus extra
1 tsp.	paprika
1	jalapeño, minced (optional)
1 tsp.	Worcestershire sauce
	zest from 1 lemon
	juice from ½ lemon
4 oz.	aged Gruyere, shredded and divided in half
¼ cup	freshly grated Parmigiano Reggiano cheese, divided in half
	toast points, tortilla chips, or toasted pita bread for dipping

Preheat oven to 425 degrees.

Bring a medium-sized pot of salted water to a boil over high heat.

While waiting for water to boil, preheat a sauté pan over medium heat for 2 minutes. Melt ½ tablespoon butter in preheated pan and add arugula. Season with a pinch of kosher salt and freshly cracked black pepper. Sauté arugula until completely wilted—usually 4 to 5 minutes—stirring often. Remove from heat and let cool for 10 minutes. Drain arugula with a towel, wringing out as much moisture as possible.

Add frozen artichoke hearts to a pot of boiling water and boil for 2 minutes. Drain artichoke hearts in a towel and blot out any excess moisture.

Combine arugula and artichoke hearts in a large mixing bowl with remaining ingredients (but only *half* of Gruyère and parmigiano cheese—the other half will be used for the topping). Using a rubber spatula, stir until well mixed and evenly distributed. Adjust seasoning to taste with kosher salt and freshly cracked black pepper.

Spoon dip into a baking dish and top with remaining cheese.

Bake dip at 425 degrees for 20 to 30 minutes or until cheese is bubbly and a light golden brown. Remove from oven and let cool for 10 minutes before serving.

Serve hot with toast points, pita bread, or tortilla chips for dipping.

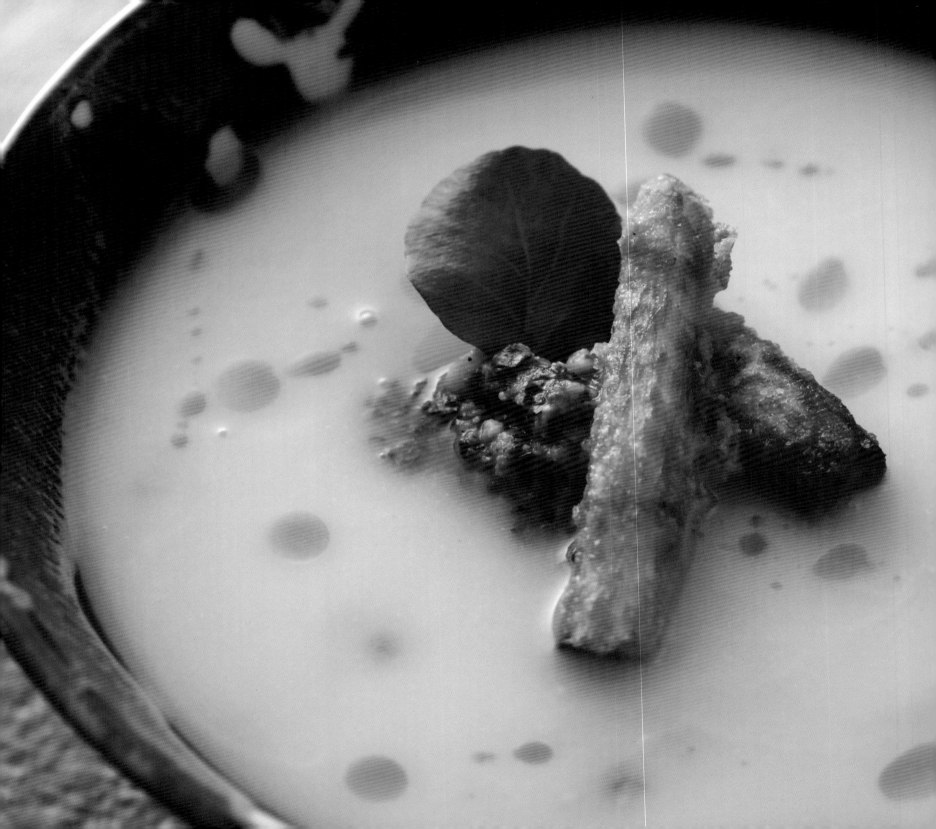

Truffled White Asparagus Soup

with Watercress Pesto

Although white asparagus has a delicate flavor, the truffle oil and watercress pesto in this dish are mild enough not to overwhelm or mask its delicateness. To keep this soup vegetarian, use vegetable stock or water rather than chicken stock. If you choose to use water, make sure you adjust the seasoning in the soup accordingly.

TRUFFLED WHITE ASPARAGUS SOUP

Soup:

1 Tbsp.	butter
1	yellow onion, peeled & diced
2	cloves garlic, minced
1½ lbs.	white asparagus, stalks trimmed and cut in 2-inch pieces, tips reserved
5 cups	chicken or vegetable stock, plus extra
3	sprigs thyme, tied together with butcher's twine
1	bay leaf
1½ tsp.	high-quality truffle oil, plus extra for garnishing
	juice from ½ lemon
	kosher salt
	freshly cracked black pepper

Batter:

⅓ cup	flour
1 tsp.	cornstarch
½ tsp.	baking soda
¼ tsp.	kosher salt
¼ tsp.	freshly cracked black pepper
½ cup	water
	peanut oil for frying

Watercress Pesto:

See Page 243

Preheat a medium-sized pot over medium heat.

Once pan is heated, melt butter and add diced onion. Sweat until translucent—about 10 minutes—stirring occasionally. Add garlic and white asparagus stalks and sauté for another 3 to 4 minutes, stirring frequently. Next, add chicken stock, thyme sprigs, and bay leaf. Raise heat to medium-high and bring to a boil. Reduce heat and simmer for 25 to 30 minutes or until asparagus stalks are quite tender.

Remove thyme sprigs and bay leaf. Transfer soup to blender. Carefully blend until very smooth. (*Note: If desired, strain the soup through a fine mesh sieve or chinois for an even silkier texture.*) Return soup to pot. If consistency of soup is thinner than desired, simply simmer until it thickens slightly; if it's thicker than desired, thin out with more stock. Stir in truffle oil and lemon juice. Season to taste with kosher salt and freshly cracked black pepper.

BATTER-FRIED ASPARAGUS TIPS

While soup is simmering, preheat peanut oil to 350 degrees in a deep fryer filled according to the manufacturer's directions.

In a mixing bowl, whisk together batter ingredients. Coat reserved asparagus tips in batter. Carefully add tips to hot oil and fry until golden—1 to 2 minutes. Remove from oil and drain on a paper towel.

To serve, ladle soup into a bowl and top with a dollop of watercress pesto, 2 or 3 fried asparagus tips, a watercress leaf, and a few drops of truffle oil.

Alaskan Halibut

with Mango-Banana Salsa and Brussels
Sprout Leaf and Macadamia Nut Salad

I suggest using a slightly under-ripe banana for this salsa because I like the little bit of the "green" flavor it adds in contrast to the sweet mango. If you only have yellow bananas on hand, it will still make for a great salsa.

BRUSSELS SPROUT LEAF & MACADAMIA NUT SALAD

Salad:

25	brussels sprouts
⅓ cup	salted macadamia nuts, roughly chopped
	kosher salt
	freshly cracked black pepper

Vinaigrette:

1 Tbsp.	freshly squeezed orange juice
	juice from 1 lime
1	clove garlic, minced
1 Tbsp.	minced fresh jalapeño
1 Tbsp.	fresh cilantro, minced
2 tsp.	Dijon mustard
¼ tsp.	kosher salt, plus extra
¼ tsp.	freshly cracked black pepper, plus extra
2 Tbsp.	canola oil, or other flavorless oil

Halibut:

½ cup	balsamic vinegar
3 Tbsp.	canola or flavorless peanut oil
4	(4 to 6 oz.) Alaskan Halibut filets, about 1½-inches thick
1 tsp.	flour, for dusting
	kosher salt
	freshly cracked white pepper (optional)

Mango-Banana Salsa:

See Page 235

Separate individual leaves of brussels sprouts into a large bowl, discarding cores and stems.

Whisk together all vinaigrette ingredients except oil in a separate mixing bowl. While whisking continuously, slowly drizzle oil into mixture to form an emulsified vinaigrette.

Pour vinaigrette over brussels sprout leaves. Toss to coat and season to taste with kosher salt and freshly cracked black pepper. Allow salad to sit in dressing for at least 20 minutes. Toss again and adjust seasonings to taste with kosher salt and pepper. Add macadamia nuts, toss, and serve immediately.

ALASKAN HALIBUT

Heat balsamic vinegar in small saucepan over medium heat until reduced by half. Remove from heat and set aside for plating.

Heat a large sauté pan with 3 tablespoons canola oil over medium-high heat until oil starts to ripple but before it starts to smoke.

While pan is heating, liberally season both sides of each fillet with kosher salt and white pepper. Lightly dust both sides of each filet with a small amount of flour and rub to evenly coat in an invisible layer. (*Note: The sole purpose of the flour is to help keep the fish from sticking to the pan and form a nice crust, not to add any flavor or visible coating. If you are on a restrictive diet, feel free to omit this step.*)

Once the pan is heated, sear fish, top-side down, over medium-high heat until a golden crust forms and the fish releases itself from the pan—about 5 minutes. (*Note: If fish filets stick to the pan when you attempt to flip them, they need to cook longer on that side.*) Turn filets and sear other side for another 5 minutes until just cooked through. Do not overcook.

Remove from heat. To serve, pile a bed of brussels sprout macadamia nut salad in the middle of each plate. Place 1 halibut filet on top of the salad. Spoon mango-banana salsa over fish and scatter around plate. Drizzle with balsamic vinegar reduction.

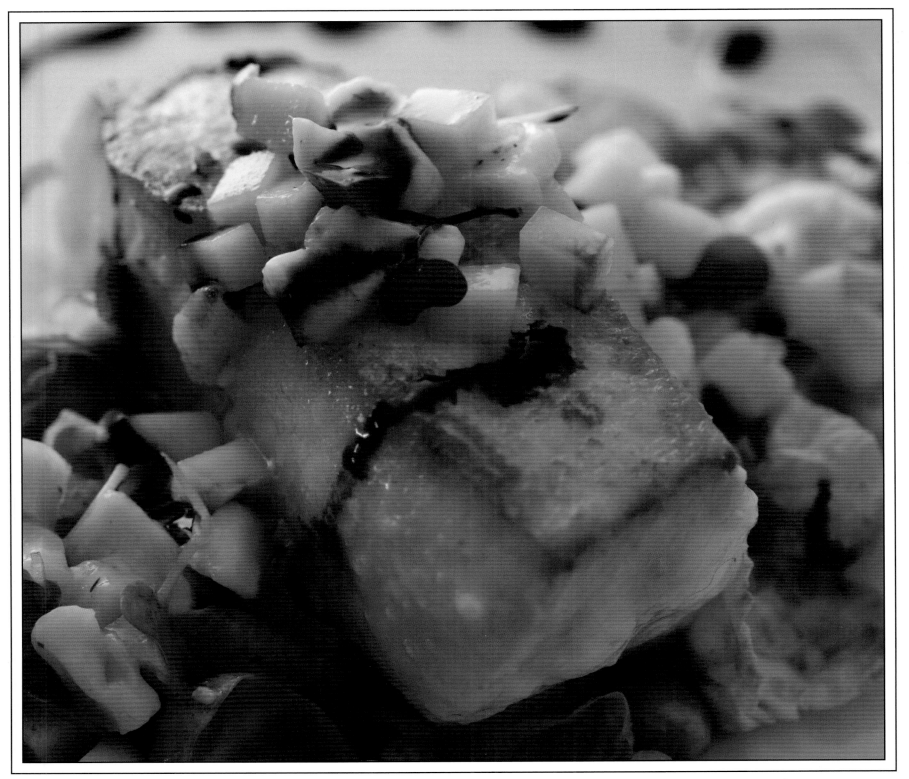

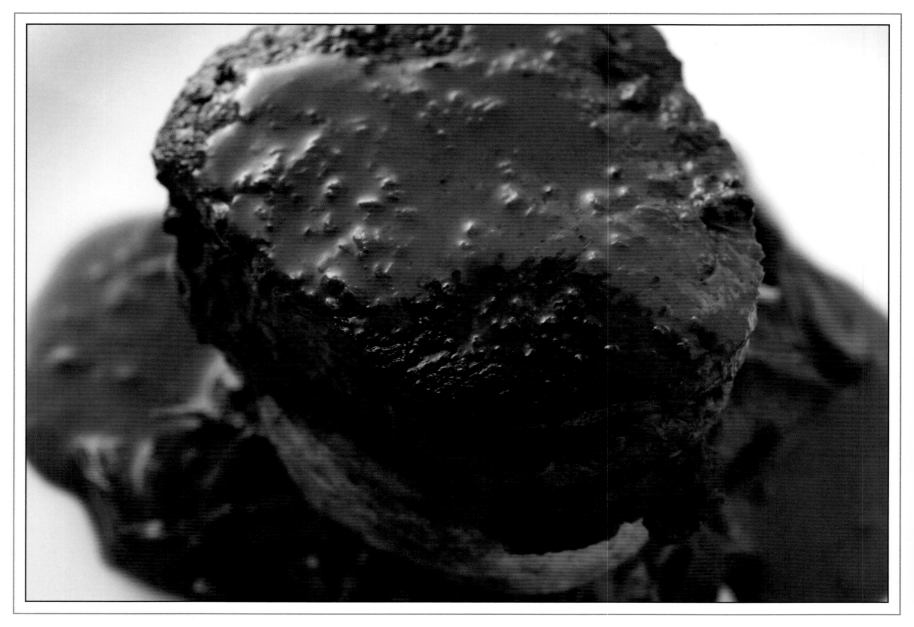

Buffalo Filet Mignon

with Creamy Horseradish-Red Wine Sauce, Buttery Roasted Potatoes, and Sautéed Spinach

Buffalo, also called bison, is a much healthier red meat option than beef due to its low fat and cholesterol content. Because the flavors are very similar, if you don't like buffalo or you can't find it in your area, you can always substitute beef for this recipe.

Creamy Red Wine and Horseradish Sauce

2 cups	Cabernet Sauvignon wine
2 cloves	garlic, peeled and smashed
1 tsp.	whole black peppercorns, smashed
3	sprigs thyme
2 Tbsp.	prepared horseradish
⅓ cup	heavy cream
	kosher salt
	freshly cracked black pepper

Buffalo Filet Mignon

4	buffalo filet mignon steaks (1¼-inches thick, approximately 6 oz. each)
	butcher's twine
	kosher salt
	freshly cracked black pepper
2 Tbsp.	canola oil
1 Tbsp.	butter

Sautéed Spinach

1 Tbsp.	butter
2 cloves	garlic, minced
1 lb.	baby spinach
	kosher salt
	freshly cracked black pepper

Buttery Roasted Potatoes

See Page 228

CREAMY RED WINE & HORSERADISH SAUCE

Add red wine, garlic, cracked whole peppercorns, and thyme sprigs to a saucepan and place over medium-high heat. Reduce wine until there is only about ¾ cup of liquid left. Strain wine reduction through a fine mesh sieve and return strained reduction to pan. Add horseradish and heavy cream to reduction, and simmer over medium heat until thickened slightly—about 5 minutes—stirring occasionally. Remove from heat and adjust seasoning to taste with kosher salt and freshly cracked black pepper.

BUFFALO FILET MINION

Preheat oven to 400 degrees.

Preheat a large sauté pan over medium-high heat until very hot—at least 3 minutes.

Tie each steak with two pieces of butcher's twine about ¼ inch from each end. (*Note: Tying the steaks will give them a more even shape and allow for more even cooking.*)

Season steaks liberally on all sides with kosher salt and freshly cracked black pepper.

Add canola oil and butter to preheated pan. Swirl pan to help butter melt and to prevent oil from burning. Once butter has melted and oil is hot, sear the filets over high heat until a nice brown crust forms—2 to 3 minutes. Flip and sear for another 2 to 3 minutes until other side has a similar crust.

Transfer filets to a baking sheet. Roast filets in preheated oven until internal temperature reaches 130 to 135 (medium rare)—typically 4 to 7 minutes, depending on thickness of filets. Do not overcook. Due to the extremely low fat content in buffalo, overcooking will lead to tough, dried-out meat.

Remove filets from oven and let rest for 5 minutes before removing twine.

To plate, place a scoop of sautéed spinach (see below) onto plate. Layer a slice of roasted Yukon gold potato onto spinach and top with filet. Spoon creamy red wine horseradish sauce over buffalo. Repeat with remaining filets and serve immediately.

SAUTÉED SPINACH

Preheat a 5-quart pot over medium heat for 3 minutes. Melt butter and sauté garlic for about 60 seconds, stirring constantly until garlic releases aroma. Add spinach to pan and sauté until wilted—3 to 5 minutes—tossing with tongs to assist in wilting process. Season to taste with kosher salt and freshly cracked black pepper. Serve immediately, draining off liquid before plating.

Shrimp and Roasted Garlic Cheese Grits

with Smoky Roasted Red Pepper Sauce

If you have any of the smoky roasted red pepper sauce leftover after this meal, save it and use it as a dipping sauce for grilled cheese the next day—it's *way* better than tomato soup.

ROASTED GARLIC CHEESE GRITS

Roasted Garlic Cheese Grits:

2 cups	whole milk
2 cups	water
1 tsp.	kosher salt, plus extra
½ tsp.	freshly cracked black pepper, plus extra
1 cup	yellow corn grits
	cloves from 1 bulb of roasted garlic, mashed (see page 240)
4 oz.	sharp cheddar cheese, shredded

Shrimp:

2 Tbsp.	extra virgin olive oil
1½ lbs.	jumbo shrimp, peeled and deveined
	kosher salt
	freshly cracked black pepper

Smoky Roasted Red Pepper Sauce:

See Page 241

Heat milk, water, kosher salt, and black pepper in a small pot over medium-high heat. Bring liquid almost to a boil, stirring occasionally and scraping bottom of the pot so milk doesn't burn. (*Note: just before the milk begins to boil, it will begin to froth up. You don't want the milk to reach a full boil, or the milk solids will separate, so keep a watchful eye on the pot!*) While whisking constantly to prevent clumping, add grits. Reduce heat to low and simmer, stirring frequently, until grits have absorbed liquid and are tender, about 15 minutes.

Add mashed roasted garlic and shredded cheddar cheese to pot. Stir until cheese melts and is fully incorporated. Adjust seasonings to taste with kosher salt and freshly cracked black pepper. (*Note: grits can handle a liberal amount of salt, but because the cheese is also salty, start with a small amount of salt and taste after each addition to reach the perfect seasoning levels. Under-seasoning is the reason most people don't like grits, so this is an important step, as seasoning always is.*) Serve immediately.

SHRIMP

Prepare grill for high heat and let grates get very hot.

Drizzle oil over peeled shrimp and toss to coat. Liberally season the shrimp with kosher salt and freshly cracked black pepper, tossing to coat.

Grill shrimp for 1½ to 2 minutes until charred, then flip and grill for another 1½ to 2 minutes until just cooked through and opaque in the middle. Remove from heat and serve immediately

ASSEMBLY

Divide grits evenly among 4 large bowls or plates. Top grits with smoky roasted red pepper sauce. Pile equal portions of grilled shrimp on top of sauce. If desired, garnish with a few thyme leaves for extra color. Makes 4 large portions.

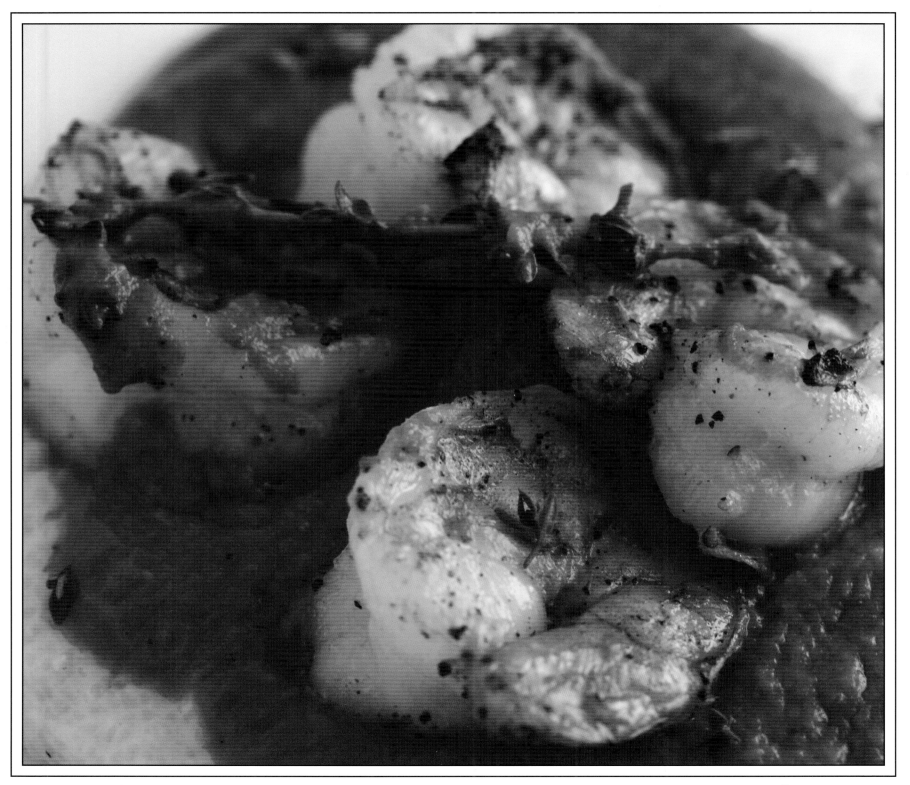

Jerk Marinated Grilled Tri-Tip

with Pineapple-Habanero Salsa

As soon as pineapple season starts in March, I jump at the chance to cooking and baking with it. Sweet, tangy ripe pineapple makes the perfect salsa to pair with this jerk marinated tri-tip.

JERK MARINATED GRILLED TRI-TIP

Marinade:

	juice from 1 lime
	juice from 1 tangerine
½ cup	fresh pineapple
5	green onions
4	garlic cloves, peeled, chopped
2 tsp.	dried thyme
1–2	habanero chile with seeds, stem removed
1½ tsp.	ground allspice
1	½-inch thick slice fresh ginger, peeled
1 tsp.	ground cinnamon
½ tsp.	ground nutmeg
¼ tsp.	ground cloves
2 tsp.	salt
2 tsp.	ground black pepper
2 tsp.	(packed) dark brown sugar
2 Tbsp.	dark rum

Tri-Tip

1	tri-tip roast (approximate 2 lbs.)
	kosher salt
	freshly cracked black pepper

Blend all marinade ingredients in a blender or food processor until smooth.

Pour marinade over tri-tip in a resealable plastic bag, tossing to coat. Seal bag, removing as much air as possible to emulate a vacuum seal. Marinate tri-tip in the refrigerator for 6 to 24 hours. Remove tri-tip from refrigerator 1 hour before grilling.

Prepare grill for medium-high heat. Remove tri-tip from marinade and season on all sides with kosher salt and freshly cracked black pepper. Grill over direct heat for approximately 30 minutes or until an instant-read digital meat thermometer reads 130 degrees for medium-rare. (*Note: The steak will continue to cook after it's removed from the grill during the resting process.*) If steak is a true triangular cut, flip the meat twice (every 10 minutes or so) to make sure that each side gets the same amount of cooking time. If steak is flatter, flip meat once after about 15 minutes. Remove tri-tip from grill and cover loosely in an aluminum foil tent. Let rest for at least 10 minutes before slicing thinly against the grain.

Continued on Next Page

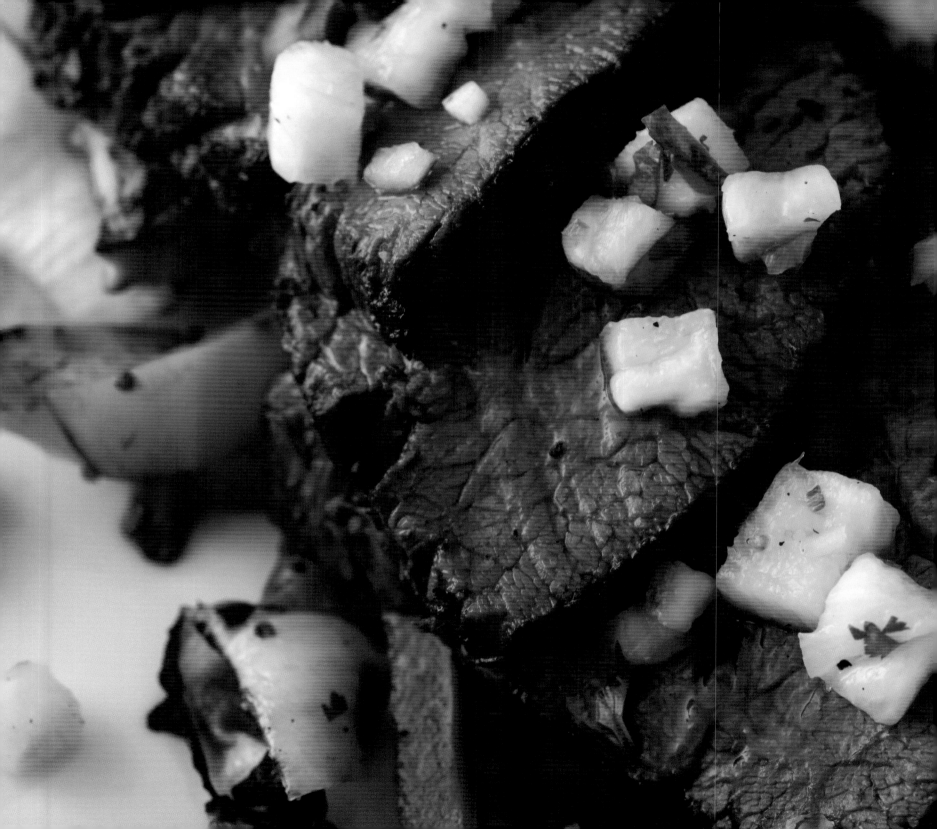

Grilled Peppers and Onions

1   yellow pepper, seeds and stem removed and cut in quarters

1   red pepper, seeds and stem removed and cut in quarters

1   sweet yellow onion, peeled and cut in ½-inch thick round slices

1 tsp.   canola oil, or other flavorless oil

1 tsp.   ground cumin

    kosher salt

    freshly cracked black pepper

2 Tbsp.   fresh cilantro, roughly chopped

    juice from ½ lime

Pineapple-Habanero Salsa

1 cup   fresh pineapple, diced into small cubes

1 tsp.   (or less) fresh habanero, seeds and veins removed, minced

2 Tbsp.   fresh cilantro

1   small clove garlic, minced

    juice from ½ lime

    kosher salt

    freshly cracked black pepper

Prepare grill for medium-high heat.

Toss the pepper quarters and onion slices with canola oil then evenly season all sides with ground cumin, kosher salt, and freshly cracked black pepper.

Grill seasoned peppers and onions over medium-high heat, with peppers lying outer skin-side down first, for 4 to 5 minutes until charred. Flip and grill for another 4 to 5 minutes. Remove from heat and let cool slightly. Slice peppers into strips (julienne) and cut onion rings in half and separate into strips. Toss onion strips and peppers with cilantro and lime juice. Adjust seasoning to taste with kosher salt and freshly cracked black pepper.

PINEAPPLE-HABANERO SALSA

Combine first 5 ingredients in a small bowl. Toss to evenly distribute and season with kosher salt and freshly cracked black pepper to taste. (*Note: Always use caution when handling habanero peppers. If you have sensitive skin, use glove.*)

Glazed Corned Beef

with Parsnip Cakes and Collard-Cabbage Slaw

Growing up, my dad would make corned beef, cabbage, and potatoes every St. Patrick's day. He would dance around singing "On Saint Paddy's Day night, on Saint Paddy's Day night . . . we'll all get together on Saint Paddy's Day night." It was a tradition that I loved and one that I still practice. Every year, I change up how I serve my corned beef and cabbage, but when March 17 rolls around, you can be sure I'm eating some version of this dish.

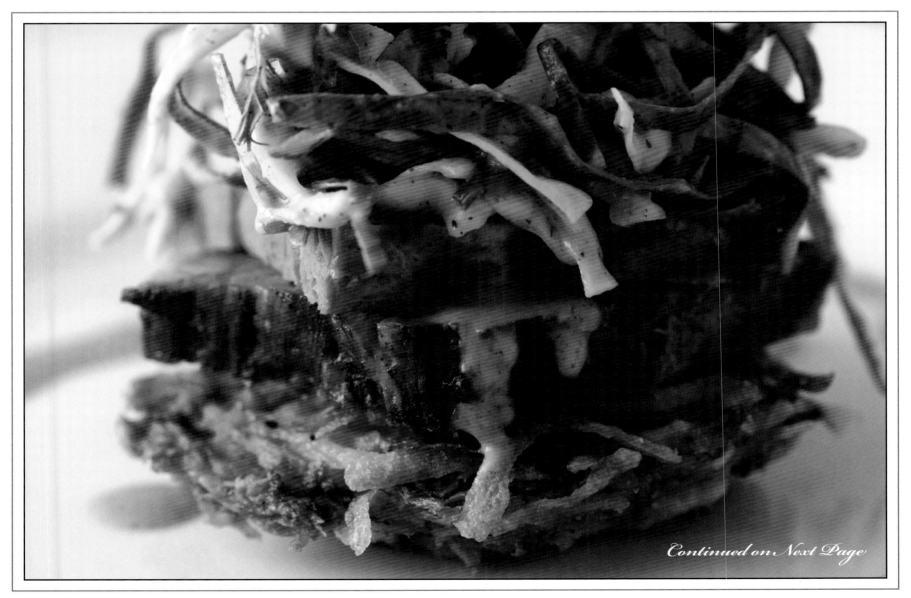

Continued on Next Page

Brine:

8 cups	water
1½ cups	coarse kosher salt
1 cup	(packed) brown sugar
1½ Tbsp	Insta Cure no. 1 (optional)
¼ cup	pickling spices
1 cup	ice

| 1 | (approximately. 6 lb). flat-cut beef brisket, trimmed with some fat remaining |

Corned Beef:

1	uncooked corned beef brisket, store-bought or homemade (see recipe above)
4	bay leaves
1 Tbsp.	coriander seeds
2	whole allspice
1	dried chile de Árbol
1	whole clove
1	whole star anise
1 Tbsp.	whole black peppercorns
1 tsp.	brown mustard seeds

For the glaze/sauce:

1 cup	stout beer
⅔ cup	spicy brown mustard
3 Tbsp.	honey
3 Tbsp.	heavy cream
1½ Tbsp.	sherry vinegar
	kosher salt
	freshly cracked black pepper

BRINE

While stirring continuously, heat all brine ingredients *except* ice in a large pot over high heat until all salt and sugar has been dissolved. Remove brine from heat and add ice. Cool to at least room temperature before submerging meat in the brine. Brine meat, refrigerated, for 4 days. Remove meat from brine and rinse before cooking.

Insta Cure No. 1 is the ingredient that will give your corned beef it's typical vibrant pink color. It is a compound of sodium nitrate and salt that is used when curing and smoking meats to prevent botulism. For this recipe, the meat is only in the brine for a short time and Insta Cure isn't necessary for food safety purposes. If you choose not to include the Insta Cure No. 1 in your brine, do not be concerned if your meat turns gray—it is a natural reaction to the brine. Insta Cure No. 1 can be purchased online from http://www.sausagemaker.com in 8-ounce, 1-pound, and 5-pound packages.

CORNED BEEF

Braise beef: Rinse off brined corned beef brisket, regardless of whether you brined your own. Be sure to discard any spices that may stick to the meat. Place corned beef into a large, wide stock pot and cover with 2 inches water. Add remaining brisket seasonings and bring to boil over high heat. Cover and reduce heat to medium-low. Simmer for about 2½ hours or until tender.

Preheat oven to 275 degrees.

Remove corned beef from water and drain on a plate for about 5 minutes. Place on an aluminum foil-lined sheet pan and brush all sides with mustard-stout glaze (see below). Cook corned beef at 275 degrees for 45 to 60 minutes until glaze has set and just begins turning golden. Remove from oven and let rest for 10 minutes before cutting. Slice thin against grain of meat.

GLAZE

In a large saucepan over medium-high heat, reduce 1 cup stout beer until only ½ cup remains. (*Note: It is important to use a large pan because the beer will foam up heavily during the reduction process.*)

Once beer has been reduced, add mustard and honey to beer reduction. Whisk to combine thoroughly. Reserve half of mustard mixture to use as a glaze for corned beef.

Add cream and vinegar to remaining mustard mixture, whisking until thoroughly combined.

Two-thirds of this sauce will be used for the slaw and the rest will be used as a garnish during plating.

Collard-Cabbage Slaw:

1	head green cabbage, finely shredded
2 cups	raw collard greens, finely shredded
3	green onions, thinly sliced
3 Tbsp.	fresh dill, minced
	kosher salt
	freshly cracked black pepper

Parsnip Cakes

2	large parsnips, peeled, grated, and wrung dry of any excess moisture
2	medium red potatoes, peeled, grated, and wrung dry of any excess moisture
3	cloves garlic, minced and mashed into a paste
1	egg, beaten
¼ tsp.	freshly cracked black pepper
½ tsp.	kosher salt, plus extra
	canola or peanut oil for frying

Combine all ingredients for slaw in a large bowl. Add two-thirds of the creamy mustard-stout sauce and toss to coat thoroughly. Season to taste with kosher salt and freshly cracked black pepper. Chill slaw in the refrigerator for at least 1 hour before serving to allow flavors to marry and collards and cabbage to wilt slightly. Remove from refrigerator right before serving, stir, and taste again. Adjust seasonings one more time, if desired, with more kosher salt and freshly cracked black pepper.

PARSNIP CAKES

In a large sauté pan over medium to medium-high heat, preheat approximately ¼-inch canola or peanut oil until hot but before it begins to smoke.

While oil is heating, prepare parsnip cakes for frying. Toss together all ingredients for parsnip cakes in a mixing bowl. Form parsnip mixture into four patties, wringing out any excess moisture as you go. (*Note: The parsnip cakes will be loose but will hold their shape once cooked partially.*) Place one patty at a time onto a metal spatula and carefully slide parsnip cake into the hot oil. Space cakes evenly around the pan so that none of them are touching. Allow patties to cook undisturbed until bottom is golden brown— usually 7 to 9 minutes. Carefully flip cakes until other side is golden—usually 7 to 8 more minutes. (*Note: If the cakes appear to be sticking to the pan, they are not ready to flip and need to be cooked longer.*) Remove from pan and drain on paper towels. Sprinkle lightly with kosher salt.

To serve, place one parsnip cake in the middle of a plate. Next, layer several slices of corned beef over the parsnip cake and top with a mound of slaw. Drizzle reserved creamy mustard-stout sauce around the plate. Repeat process three more times for a total of four servings.

Parsnips can be hard to grate, so be very careful if grating by hand. It's best to use a food processor with a grating attachment, if you have one.

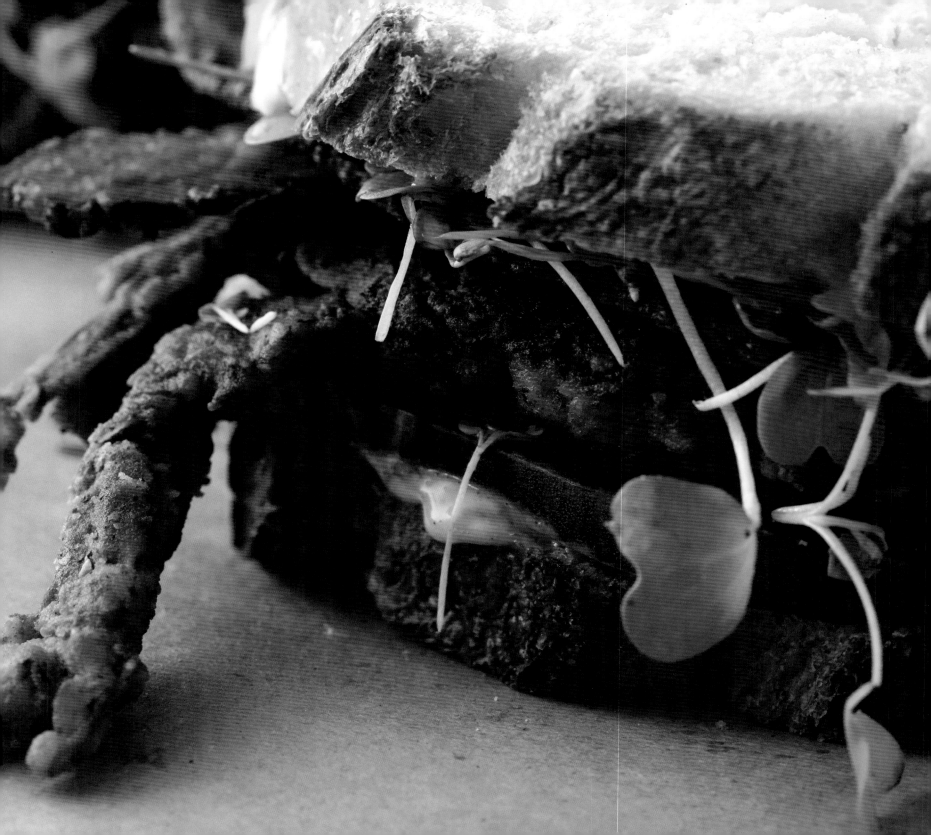

Soft Shell Crab BLT

In the Gulf of Mexico, soft shell crab season starts in early April and lasts through October. Because soft shell crabs are one of my favorite proteins, I start looking for them as soon as they become available so we can enjoy the season as long as possible.

SOFT SHELL CRAB BLT

Soft-Shell Crab:

1 cup	flour
2 tsp.	kosher salt
1 tsp.	sweet paprika
½ tsp.	freshly cracked black pepper
½ tsp.	granulated garlic
1 cup	buttermilk
4	soft shell crabs, cleaned (see note)
3 Tbsp.	butter
2 Tbsp.	canola or peanut oil

Sandwiches:

	Tarragon Aioli (see page 75).
8	slices of good sourdough bread, warmed in the oven
2	medium-sized ripe heirloom tomatoes, sliced
8 to 12	slices thick-cut bacon, cooked
	micro-greens, watercress, mache, spring mix or any lettuce you desire

Preheat a large sauté pan over medium to medium-high heat.

Whisk to combine first 5 ingredients for crab in a small bowl. Place buttermilk in a separate bowl for dipping. Coat each soft-shell crab, one at a time, in flour mixture first and then dip crab into buttermilk to coat completely. Dip crab back into flour mixture to coat once more and set aside. Repeat coating process with all crabs

Add butter and canola oil to preheated pan. Once butter has melted and oil is hot, arrange soft-shell crabs in pan, top-down. Sauté until golden—usually 4 to 5 minutes. Flip and continue sautéing for another 4 to 5 minutes until both sides are golden and crab is cooked through. If necessary, avoid overcrowding by cooking in batches. Remove crabs from pan and drain on paper towels.

Assemble sandwiches:

For each sandwich, smear tarragon aioli evenly over one side of two slices of oven-warmed bread. Layer tomato slices, 1 soft-shell crab, and 2 to 3 slices of bacon on top of one aioli-coated slice of bread, aioli-side down. Add a handful of micro greens (or your lettuce of choice) and top with remaining slice of bread, aioli-side down. Repeat this process three more times for a total of 4 sandwiches.

To clean soft shell crabs, begin by cutting off a ½-inch section from the crab around the eyes and mouth. To clean out the cavity, either gently squeeze directly behind the cut you made, or carefully swipe your finger inside of the incision and scrape out all of the "mustard" and guts. Next, lift up one of the pointed ends of the shell and remove and discard the gills. Repeat the process on the other side of the crab. Flip the crab over and cut off the little flap known as the "apron." Rinse the crabs and pat dry. Do not clean the crabs until ready for immediate use.

Lamb Kebab Pita Sandwiches

with Minted Black-Eyed Pea Hummus

The black-eyed peas in the hummus add a distinctly earthy flavor to the sandwich. Fortunately you will not need to use all of the hummus on the sandwiches and can devour the rest as a dip with any spare pita bread or tortilla chips.

LAMB KEBAB PITA SANDWICHES

Marinade:

	juice from 2 lemons
¼ cup	extra virgin olive oil
½ tsp.	chile powder
1 tsp.	granulated garlic
½ tsp.	granulated onion
½ tsp.	smoked paprika
¼ tsp.	ground cinnamon
1 tsp.	dried oregano
1 tsp.	kosher salt, plus extra
½ tsp.	freshly cracked black pepper, plus extra

Lamb Kebabs:

2 lbs.	boneless leg of lamb, cut into about 1½-inch cubes
	skewers (if wooden—soak in water for at least 1 hour)
	kosher salt
	freshly cracked black pepper

Pita Sandwiches:

4	whole pitas
	Minted Black-eyed Pea Hummus (see page 236)
	mache or any other greens you like
	sautéed onions and peppers
1	recipe Lamb Kebabs
4 oz.	crumbled feta

Whisk together all marinade ingredients in a small bowl. Pour marinade over lamb cubes in a resealable bag. Seal bag, removing as much air as possible to emulate a vacuum seal. Marinate, refrigerated, for at least 2 hours and up to 12 hours.

Prepare grill for high heat and preheat oven to 350 degrees.

Skewer marinated lamb cubes, leaving a ¼-inch space between each piece of meat.

Lightly sprinkle all sides of kebabs with kosher salt and freshly cracked black pepper. Grill over direct high heat for 2 minutes on all sides—8 minutes total. Remove from heat and let lamb cool for 5 minutes before removing from skewers.

Heat pitas in oven for 5 minutes or until warmed through and soft.

To assemble sandwiches, place a square piece of parchment or aluminum foil onto a cutting board and position one pita round halfway onto parchment paper or foil, leaving half of the pita overlapping onto the cutting board.

Smear hummus all over the top of one side of pita. Spread a handful of mache down the center of the pita. Layer sautéed onions and peppers and 4 to 5 cubes lamb over the mache. Sprinkle 1 ounce crumbled feta over the lamb. Bring the sides of the pita together to form a closed sandwich with gaping ends. Wrap the parchment or aluminum foil tightly around the sandwich, twisting the end of the paper or foil where the sandwich ends and tucking it under to hold it together. Repeat sandwich-making process three more times for a total of four sandwiches.

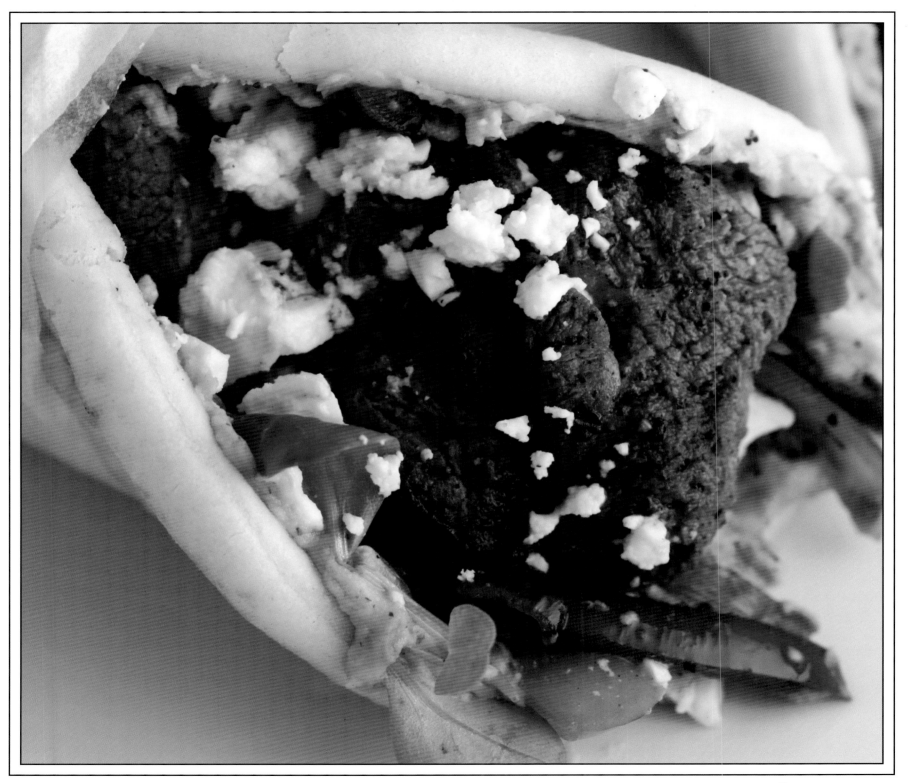

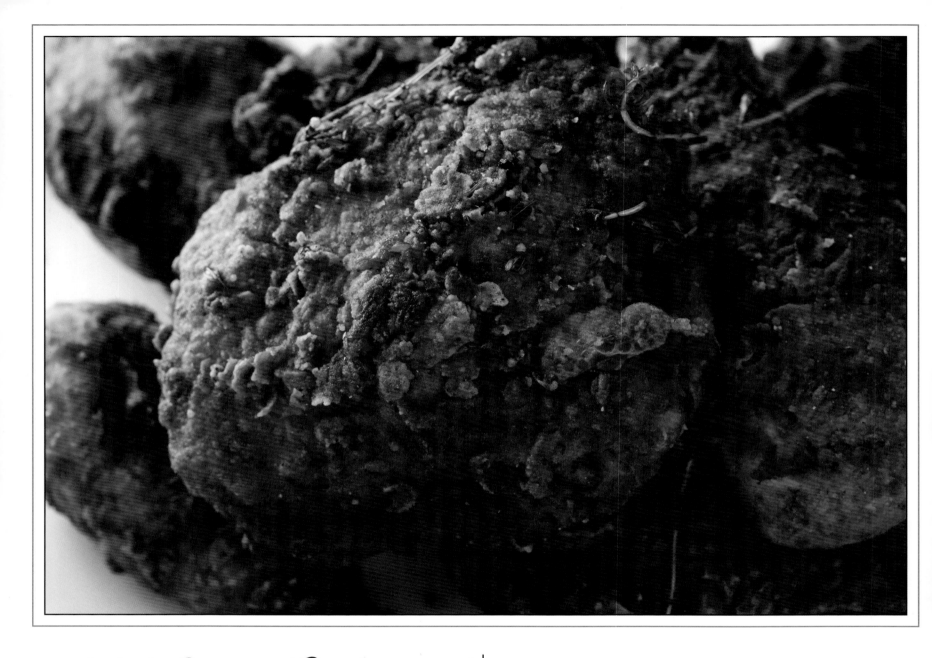

Herbed Buttermilk Marinated Fried Chicken

Garnished with Fried Herbs

I try to only make fried chicken for special occasions because I don't have the self-control not to devour a whole pile of it! Also, I'm not giving any side dishes for this meal because, really, what more do you need other than fried chicken?

HERBED BUTTERMILK MARINATED FRIED CHICKEN

Marinade:

1 quart	buttermilk
¼ cup	vinegary hot sauce, like Texas Pete or Crystal brand
6	sprigs fresh thyme
3	sprigs fresh rosemary
6	cloves garlic, peeled and mashed
6	sage leaves
1½ Tbsp.	kosher salt
½ Tbsp.	freshly cracked black pepper
½ tsp.	ground cayenne
4 lbs.	chicken parts, whatever you like— breast, wings, thighs, drumsticks

For dredging:

3 cups	flour
2½ Tbsp.	kosher salt
1 Tbsp.	freshly cracked black pepper
1 Tbsp.	(heaping) sweet paprika
1½ tsp.	ground cayenne
1 Tbsp.	granulated or powdered garlic

For frying:

12 cups	peanut oil

For garnish:

sprigs of thyme

fresh sage leaves

In a large mixing bowl, whisk together all marinade ingredients. Add chicken parts to marinade, pushing all the chicken beneath the surface of the liquid. Marinate for 12 to 24 hours, covered and refrigerated. (*Note: If you weren't able to be completely submerged in the marinade, toss the chicken 3 or 4 times while marinating so that everything has a chance to soak evenly.*)

Remove chicken from marinade and pat dry with paper towels, removing any pieces or garlic or herbs.

Strain leftover buttermilk marinade through a fine mesh sieve into a large bowl and discard solids. You will use remaining seasoned buttermilk to dredge chicken.

In a separate bowl, whisk together all dry ingredients for dredging until well mixed.

Line a sheet pan with parchment or wax paper.

Working with one piece of chicken at a time, first dredge dry chicken into flour mixture and toss to coat; second, dip into buttermilk and coat completely; finally, dredge chicken once again in flour to coat on all sides. Remove from flour and place on parchment-lined sheet pan. Repeat process with remaining chicken. (*Note: Arrange the coated chicken so that none of the pieces are touching one another on the sheet pan. If necessary use two lined sheet pans.*)

Chill chicken on sheet pans in the refrigerator for 1½ hours. Remove from refrigerator and let sit at room temperature for 20 minutes before frying.

Either fill a deep fryer with the peanut oil to fill line and set oil temperature to 320 degrees OR preheat oil in a large pot to 320 degrees. Use a candy/deep frying thermometer to constantly watch oil temperature. (*Note: It is important to maintain an oil temperature of about 320 degrees—anywhere from 315 to 325 will be fine. Frying at a temperature higher than 330 will cause the coating to burn before the chicken is cooked through. Frying at a much lower temperature will cause the chicken to be greasy and soggy by the time it's done. If your deep fryer does not allow you to change the temperature, only use it if the manufacturer's set temperature falls between 315 and 330.*)

Fry chicken in batches of all dark or white meat at a time. Do not overcrowd the pot or fryer—fry only 3 or 4 pieces at a time. Fry chicken until just cooked through—8 to 9 minutes for breasts and wings and 13 to 14 minutes for thighs and drumsticks—turning once, halfway through. Remove from heat and let drain on paper towels. Repeat frying process in batches with remaining chicken.

After removing final batch of chicken from oil, *carefully* add sprigs of fresh thyme and sage leaves to oil and fry for about 15 seconds. Remove with a spider and drain on paper towels. (*Note: Because of the high water content in herbs—especially thyme—the oil will splatter and pop furiously when the herbs are first added. Be very careful, because hot oil can cause serious burns.*)

To plate, stack chicken onto a platter and sprinkle with fried herbs. Serve immediately.

Grilled Ribeye

with Lime-Scented Quinoa and Roasted
Jalapeño Vinaigrette

Quinoa (pronounced *Keen-Wah*) is the Incan super-grain that arrived in the U.S. during the 1980s and gained popularity in the mid-2000s. As a complete protein, ancient Incas referred to Quinoa as the "mother grain" and would fuel their armies with "war-balls"—a mixture of Quinoa and fat.

Ribeye steak:

4	cloves garlic, minced then mashed into a paste
¼ cup	freshly squeezed lime juice
½ tsp.	freshly cracked black pepper, plus extra
2	boneless ribeyes, trimmed of most outer fat (approximately 10 oz. each and cut 1-inch thick)
	oil, for brushing
	kosher salt

Quinoa:

2 cups	water
	zest of 1 lime
1½ tsp.	kosher salt
1 cup	Quinoa
	juice from ½ lime
2 Tbsp.	(packed) fresh cilantro, chopped

Garnish:

2	roasted jalapeños, seeds and stem removed, julienned (see page 239)
8–10	medium-sized strawberries, trimmed and cut in quarters
2 oz	cotija cheese, crumbled

Roasted Jalapeño Vinaigrette

See Page 240

Combine garlic paste, lime juice, and ½ teaspoon freshly cracked black pepper in a large resealable bag. Add ribeyes to lime marinade. Toss to coat, making sure marinade is touching all surfaces of both steaks. Seal bag, removing as much air as possible to emulate a vacuum seal. Let the steaks marinate, chilled, for about 1 hour.

While steaks are marinating, prepare Quinoa. Add water, lime zest, and kosher salt to a saucepan and bring to boil over high heat. Once water has reached a boil, stir in Quinoa. Reduce heat to low and simmer uncovered, stirring occasionally, for about 20 minutes or until Quinoa have popped and are tender. (*Note: All of the water will not necessarily absorb into the grain. Taste to check for doneness.*) Strain Quinoa through a fine mesh sieve, and return to saucepan. Remove saucepan from heat and continue with the meal preparation.

Preheat grill for medium-high heat. (*Note: If using a charcoal grill, light coals before you begin the Quinoa so that the grill is ready when you need it.*)

Remove steaks from marinade, scraping away any clinging garlic. (*Note: The garlic will burn easily and cause a bitter flavor.*) Brush steaks with oil. Season all sides of steaks liberally with kosher salt and more freshly cracked black pepper, if you like a peppery steak.

Grill steaks over direct heat, flipping only once, for 4 to 5 minutes per side, 8 to 10 minutes total, or until you reach an internal temperature of 125 to 130 degrees for medium-rare doneness. Let rest for 5 minutes before slicing. (*Note: While resting, the internal temperature will continue to rise about 5 degrees. Cooking times will vary depending on the thickness of the steak. A thicker steak will require an extra minute or two per side to reach medium-rare, whereas a thinner steak will require a minute or two less.*)

While steak is resting, add chopped cilantro and lime juice to the slightly cooled Quinoa. Stir to incorporate.

Thinly slice steaks against the grain. To serve, spoon Quinoa in the center of four plates. Top Quinoa with sliced steak. Scatter julienned roasted jalapeños and strawberry pieces around the plates. Drizzle with roasted jalapeño vinaigrette, and finish by sprinkling .5 ounces crumbled cotija over each plate.

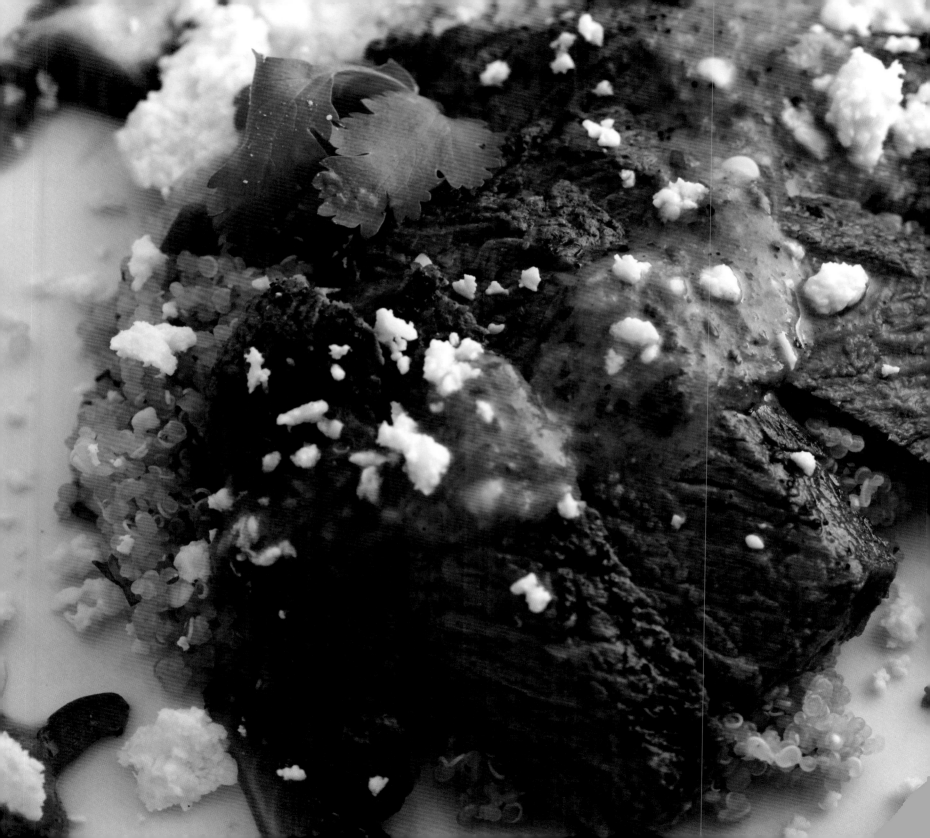

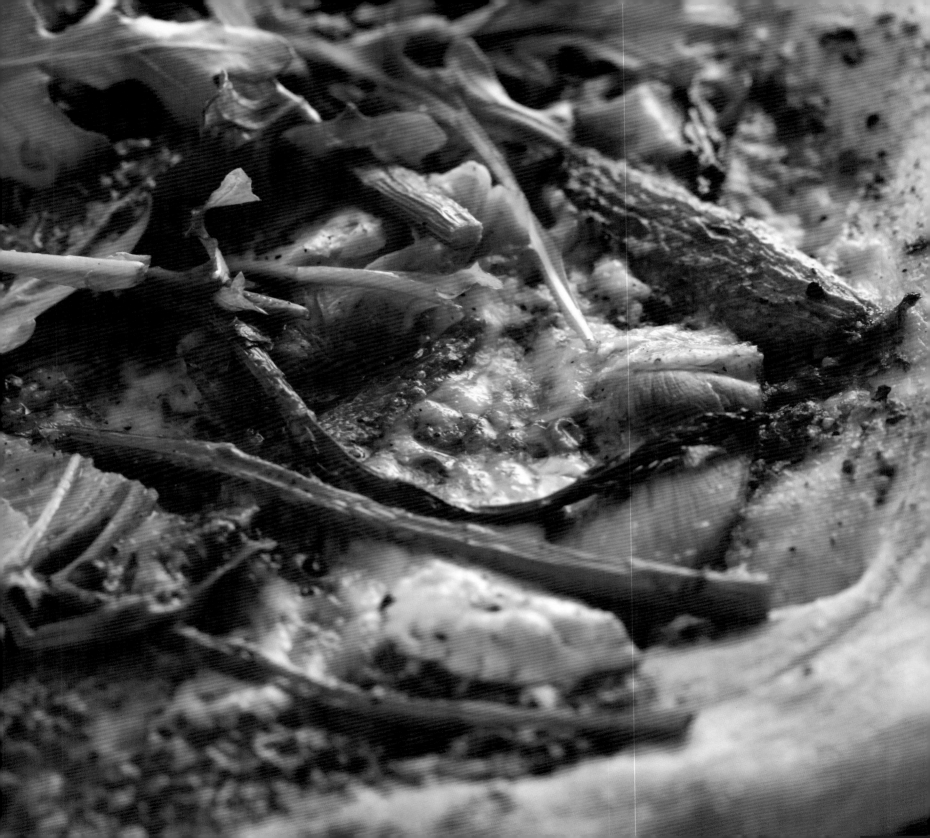

Spring Veggie Pizza

with Artichokes, Asparagus, Roasted Carrots and
Arugula Pesto

I know it's unusual for carrots to make an appearance on pizza, but once you taste this, you will no longer question my sanity.

Spring Veggie Pizza:

4	young carrots, peeled & trimmed
1 tsp.	olive oil
	kosher salt
	freshly cracked black pepper
1 cup	frozen artichoke hearts
½ recipe	Pizza Crust (see page 237; full recipe makes enough dough for 2 pizzas)
1 recipe	Arugula Pesto (see page 228)
4 oz.	buffalo mozzarella, roughly chopped
10	skinny spears asparagus, fibrous stalks trimmed
⅓ cup	fresh spring peas
2 oz.	herbed chevre, crumbled
	olive oil, for brushing the crust

Salad:

1 Tbsp.	red wine vinegar
¼ tsp.	granulated garlic
¼ tsp.	onion powder
¼ tsp.	freshly cracked black pepper, plus extra
¼ tsp.	kosher salt, plus extra
1 tsp.	Dijon mustard
2 Tbsp.	extra virgin olive oil
3 cups	arugula, washed & trimmed

Preheat oven to 400 degrees.

Toss whole carrots with 1 teaspoon olive oil and season with kosher salt and freshly cracked black pepper. Bake on a sheet pan at 400 degrees for 40 minutes, tossing after 20 minutes to caramelize both sides. Remove from oven and let cool until able to handle. Slice carrots in half, lengthwise. Increase oven temperature to 500 degrees or as high as your oven will heat.

Bring a medium-sized pot of water to a boil. Add frozen artichokes and boil for 1 minute. Drain thoroughly in a mesh sieve. Pat dry with paper towels

Prepare pizza crust according to recipe. Once dough has been shaped and is ready for topping, spread Arugula Pesto evenly over the crust. Sprinkle buffalo mozzarella evenly over pesto. Next, arrange roasted carrot halves, artichoke hearts, asparagus spears, and fresh peas around pizza. Sprinkle with crumbled herbed chevre. Brush outer edge of crust with olive oil. Sprinkle pizza with freshly cracked black pepper.

Bake pizza in *super hot* oven. Bake until bottom of crust is crispy and golden and the cheese is bubbly and golden in spots—10 to 15 minutes. Remove from oven.

While pizza is baking, prepare salad. Whisk together first 6 salad ingredients. While whisking continuously, drizzle in olive oil to form an emulsified vinaigrette. When pizza has finished baking, add arugula leaves to vinaigrette and toss to coat.

Top hot pizza with dressed arugula leaves. Slice using a pizza slicer and serve immediately.

Turkey Meatballs:

2	slices white sandwich bread
⅓ cup	buttermilk
½ tsp.	granulated garlic
½ tsp.	onion powder
⅓ cup	freshly grated Parmesan cheese
¼ tsp.	dried oregano
¼ tsp.	dried thyme
¼ tsp.	dried basil
1 tsp	kosher salt
½ tsp.	freshly cracked black pepper
1 lb.	ground turkey

Cremini, Artichoke, and Tomato Sauce:

1 Tbsp.	olive oil
12	cremini mushrooms, thickly sliced
3	cloves garlic, minced
¼ tsp.	crushed red pepper flakes (optional)
1 can	crushed San Marzano tomatoes
2 tsp.	(packed) brown sugar
1 tsp.	anchovy paste or 3 minced anchovy filets
¼ tsp.	dried oregano
1	sprig fresh thyme
1	inch sprig of fresh rosemary
½ cup	fresh basil leaves, torn
¼ cup	water
8 oz.	frozen artichoke hearts
	kosher salt
	freshly cracked black pepper, to taste
	al dente spaghetti, cooked according to package

Preheat oven to 450 degrees.

In a large mixing bowl, toss sandwich bread in buttermilk until coated. Let soak for 20 minutes until soggy. Whisk bread and buttermilk until mixture breaks down into paste. Add remaining ingredients except turkey and whisk to combine thoroughly. Add ground turkey to bowl. Using your hands, work seasoned bread paste into turkey meat until thoroughly incorporated.

Again, using your hands, roll turkey mixture into 16 evenly sized meatballs. Place meatballs onto a baking sheet or into a mini-muffin tin. (*Note: Using a muffin tin will help the meatballs keep their round shape during the cooking process but is not necessary. If you do use a muffin tin, place it on a baking sheet to catch any juice that may run off during the cooking process.*) Bake meatballs at 350 degrees for 25 to 30 minutes until just cooked through.

CREMINI, ARTICHOKE, AND TOMATO SAUCE

Heat olive oil in large sauté pan over medium-high heat. Once oil ripples with heat, add cremini mushrooms. Sprinkle with kosher salt and freshly cracked black pepper. Stir. Sauté over medium-high heat until caramelized and cooked through—about 10 minutes—stirring occasionally.

Add garlic and crushed red pepper flakes to caramelized cremini mushrooms. Sauté, stirring constantly for 30 to 60 seconds. Do not let garlic brown, or sauce will be bitter. Add next 8 ingredients, stirring to combine thoroughly. Reduce heat to low and simmer for 15 minutes, stirring occasionally. Add frozen artichokes to sauce and simmer for another 10 minutes until sauce thickens and artichokes are cooked through. If sauce gets too thick, simply add a small amount of water until desired consistency is reached. Adjust seasoning to taste with kosher salt and freshly cracked black pepper.

Add cooked meatballs to sauce and simmer for another 3 to 4 minutes. Serve over spaghetti prepared al dente according to directions on the package and garnish with freshly grated Parmesan cheese.

Hearty Spaghetti and Turkey Meatballs

with Cremini and Artichoke Tomato Sauce

Who doesn't have a soft spot in their heart for spaghetti and meatballs? In this version, we're using ground turkey for the meatballs, but if you prefer, you can always substitute ground beef or pork in place of the turkey.

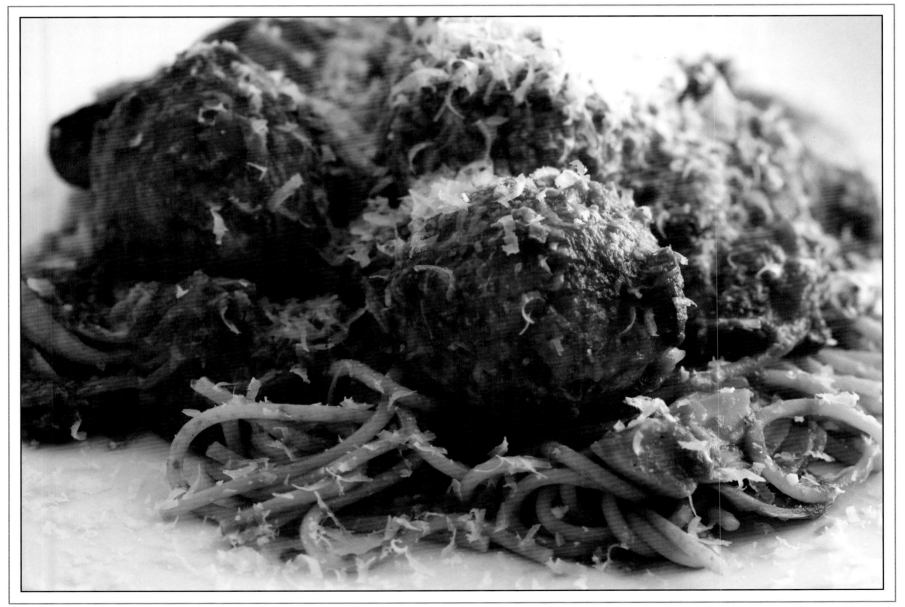

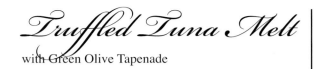

Truffled Tuna Melt

with Green Olive Tapenade

Truffle oil and canned tuna are a magical combination. Once you've eaten a truffled tuna salad sandwich without any trace of mayonnaise, you'll wonder why it isn't a more popular way to fix this old school dish.

Tuna Salad:

2 tsp.	extra virgin olive oil
1	bulb fennel, trimmed and diced
1	clove garlic, minced
2 cans	tuna in oil, drained
2 tsp.	truffle oil
	juice from ½ large lemon
2 Tbsp.	parsley, chopped
¼ tsp.	freshly cracked black pepper, plus extra
¼ tsp.	kosher salt, plus extra

Sandwiches:

8	(½-inch thick) slices crusty olive or sourdough bread
4 oz.	Manchego cheese, grated
	green olive tapenade
2	ripe yellow tomatoes, thinly sliced
2–3	roasted Piquillo peppers, julienned (can substitute any roasted red peppers)
	green leaf lettuce, separated into individual leaves

Green Olive Tapenade:

See Page 233

Preheat oven to 450 degrees.

Heat olive oil in a small sauté pan over medium heat. Once pan is hot, add diced fennel to oil. Sauté until tender, about 10 minutes, stirring occasionally. Add minced garlic and sauté for another 60 seconds, stirring continuously. Remove from heat and transfer to a mixing bowl.

Add remaining tuna salad ingredients to fennel and garlic. Stir to mix thoroughly. Adjust seasonings to taste with kosher salt and freshly cracked black pepper.

Lightly toast bread slices in oven until just beginning to brown. Remove from oven.

Place four slices of lightly toasted bread onto a sheet pan. Evenly divide the tuna salad among the four slices of toast and spread in an even layer across the bread. Top each sandwich bottom with 1 ounce of grated Manchego cheese. Place bottom half of tuna melts into preheated oven until cheese has melted— about 5 minutes.

While cheese is melting, spread 2 tablespoons of green olive tapenade onto each of the remaining 4 slices of toast.

Remove tuna melts from oven. Layer slices of yellow tomato, roasted Piquillo peppers and green leaf lettuce onto tuna melt. Top each melt with a tapenade-smeared piece of toast to complete the sandwich. Slice sandwiches in half and serve immediately.

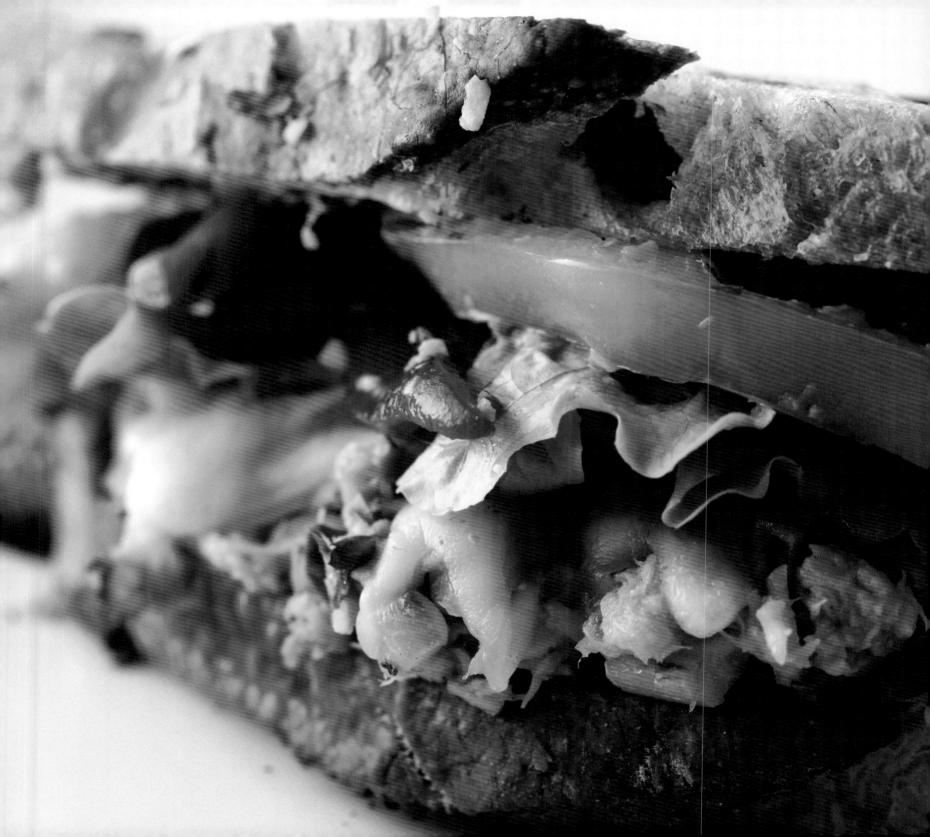

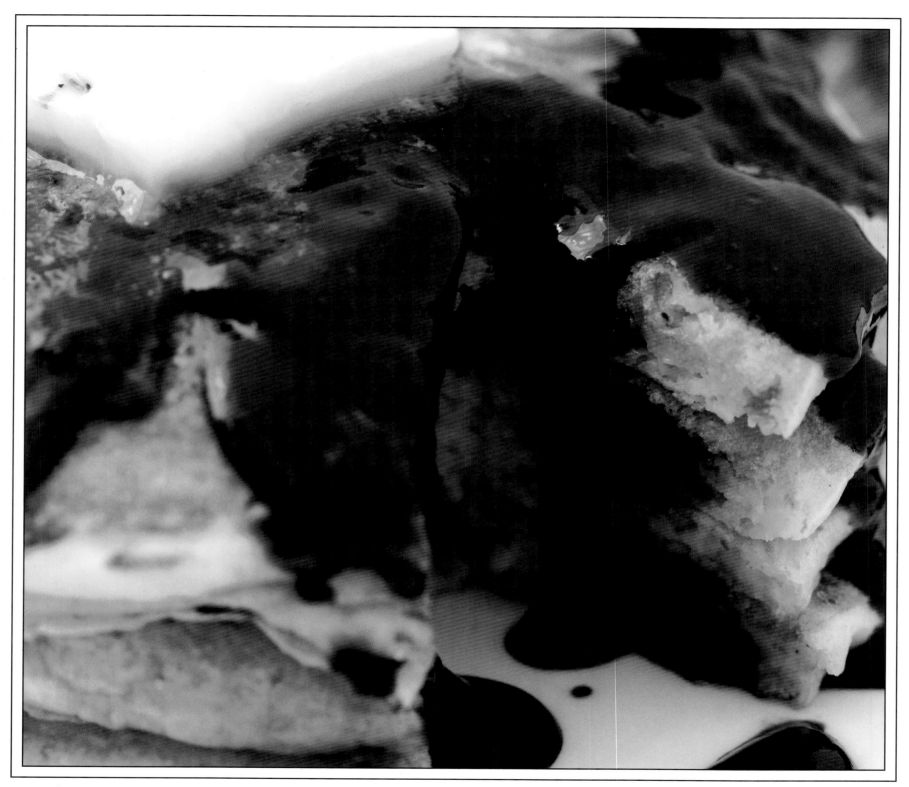

Blueberry Cornmeal Pancakes

with Blueberry–Star Anise Maple Syrup

The cornmeal in the pancakes adds a touch of texture, and the star anise in the syrup raises this above standard diner fare.

BLUEBERRY CORNMEAL PANCAKES

Pancakes

1 cup	buttermilk
1 cup	plain yogurt, *not* low or non-fat
1	egg
1 cup	flour
⅓ cup	yellow cornmeal
1 tsp.	baking powder
1 tsp.	baking soda
2 Tbsp.	(packed) dark brown sugar
¼ tsp.	kosher salt
1 cup	blueberries
1 Tbsp.	melted butter

Blueberry–Star Anise Maple Syrup

12 oz.	blueberries, rinsed
	juice from half a lemon
1	whole star-anise
8 oz.	pure maple syrup
¼ tsp.	kosher salt

butter, for serving

Preheat oven to 200 degrees.

Preheat a griddle or large non-stick pan to medium heat.

In a mixing bowl, whisk together buttermilk, yogurt, and egg.

In a separate bowl, combine flour, cornmeal, baking powder, baking soda, brown sugar, and salt. Whisk to evenly distribute ingredients. Add blueberries and stir to incorporate.

Add wet ingredients to dry ingredients and stir until just combined. (*Note: The batter will still be lumpy. Do not overwork the batter.*)

Add melted butter to batter and stir until just incorporated.

Scoop about ⅓ cup batter onto griddle or non-stick pan. Cook for about 3 minutes until bottom is golden and there are visible air bubbles in the batter. Flip pancake and cook for another 1 to 2 minutes until browned. Remove pancake from pan and place on a heat-safe plate in warming oven preheated to 200 degrees. Repeat cooking process with remaining batter. Serve warm with blueberry star-anise maple syrup and butter.

BLUEBERRY–STAR ANISE MAPLE SYRUP

Simmer all syrup ingredients in a small saucepan over medium-low heat until most blueberries have popped and syrup is a dark purple color—20 to 25 minutes—stirring frequently. Remove star anise from syrup. Transfer syrup to blender and blend on high until very smooth. For best texture, strain through a fine mesh sieve. Store chilled for up to 1 week.

Topping:

1½ cups	heavy whipping cream
1	vanilla bean pod, sliced in half lengthwise
3	Tbsp. sugar
¼	tsp. salt

Crust:

1 stick	butter, at room temperature
⅓ cup	(packed) brown sugar
	zest from 1 lime
½ tsp.	salt
⅓ cup	pignoli (pine nuts), toasted and roughly chopped
½ cup	(loosely packed) sweetened coconut flakes, roughly chopped
1 cup	flour

Filling:

3	eggs
1 egg	yolk
⅔ cup	sugar
½ tsp.	salt
1 Tbsp.	lime zest
½ cup	lime juice, freshly squeezed
⅓ cup	flour

lime zest, for garnishing

VANILLA BEAN TOPPING

Combine all topping ingredients into a small saucepan over medium-low heat. Whisk until sugar has dissolved into cream. Reduce heat to low and steep vanilla bean in cream for 15 minutes, stirring occasionally. Remove bean and carefully scrape seeds from pod with the tip of a knife. Add scraped seeds to cream, whisking to combine. Remove from heat and let cool for 20 minutes at room temperature. Cover and chill vanilla bean cream in the refrigerator until very cold—at least 4 hours but no longer than 2 days.

COCONUT-PIGNOLI SHORTBREAD CRUST

Preheat oven to 375 degrees.

Prepare crust: Using a stand mixer with whisk attachment or a mixing bowl and whisk or rubber spatula, cream butter until fluffy and light yellow. Add brown sugar, lime zest, and salt; beat until fully incorporated. Add remaining ingredients and beat until mixture resembles coarse crumbs.

Pour crust mixture into a 9½x1-inch or 10x1-inch tart pan with a removable bottom placed on a sheet pan. Using your fingers or a flat-bottomed straight-edged cup, pack the shortbread crust mixture into a compact, even layer across the bottom and up the sides of tart pan. Bake tart shell on sheet pan for 20 minutes or until crust is golden around the edges. Let cool for 10 minutes before adding lime filling.

LIME FILLING & ASSEMBLY

While crust is cooling, prepare filling:

In a medium mixing bowl, beat whole eggs and egg yolk with a whisk. Add sugar, salt, and lime zest. Beat until fully incorporated. Whisk in lime juice. Add flour and whisk until smooth and fully incorporated.

Pour filling into slightly cooled tart shell and bake for another 15 minutes, or until tart has set and filling is firm. Remove from oven and cool completely before proceeding.

Whip cream: Pour chilled vanilla bean whipping cream into bowl of a stand mixer. Using the whisk attachment, whip cream on medium speed until cream can hold stiff peaks. If beating by hand, whisk vigorously until whipped cream holds stiff peaks.

Pour whipped cream over cooled tart and spread into an even layer. Using a Microplane or fine grater, garnish top of tart with a dusting of lime zest. Chill for at least 2 hours until ready to serve. Tart can be made up to 2 days in advance if stored chilled.

Tangy Lime Tart

with Coconut-Pignoli Shortbread Crust

The toasted pine-nut shortbread crust is really what sets this lime tart apart from similar lime desserts. While key limes have a great flavor, they can't always be found as ripe and juicy year-round like Persian or Tahitian limes (the standard grocery store variety). Plus, key limes require a LOT more work to get the same amount of juice. For these reasons, the typical grocery store variety lime will work perfectly for this recipe.

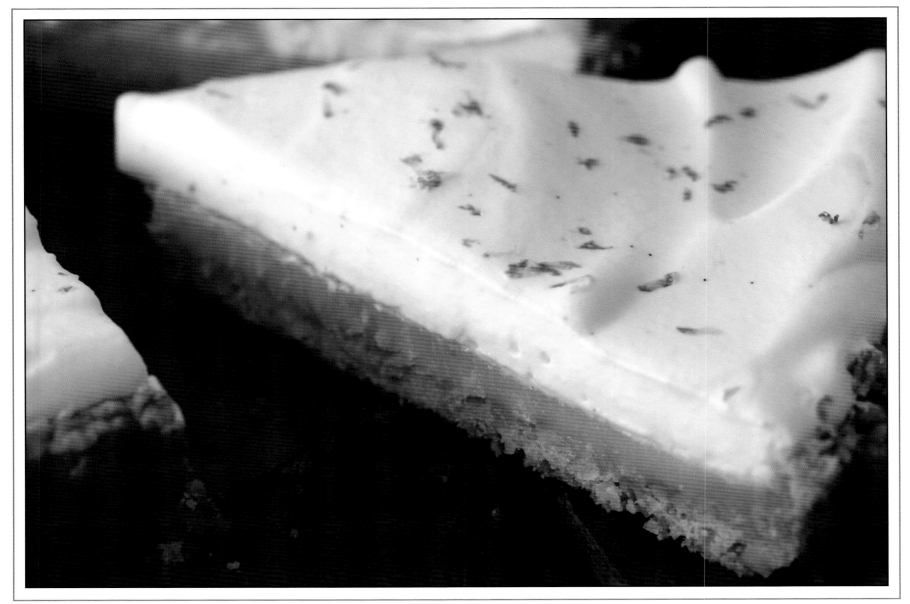

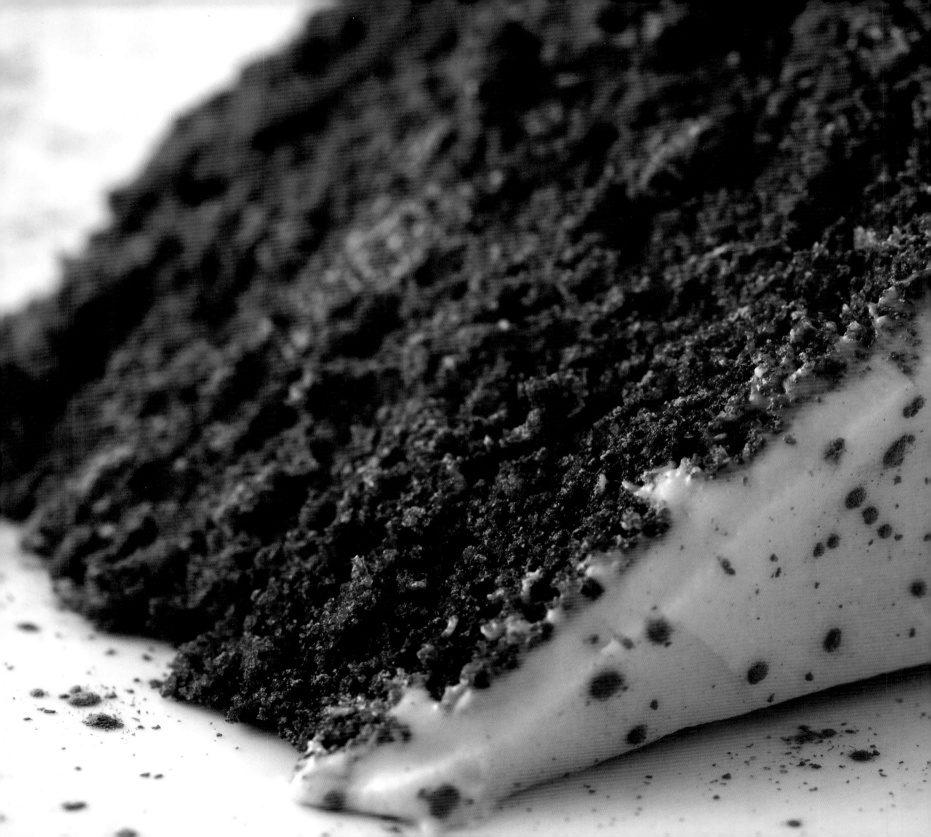

Carbomb Cake

Perfect for St. Patrick's Day, the flavors for this cake are pulled from the classic "carbomb" cocktail that consists of a shot of Irish Whiskey topped with Bailey's, which is dropped into half of a glass of Guinness stout. Traditionally the cocktail is chugged, but I don't suggest chugging this dessert. Cake just doesn't go down as smoothly as liquid.

CARBOMB CAKE

Carbomb Cake

1 cup	cocoa powder, Valrhona if possible, plus extra for dusting
1 cup	buttermilk
¾ cup	Guinness beer
2¾ cups	cake flour
1 tsp.	baking soda
½ tsp.	salt
1½ cups	(3 sticks) butter, at room temperature
2¼ cups	granulated sugar
1 Tbsp.	pure vanilla extract
4	eggs

Bailey's Buttercream

See Page 228

Irish Whiskey Ganache:

See Page 234

Preheat oven to 350 degrees.

Grease two 9-inch cake pans with butter and line bottom of pans with parchment paper. Grease parchment with butter and dust pans with flour or cocoa powder, shaking out any excess powder.

In a small mixing bowl, slowly add buttermilk to cocoa powder while continuously whisking until all buttermilk has been added and cocoa powder has dissolved into buttermilk. Add Guinness to cocoa mixture. Whisk to combine thoroughly. Set aside.

Sift together flour, baking soda, and salt. Set aside.

In a separate mixing bowl, beat butter until fluffy. Add sugar and vanilla and beat until fully incorporated and fluffy. Add eggs one at a time and beat until each egg is fully incorporated before adding next egg.

Add cocoa mixture to butter mixture and beat until fully incorporated.

Add sifted dry ingredients to butter-cocoa mixture. Stir until just incorporated. (*Note: Do not overwork the batter or the cake will be tough and dense.*) Divide cake batter evenly into prepared cake pans.

Bake cakes at 350 degrees for 30 to 35 minutes until a toothpick inserted into center of cake comes out clean, with only a few crumbs but no batter.

Cool cakes in pans completely—at least 1½ hours—on a wire rack. Slide a knife around edge of cake to loosen, and then invert the cakes onto a plate. Carefully remove parchment paper.

To assemble cake:

Place one cake on serving dish, bottom-side up. Line dish with strips of parchment paper tucked underneath bottom of cake to prevent serving dish from getting dirty during frosting process. Carefully spread ganache over top of cake in an even layer. Place second cake on top of ganache layer. Evenly coat top and sides of cake with the butter-cream frosting. Dust with cocoa powder to garnish and remove parchment strips. Serve at room temperature. If making ahead of time, keep cake chilled, but bring to room temperature before serving.

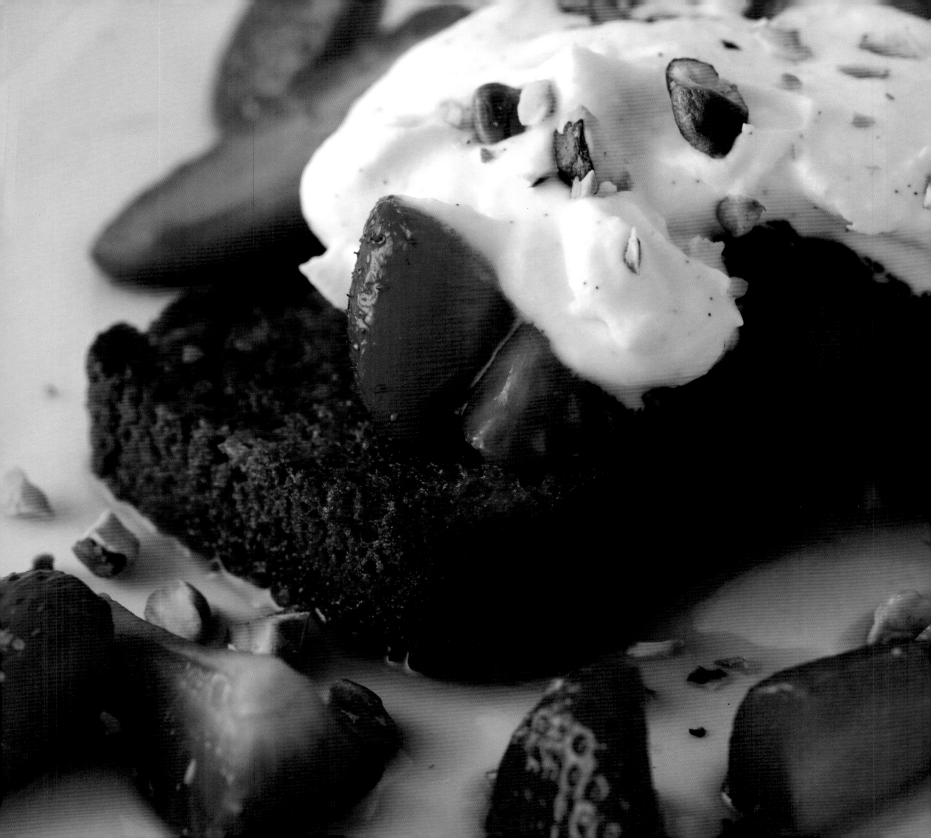

Strawberry "Shortcake"

with Cardamom Strawberry Pistachio Bread &
Vanilla Bean Whipped Cream

Everybody loves strawberry shortcake. Here, strawberries are also incorporated into a cardamom quick bread that is then brushed with butter and seared before being topped with the traditional macerated berries and whipped cream.

Strawberry Pistachio Cardamom Bread

2 cups	strawberries, hulled and roughly chopped
½ cup	sour cream
2 cups	flour
½ tsp.	baking soda
½ tsp.	baking powder
1 tsp.	ground cardamom
½ tsp.	ground cinnamon
½ cup	(1 stick) butter, at room temperature
1 cup	brown sugar
¼ tsp.	salt
3	eggs
1 tsp.	good vanilla extract
½ cup	unsalted, shelled pistachios, roughly chopped

To Plate:

4	(1-inch thick) slices of strawberry-pistachio-cardamom bread
3–4 Tbsp.	butter, softened to room temperature
	shelled pistachios, roughly chopped

Macerated Strawberries:

See Page 235

Vanilla Bean Whipped Cream:

See Page 243

Preheat oven to 350 degrees with a rack in center position. Grease a 9x5-inch glass or ceramic loaf dish with butter and flour. Set aside.

In a blender, blend strawberries and sour cream until smooth. Set aside.

Sift together flour, baking soda, baking powder, cardamom, and cinnamon. Set aside.

Using a stand mixer with whisk attachment or a large mixing bowl with a whisk, beat together softened butter, brown sugar, and salt until fluffy. Add eggs to butter one at a time, beating until fully incorporated before adding next egg. Scrape down sides of bowl as necessary. Once eggs have been incorporated, whisk in vanilla.

Add one-third of flour mixture, beating until flour is mostly incorporated, and add half of strawberry puree, scraping down sides of bowl after each addition. Beat until just incorporated. Alternate adding flour and puree in 3 more additions, ending with last addition of flour. Whisk in each addition until just barely incorporated. (*Note: It's important not to overwork the batter or else the bread will be dense and tough.*)

Gently fold pistachios into batter. Pour batter into prepared loaf pan. Bake at 350 degrees for 60 to 75 minutes, or until a toothpick inserted into middle of

loaf comes out clean. Remove from oven and let cool on a wire rack. To remove from pan, gently run knife around outside of loaf. Place a plate over pan, invert loaf onto plate, and then turn loaf right side up. Slice 4 1-inch pieces of strawberry bread.

Heat a sauté pan over medium-high heat.

While pan is heating, slather a thin layer of softened butter on both sides of each slice of strawberry bread. Depending on size of your pan, place either one or two slices of buttered bread into pan. Sear bread until caramelized and golden on both sides—2 to 3 minutes per side. Remove from pan and repeat process with rest of bread.

To plate individual desserts, slice one piece of grilled bread in half diagonally. Stack halves in middle of a plate. Spoon a quarter of macerated berries over the bread and around the plate, including a quarter of juice from berries. Spoon a hefty dollop of vanilla bean whipped cream over bread and garnish with a sprinkle of roughly chopped shelled pistachios.

Repeat plating to make a total of four large desserts.

Fluffy Coconut Cake

with Chunky Pineapple Filling

In general, I'm not much of a sweets eater, but when this classic Southern coconut cake is around I just can't help myself. The addition of the pineapple filling makes this cake even that much better.

Coconut Cake:

1½ cups	unsweetened coconut milk
1 cup	(loosely packed) sweetened flaked coconut
1 tsp.	pure vanilla extract
1 tsp.	coconut extract
3 cups	cake flour
1 Tbsp.	baking powder
½ tsp.	salt
14 Tbsp.	(1¾ sticks) butter, at room temperature
1¾ cup	granulated sugar
5	eggs

Chunky Pineapple Filling:

See Page 237

Vanilla Bean Whipped Cream:

See Page 243

3–4 cups	sweetened flaked coconut

Preheat oven to 350 degrees. Butter and flour two 9-inch round cake pans and line the bottoms with parchment paper. Set aside.

Blend coconut milk, flaked coconut, and coconut and vanilla extracts in a blender for 30 seconds and set aside.

Sift together flour, baking powder, and salt. Set aside.

Add butter to the bowl of a stand mixer or a large mixing bowl. With a whisk attachment or a hand mixer, beat until fluffy and light yellow. Add sugar and beat again until completely incorporated and smooth. Add eggs, one at a time, beating until each egg is fully incorporated before adding next egg. Scrape down sides of bowl as necessary throughout the cake-making process.

Add the reserved ingredients, alternating dry and wet: beat in one-third of flour until just incorporated followed by half of milk, and so on, ending with last of flour. Beat each addition only until just barely incorporated. (*Note: Do not overwork the batter. Overmixing will lead to a tough, chewy, dense cake.*)

Once all ingredients have been incorporated, divide batter equally between prepared cake pans. Bake for 30 to 35 minutes, or until the top is golden, the edges have pulled away from the sides, and a toothpick inserted into center of cake comes out clean, with only a couple of crumbs and absolutely no batter. Remove from oven and place on a wire rack to cool. Cool completely before removing from pan.

To remove from pan, run knife around edges. Place a plate over cake and invert pan. The cake should release onto the plate. Peel off parchment paper.

Assemble cake:

Place one cake onto to your serving dish. Line dish with strips of parchment paper tucked under edges of cake to keep dish clean during assembly.

Trim top of bottom layer so that cake is flat. Spread pineapple filling over cake in an even layer. Place second cake on top of pineapple filling. Frost the top and sides of layer cake liberally with whipped cream. Sprinkle flaked coconut over top and sides of cake to coat. (*Tip: An easy way to coat the sides of the cake, is to take handfuls of coconut and softly pat flakes all round the sides.*) Carefully remove parchment strips, which will likely be covered with coconut flakes and whipped cream. Try to keep the serving dish as clean as possible. Chill cake until ready to serve. Cake can be stored chilled for a few days but tastes best if eaten within the first 24 hours.

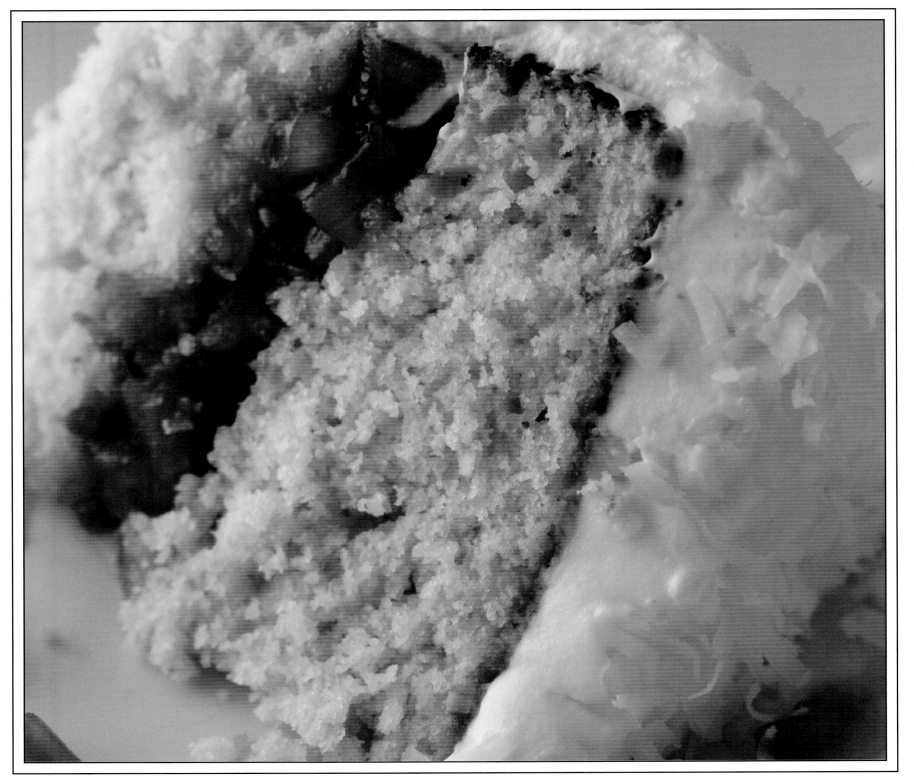

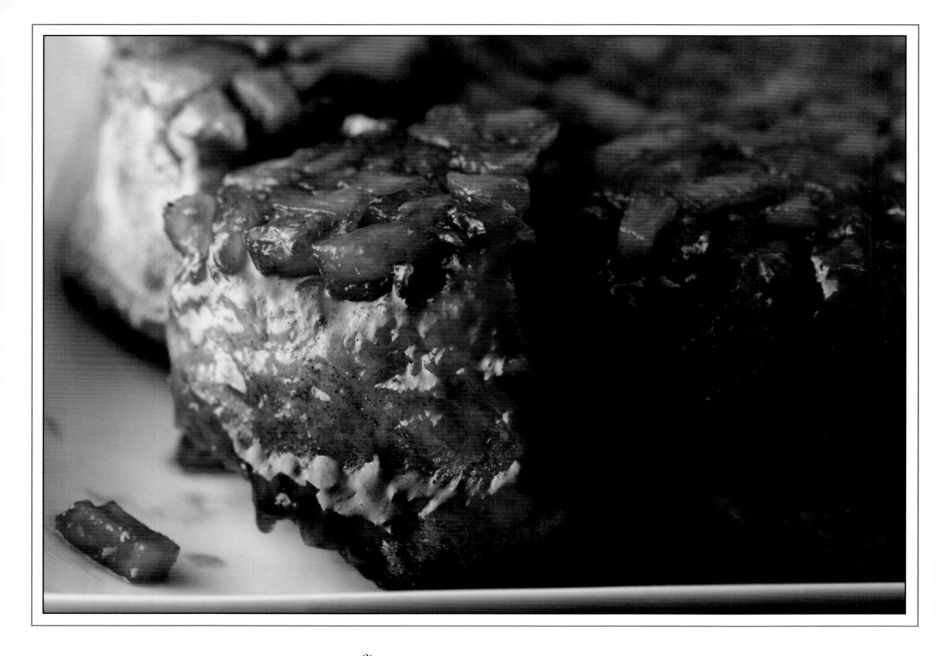

Gooey Pineapple Flambé Monkey Bread

Monkey bread in its most basic form is just cinnamon-sugar coated, pull-apart yeast bread. This version includes some brown sugar pineapple flambé to make it even more irresistible.

Dough:

2 Tbsp.	butter
¼ cup + 1 Tbsp.	sugar
½ tsp.	salt
8 oz.	sour cream
1	packet active dry yeast
¼ cup	lukewarm water, about 105 degrees
2¾–3¼	cups flour
	oil, for greasing the bowl

Topping:

3 Tbsp.	butter
½ cup	(packed) brown sugar
2 cups	fresh pineapple, peeled, cored & diced
¼ tsp.	salt
⅓ cup	bourbon
½ tsp.	ground cinnamon

Coating:

½ cup	(packed) brown sugar
¼ tsp.	salt
2 tsp.	ground cinnamon
4 Tbsp.	butter

Preheat oven to 375 degrees.

With a liberal amount of oil, grease a large, non-reactive mixing bowl for the dough to rise in. Set aside.

In a small saucepan over medium heat, melt butter for dough. Once butter has melted, add ¼ cup sugar, and salt, stirring to dissolve. Whisk in sour cream until smooth. Heat sour cream mixture until lukewarm—about 105 degrees—stirring occasionally. Remove from heat.

While sour cream mixture is heating, add warm water and 1 tablespoon sugar to yeast in a large mixing bowl and stir. Let yeast mixture set for five minutes to activate—it should begin foaming and bubbling. (*Note: If after five or so minutes the yeast does not activate, discard the mixture and start with new ingredients.*)

Add lukewarm sour cream mixture and 1 cup flour to activated yeast. Stir thoroughly. Add another 1¾ cups flour. Mix until fully incorporated. (*Note: You want the dough to be soft, but not sticky or wet. During the kneading process you will be able to incorporate more flour, so it's okay if the dough is just slightly sticky at this point. It's much harder to add liquid once the dough has been formed, so I suggest adding less flour in the beginning and working it in as you knead. I find that three cups of flour gives me the soft dough texture desired.*)

Turn dough out onto a clean surface, lightly dusted with flour. Kneed dough for 7 minutes, adding more flour as necessary if the dough is too wet and sticks to the surface. Shape dough into a ball and set aside in prepared bowl. Flip dough ball around bowl so that all sides get coated with oil. Spray a sheet of plastic wrap with cooking spray or grease with oil. Cover bowl with plastic wrap, greased-side down. Cover plastic wrap with kitchen towel. Set bowl aside in a warm, draft-free location. (*Note: I find that a spot near the preheating oven works well.*) Let dough rise until doubled in size, about 1 hour.

While dough is rising, prepare topping. Melt 3 tablespoons of butter in a large sauté pan over medium heat. Once butter has melted, add brown sugar to pan, stirring to dissolve. Add diced fresh pineapple and salt to brown sugar/butter mixture. Stir to coat pineapple. Cook for 3 minutes, stirring occasionally. Pour bourbon into to the sauté pan. Carefully light the bourbon on fire with a kitchen lighter to flambé pineapple. Once flame has died down, let pineapple mixture simmer over medium heat, stirring occasionally, for 15 to 20 minutes or until liquid reduces by a little more than half to form a thickened syrup. Remove from heat and pour into a 9-inch cake pan. Let mixture cool to room temperature.

Combine brown sugar, salt, and cinnamon for coating in a small bowl. Meanwhile, melt butter for coating in separate bowl.

Once dough has doubled in sized, pinch off 14 equally sized pieces of dough and roll into balls. Dip each ball first into the melted butter and then in the brown sugar-cinnamon mixture, tossing to coat. Arrange coated dough balls on top of pineapple flambé. Once finished, cover cake pan with greased plastic wrap and a kitchen towel and let rise another 30 minutes until almost doubled in size again.

Remove kitchen towel and plastic wrap. Place pan of monkey bread onto a large baking sheet lined with foil to catch any brown sugar syrup that might drip over the edge during the baking process. Place the baking sheet onto the center rack of a preheated 375 degree oven. Bake monkey bread for 20 to 25 minutes until golden and bubbly. Remove from oven and let cool for 20 minutes on a wire rack.

Slide a table knife around the edge of the pan to help release the dough from the sides. Place a large plate over the cake pan. Invert the monkey bread onto the plate and carefully lift up to unveil. Use a rubber spatula to transfer any of the pineapple syrup that remains in the pan to the monkey bread. Serve immediately and devour!

Strawberry Sorbet Prosecco Float

Strawberries are the perfect complement for sparkling wine or champagne. Here Prosecco, an Italian sparkling wine, is mixed with fresh strawberry sorbet to create the perfect cocktail "float" for brunch, lunch, or after dinner. That's the joy of sparkling wine—it goes with any time of day.

Sorbet:

1 cup	sugar
1 cup	water
½ tsp.	salt
1 quart	fresh ripe strawberries, hulled
	juice from ½ lemon

For the cocktail:

Prosecco or dry sparkling wine or Champagne

strawberries, sliced half-way up the middle for garnish

Special Equipment: Ice Cream Machine

STRAWBERRY SORBET PROSECCO FLOATS

Make sorbet: Stir sugar, water, and salt together in a small pot over medium-high heat. Bring to a simmer and dissolve sugar into the water to form a simple syrup. Remove from heat.

Add strawberries, lemon juice, and simple syrup to a blender and puree until very smooth. Strain sorbet base through a fine mesh sieve twice to remove any pulp or seeds. Chill, covered, in refrigerator for at least 6 hours and up to 2 days. Once chilled, transfer sorbet base to an ice cream machine and freeze according to manufacturer's directions. Transfer frozen sorbet to an airtight container. Freeze for at least 2 hours before serving and up to 2 days.

To serve, pour Prosecco over a scoop of sorbet in a wine glass. Garnish rim with a fresh strawberry.

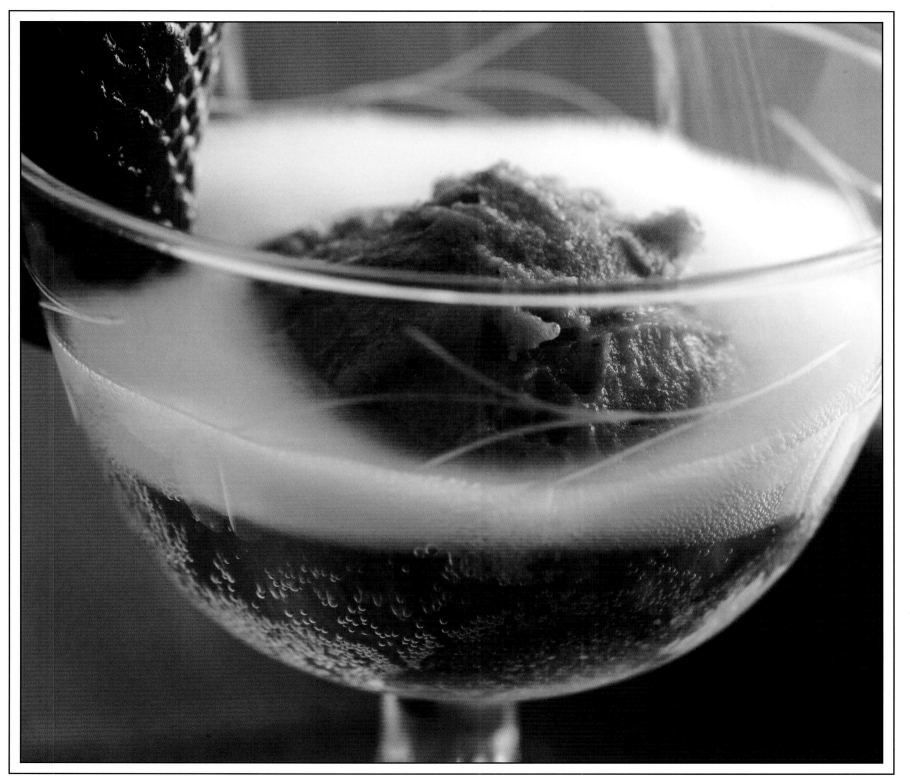

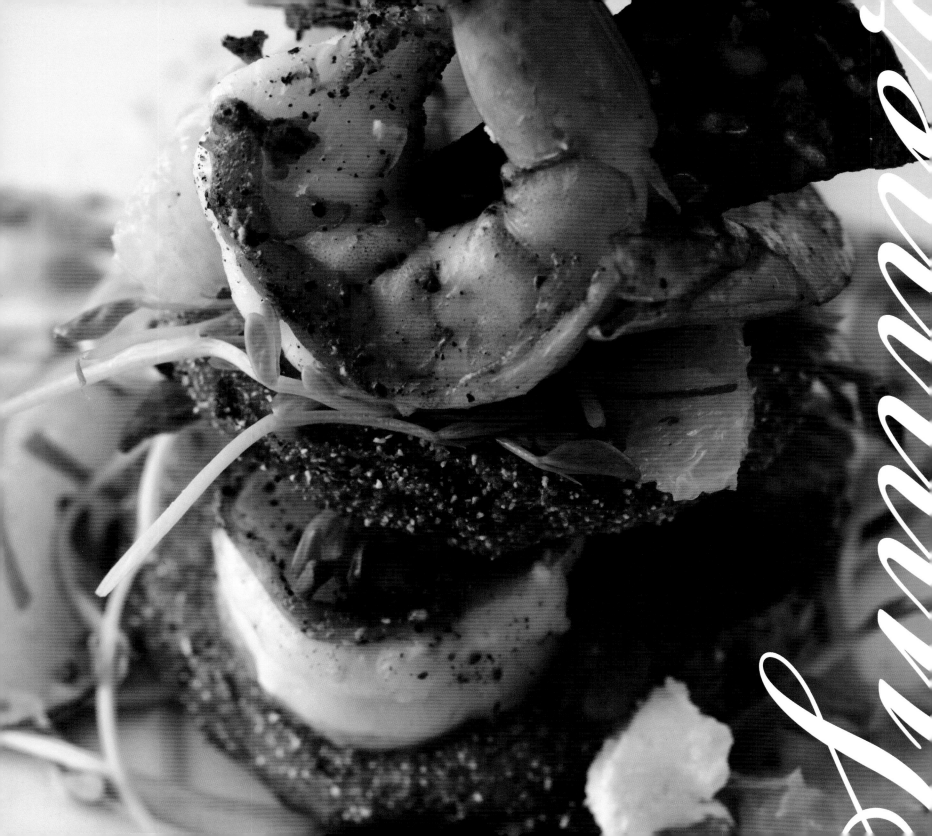

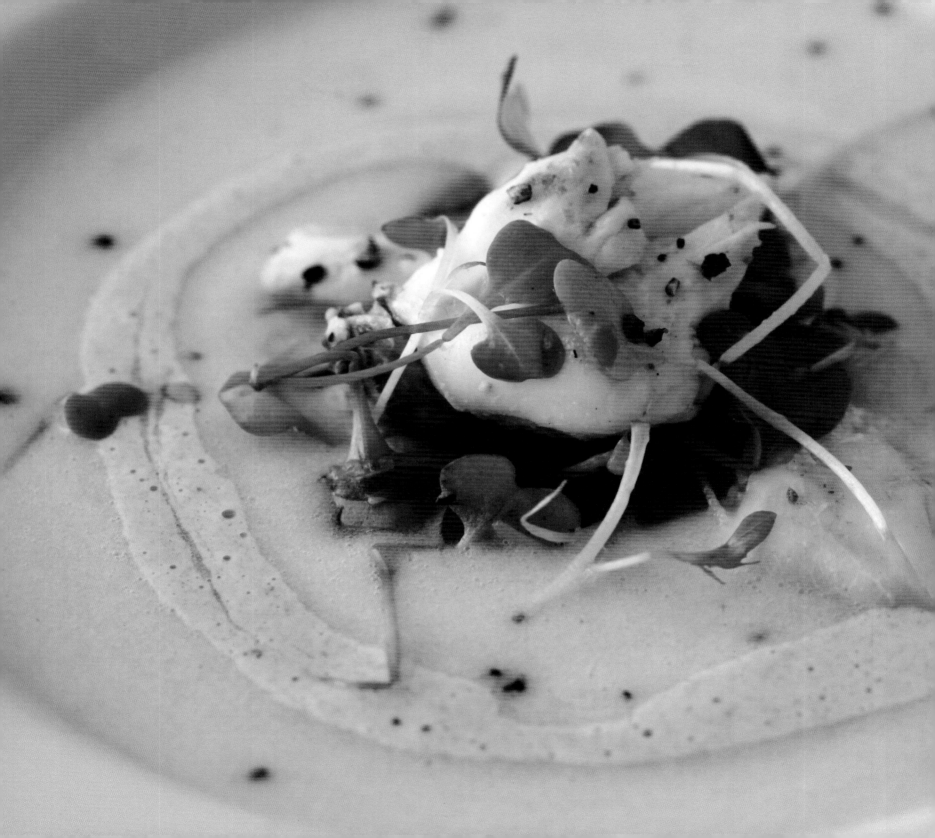

Silky White Corn Soup
with Chilled Crab, Roasted Poblano, and Corn Garnish

The perfect dish to begin a mid-summer's dinner party, this silky corn soup is extremely simple and is focused on the pure flavor of fresh, sweet white corn.

CORN SOUP

For the soup:

5 ears	sweet white corn, like Silver Queen, shucked and cleaned of any remaining corn silk
1 bulb	roasted garlic, separated into cloves (see page 240)
	juice from ½ lime
	kosher salt
	freshly cracked black pepper
	water

For the garnish:

½ cup	cooked lump crab meat, chilled
1 ear	sweet white corn, shucked and cleaned of silk
1	roasted poblano chile (see page 239) peeled, seeds and stem removed, and diced
	juice from ½ lime
½ cup	micro greens
2	slices bacon, cooked crispy & crumbled
	kosher salt
	freshly cracked black pepper
1 recipe	Roasted Poblano Crème Fraîche

Roasted Poblano Crème Fraîche

1	roasted poblano chile (see page 239)
½ tsp.	oil
⅓ cup	crème fraîche
	juice from 1 lime
¼ tsp.	kosher salt, plus extra

Add 6 ears of corn (5 for soup and 1 for garnish) to a pot of boiling water. Boil for 3 minutes, stirring once or twice. Remove ears from water. Allow water to continue to boil.

Once the corn is cool enough to handle, cut kernels from cobs, reserving the cobs. Reserve kernels from 1 ear of corn for garnish in a separate bowl. Place remaining kernels into blender.

Place reserved cobs back into pot of boiling water for 30 minutes to make a quick corn stock.

Add roasted garlic cloves, lime juice, 1 teaspoon kosher salt, ¼ teaspoon freshly cracked black pepper, and about 2 cups of corn stock to blender with corn. Puree until as smooth as possible—3 to 4 minutes depending on the blender. Strain soup through a fine mesh sieve or chinois over a large bowl or pot. Discard any solids and strain soup a second time to ensure a silky smooth texture. Adjust seasoning with kosher salt and freshly cracked black pepper as desired.

Finish garnish: Add lump crab meat, diced roasted poblano, lime juice, micro greens, and crumbled bacon to reserved corn kernels and toss. Season to taste with kosher salt and freshly cracked black pepper.

To plate, ladle soup into a bowl. Drizzle roasted poblano crème fraîche (see below) in a circle around soup. Place heaping spoonful of the crab-corn-chile garnish in the middle of the soup. Serve immediately.

ROASTED POBLANO CRÈME FRAÎCHE

Remove stem and seeds from roasted poblano chile and discard. Blend chile with remaining ingredients until very smooth. Adjust seasoning to taste with more kosher salt. Store chilled until ready for use.

Grilled Summer Vegetable Salad

with Buffalo Mozzarella and Classic Basil Pesto

A caprese salad (fresh mozzarella, basil leaves, and tomato slices) is perhaps the epitome of a perfect summer salad. This dish takes those flavors and expands on them by adding grilled summer squash and turning the basil into pesto. Although we suggest serving this as the opening salad course, I would happily eat the entire dish for my full meal.

GRILLED VEGETABLE SALAD

Grilled Vegetable Salad:

2	zucchini, stems cut off and discarded
2	yellow squash, stems cut off and discarded
1	red bell pepper, cut in ½, stem and seeds removed
12	cherry tomatoes
	extra virgin olive oil
	kosher salt
	freshly cracked black pepper
1	recipe Basil Pesto
	buffalo mozzarella, cut in slices

Classic Basil Pesto:

1 large	(or 2 small) clove(s) garlic
2 Tbsp.	pine nuts
1½ cups	(packed) basil leaves
	juice from 1 lemon
3–4 Tbsp.	extra virgin olive oil
¼ cup	freshly grated Parmesan cheese
	kosher salt
	freshly cracked black pepper

Prepare grill for high heat.

Using either a mandoline or a sharp knife, carefully slice zucchini and yellow squash in long, thin (¼-inch) slices.

Place zucchini and yellow squash slices onto a sheet pan with red pepper halves and cherry tomatoes. Drizzle with olive oil and toss to coat, being careful not to break squash slices. Sprinkle liberally with kosher salt and freshly cracked black pepper. Toss again to evenly distribute seasonings.

Grill veggies in a single layer over high direct heat until charred—1 to 2 minutes per side. Once grill marks have been charred into both sides, remove from grill. When veggies are cool enough to handle, julienne the red bell pepper. Slice squash in half widthwise and then once lengthwise so that squash pieces are approximately same size and length of bell pepper strips. Place all grilled veggies into a bowl with ¼ cup basil pesto (see below). Toss to coat. Plate veggies in a pile with slices of buffalo mozzarella distributed throughout. Drizzle with extra pesto.

CLASSIC BASIL PESTO

Process first 4 ingredients in a food processor. While the food processor is running, drizzle in olive oil and process ingredients until minced thoroughly. Turn off the machine and scrape down sides of bowl. Add the Parmesan cheese and process until incorporated, adjusting seasoning to taste with kosher salt and freshly cracked black pepper. If pesto is thicker than desired, simply add more olive oil. Pulse to incorporate. For a brighter pesto add more lemon juice.

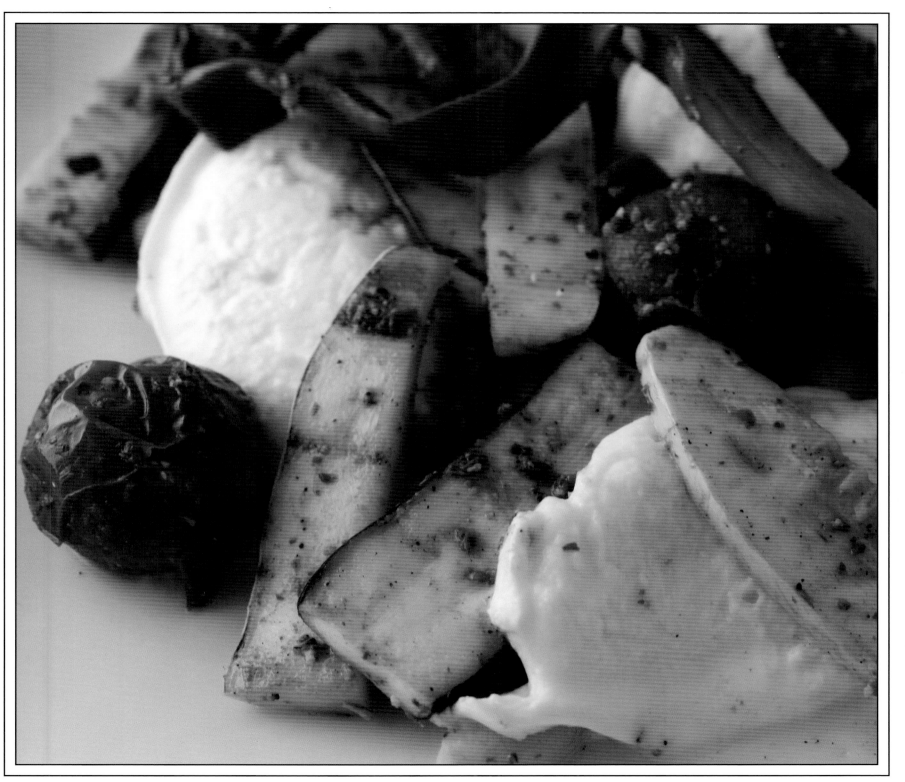

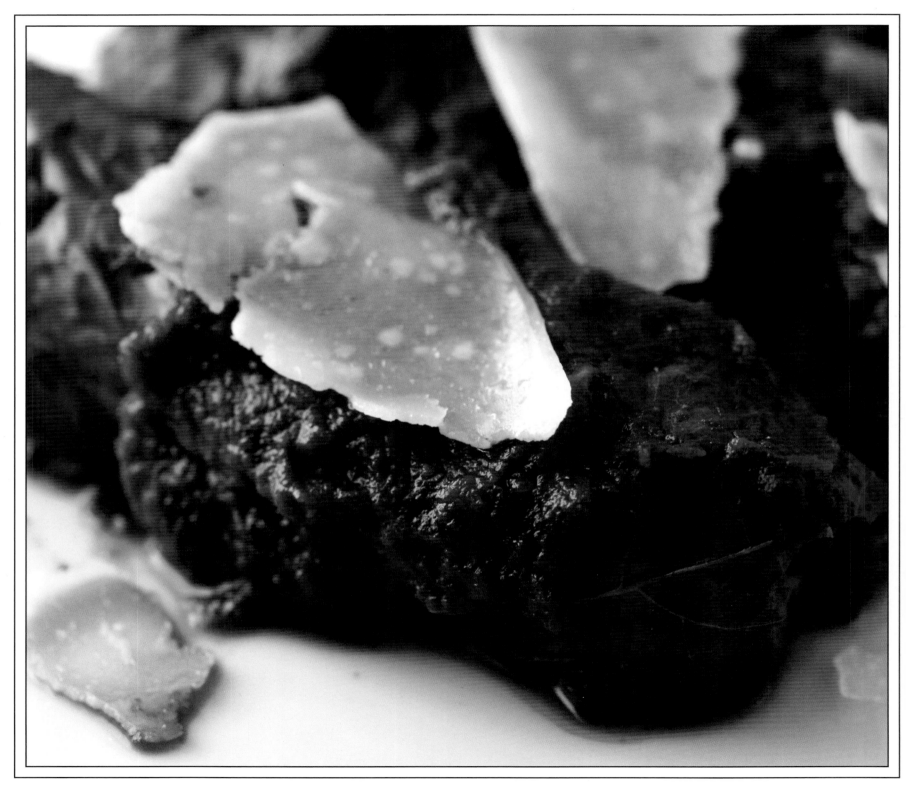

Shrimp, Eggplant, and Wild Mushroom-Stuffed Grape Leaves

with Ancho-Tomato Sauce

The ancho chiles in the tomato sauce for these stuffed grape leaves add some roasty notes to the dish that play well with the cumin and chile powder found in the stuffing. Once cooked, grape leaves can be stored in the fridge for up to 2 days and eaten either hot or cold.

STUFFED GRAPE LEAVES

Stuffed Grape Leaves

1	medium sized eggplant, peeled, stem trimmed and cut in ½-inch cubes
1	cup water
½ cup	long grain white rice
2	Tbsp. extra virgin olive oil
5	shiitake mushrooms, diced
1	portabella mushroom, stem removed and diced
	kosher salt
	freshly cracked black pepper
½ tsp.	ground cumin
½ tsp.	ground chile powder
½ tsp.	dried thyme
3 Tbsp.	sherry vinegar
3	green onions, thinly sliced
¾ lb	shrimp, peeled, deveined and roughly chopped
⅓ cup	freshly grated Parmesan cheese
1	jar brined grape leaves, drained and separated (about 18 to 20 leaves for this dish)
	kosher salt
	freshly cracked black pepper
1 recipe	Ancho-Tomato Sauce (see page 227)
	Parmesan cheese, for garnish

Toss eggplant in a bowl with 1 teaspoon kosher salt. Set aside salted eggplant for 1 hour. Rinse with water and squeeze to drain.

Preheat oven to 350 degrees.

Cook rice: Bring 1 cup of water to a boil in a small saucepan with tight-fitting lid over high heat. Once boiling, stir in a liberal pinch of salt and ½ cup rice. Cover with lid and reduce heat to low. Cook for 20 minutes and then remove from heat. Let rice steam inside saucepan for another 10 minutes. Do not remove lid during cooking and steaming process. Fluff with a fork and set aside in a large mixing bowl.

Heat 1 tablespoon olive oil in a large sauté pan over medium-high heat. Once pan and oil are hot, add shiitake and portabella mushrooms. Sprinkle with a pinch of kosher salt, freshly cracked black pepper, and half of the cumin, chile powder, and dried thyme. sauté seasoned mushrooms, stirring occasionally until mushrooms have caramelized and cooked through—8 to 10 minutes. Deglaze pan with 1 tablespoon sherry vinegar, scraping up any bits stuck to bottom of pan. Add mushrooms to bowl with rice.

Heat 1 tablespoon olive oil in same sauté pan used to cook mushrooms and place over medium heat. Once hot, add eggplant and sprinkle with black pepper and remaining cumin, chile powder, and dried thyme.

Stir. Sauté until cooked through and soft—about 5 minutes—stirring frequently. Remove from heat and place in bowl with rice and mushrooms.

Add the remaining sherry vinegar, green onions, shrimp, grated Parmesan, ¼ teaspoon freshly cracked black pepper and ½ teaspoon kosher salt to mixing bowl with rice and sautéed vegetables. Stir to thoroughly combine.

Lay one grape leaf out flat on a clean surface with the stem closest to you and the tips of the leaves farthest from you. Place ¼ cup rice-vegetable filling in a horizontal log across middle of the leaf. Fold in sides and then wrap stem end over stuffing, tucking it under and rolling leaf up into a tightly-packed log like a burrito. Place stuffed grape leaf, seam-side down, in a glass or ceramic baking dish. Repeat this stuffing process until remaining stuffing has been used.

Pour Ancho-Tomato sauce evenly over stuffed grape leaves. Cover baking dish tightly with aluminum foil. Bake at 350 degrees for 40 minutes. Remove from oven and garnish with shaved Parmesan cheese before serving.

Stuffed Heirloom Tomatoes

with Wild Rice and Italian Sausage

In the middle of summer when tomato season is at its peak and your counter tops are covered with the fruits of your tomato vines, this easy and delicious recipe is a great way to work through some of those perfectly ripe tomatoes. Serve alone as an appetizer or pair them with a salad or bowl of soup to make a complete meal.

STUFFED HEIRLOOM TOMATOES

½ cup	wild rice blend
6	medium heirloom tomatoes, various types
1 Tbsp.	canola oil
½ lb	hot Italian sausage, casings removed
1	yellow onion, finely diced
4	cloves garlic, minced
	juice from 1 lemon
1	green onion, chopped
¼ cup	(packed) flat leaf parsley, chopped
3 oz.	part-skim mozzarella, shredded
	kosher salt
	freshly cracked black pepper

Preheat oven to 350 degrees.

Bring a medium-sized pot of salted water to a boil over high heat. Add wild rice and boil for 30 minutes. Strain rice and return it to empty pot. Cover and let steam for 15 minutes untouched.

Cut off top (stem-side) ¼-inch of each tomato. Carefully hollow out tomatoes by scooping out seeds and pulp from middle, trying hard not to crush or tear tomato shells. Season inside cavity of each tomato with kosher salt and freshly cracked black pepper. Set aside.

While rice is cooking, brown Italian sausage in a preheated sauté pan with 1 tablespoon of canola oil over medium-high heat until cooked through, stirring occasionally and breaking up sausage into small pieces as it cooks. Remove from pan and drain on paper towels until ready to use.

Drain off all but 1 tablespoon of oil from sauté pan used to brown sausage. Reheat pan over medium heat. Add onions to pan and stir, scraping up any browned bits on the bottom of the pan. Sauté onions until translucent, stirring occasionally—about 10 minutes. Add minced garlic to pan and sauté for another 60 seconds, stirring continuously.

Combine sautéed onions and garlic, browned sausage, cooked wild rice, lemon juice, green onions, and parsley in a mixing bowl. Adjust seasonings to taste with kosher salt and freshly cracked black pepper.

Place the seasoned and hollowed-out tomatoes onto a sheet pan, open-side up. Stuff tomatoes with equal amounts of sausage-rice mixture. Sprinkle shredded mozzarella evenly over the tops of each tomato. Bake tomatoes for 20 to 25 minutes or until cheese is golden and bubbly. Remove from oven and serve hot.

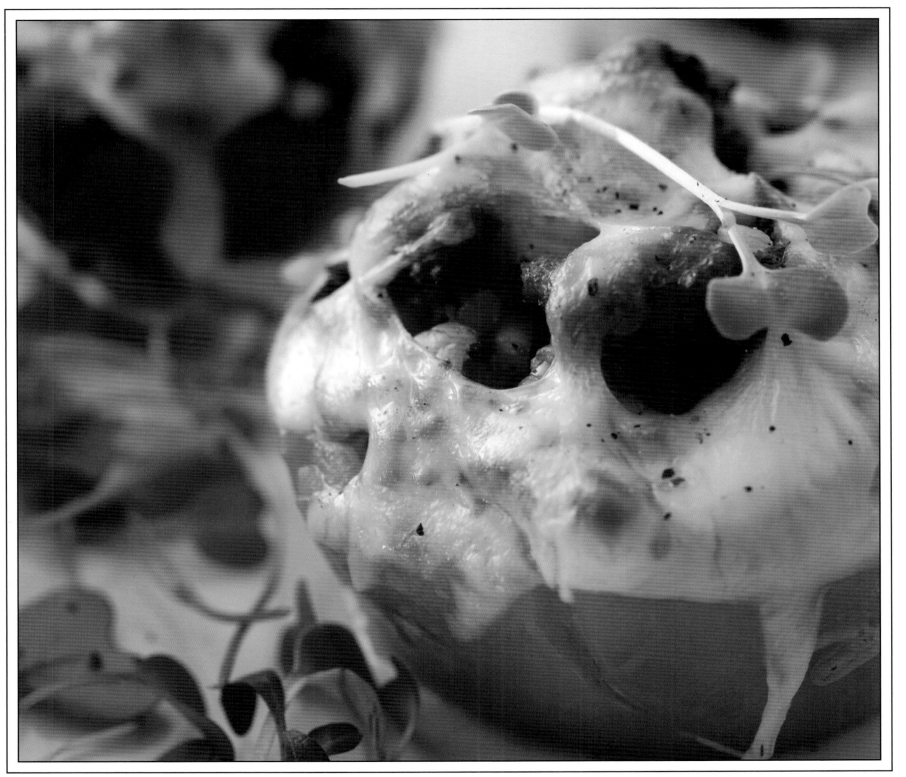

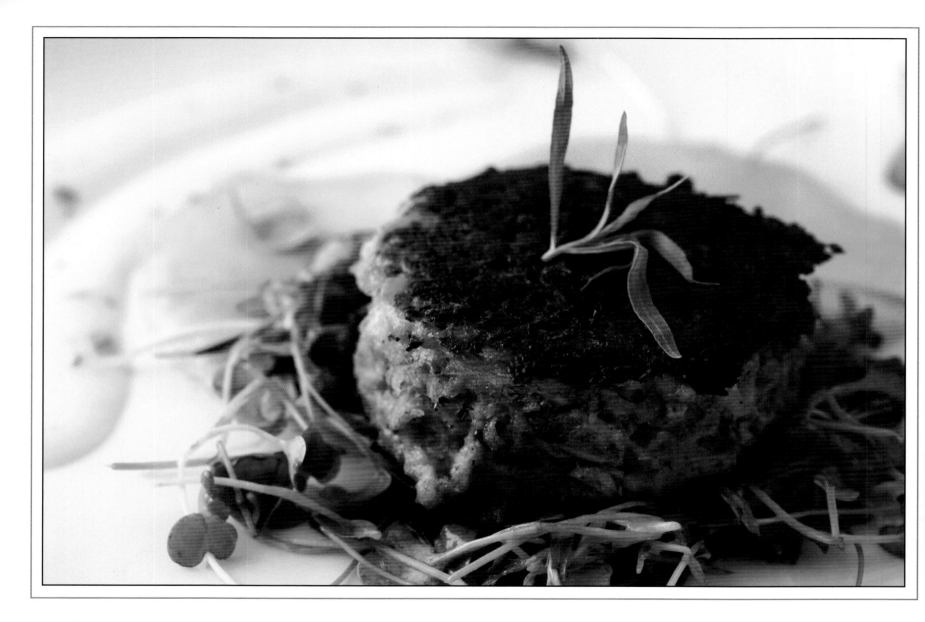

Tarragon-Macadamia Crab Cakes

with Mango & Micro Greens Salad and Tarragon Aioli

When my sister, a Chesapeake Bay–style crab cake purist, saw this dish, she said, "*Please tell me you didn't use blue crabs for this dish!*" I'm sorry, Sis, but there *are* other delicious ways to eat crab cakes than just the (incredibly tasty) ones we ate growing up. As long as the crab cake has way more crab meat than bready filling, I love introducing different flavors to shake things up. Crab and tarragon work beautifully together, and the mango and macadamia nuts give the dish an island feel.

TARRAGON-MACADAMIA CRAB CAKES

Tarragon-Macadamia Crab Cakes:

16 oz.	lump crab meat, picked over for shells
3 Tbsp.	tarragon aioli
1	egg, beaten
¼ tsp.	kosher salt
¼ tsp.	freshly cracked black pepper
¾ cup	bread crumbs
2 Tbsp.	fresh tarragon, chopped
¼ cup	macadamia nuts, chopped

2 Tbsp.	butter, divided
	chopped macadamia nuts, for garnish
	whole fresh tarragon leaves, for garnish

Mango & Micro Greens Salad:

2	mangoes (peeled, pitted, and thinly sliced)
4 cups	micro greens
2 Tbsp.	whole fresh tarragon leaves
¼ cup	red onions, shaved
1 Tbsp.	Tarragon Aioli
	kosher salt and freshly cracked black pepper, to taste

Tarragon Aioli:

1	large clove garlic, minced
2 tbsp	fresh tarragon, chopped
1 tbsp	Dijon mustard
1 tbsp	freshly squeezed lemon juice
1	egg yolk, as fresh as possible
½ tsp	kosher salt, plus extra
¼ tsp	freshly cracked black pepper, plus extra
½ cup	canola oil, or other flavorless oil

Preheat oven to 200 degrees

Place all ingredients for crab cakes into a mixing bowl. Mix well, trying not to break up any lumps of crab meat. Form crab mixture into 5 even crab cakes, using your hands to free-form or a ring mold as your guide.

Melt 1 tablespoon butter in a large sauté pan over medium-high heat. Once pan is hot and butter has melted, add 2 or 3 crab cakes to melted butter. Sauté over medium-high heat for 6 minutes or until bottom of crab cake releases from pan and edges turn golden brown. Flip and cook for another 6 minutes until golden. Transfer crab cakes to a baking sheet and keep warm in preheated oven.

Melt remaining butter in sauté pan and repeat cooking process with remaining crab cakes. (*Note: Trying to cook all of the crab cakes at the same time will overcrowd the pan and make cakes hard to flip.*) Serve crab cakes immediately.

MANGO & MICRO GREENS SALAD AND ASSEMBLY

Place equal amounts of sliced mango in a single layer onto 4 serving plates.

Toss micro greens, tarragon leaves, onions, and 1 tablespoon tarragon aioli in a large mixing bowl until aioli is evenly distributed. Adjust seasoning to taste with kosher salt and freshly cracked black pepper.

Top mango on each plate with a quarter of the dressed salad and place one crab cake on top of salad. Add a dollop of tarragon aioli next to the crab cake. Using the back of a spoon, spread aioli out in a curved swoop partially around the cake. Garnish with chopped macadamia nuts and small tarragon sprigs.

TARRAGON AIOLI

Whisk together first 7 ingredients in a large mixing bowl or add to the bowl of a food processor and pulse to combine. While continuously whisking vigorously or with the food processor running, very slowly drizzle in the oil in thin stream to form an emulsified sauce. If you note any oil beginning to pool, stop drizzling oil and continue whisking until incorporated. If the sauce breaks, start over. Adjust seasonings to taste with more kosher salt and freshly cracked black pepper. Chill for at least an hour before serving for the flavors to marry. Store chilled for up to 4 days.

Achiote Pork Loin Sandwiches

with Refried Black Beans, Fried Plantains, and Cilantro Pesto

Bright and bold Latin flavors almost instantly remind me of summer and tropical weather, which makes these sandwiches perfect for a steamy summer night.

ACHIOTE GRILLED PORK LOIN

4   boneless pork loin chops, trimmed of fat and pounded to about ⅓- to ½-inch thick

Marinade:

4   cloves garlic, peeled and minced

1 Tbsp.   achiote paste

   juice from 3 limes

1 tsp.   kosher salt, plus extra

½ tsp.   freshly cracked black pepper, plus extra

2 Tbsp.   canola oil

Whisk together first 5 ingredients for marinade. While whisking constantly, drizzle in the canola oil.

Place pounded pork chops into a resealable plastic bag. Pour marinade over the chops in the bag. Toss to ensure that all surface area of pork chops is covered in marinade. Seal bag, removing as much air as possible to emulate a vacuum seal. Marinate pork, refrigerated, for 4 to 24 hours.

Prepare grill for medium-high heat.

Once grill is hot, remove chops from marinade. Lightly season chops on all sides with kosher salt and freshly cracked black pepper. Grill over medium-high heat for 3 to 4 minutes. Flip and grill for another 3 to 4 minutes until just cooked through to an internal temperature of about 140 degrees for medium doneness.

REFRIED BLACK BEANS

Refried Black Beans:

1   slice thick-cut bacon, cut in half lengthwise

2   cloves garlic, minced

1   (15-oz.) can black beans, drained and rinsed (or 1½ cups cooked black beans)

½ tsp.   kosher salt, plus extra

¼ tsp.   freshly cracked black pepper, plus extra

½ tsp.   chili powder

½ tsp.   ground cumin

½ cup   water, plus extra as needed

Cook bacon in small saucepan over medium heat until all fat has been rendered out and bacon is crisp. Remove bacon from pan and eat. (Or give to a loved one to eat.)

Add minced garlic to rendered fat and sauté over medium heat for about 60 seconds, stirring constantly, until the aroma of sautéing garlic reaches your nose. Add remaining ingredients *except* water to pan. Sauté

beans in fat for about 3 minutes, stirring occasionally. Add water to pan and bring to a simmer. Carefully mash simmering beans with a fork or potato masher, or blend with an immersion blender until beans reach the consistency of refried beans. Gradually add more water if necessary to thin out beans to desired consistency. Adjust seasonings to taste with more kosher salt and freshly cracked black pepper.

Continued on Next Page

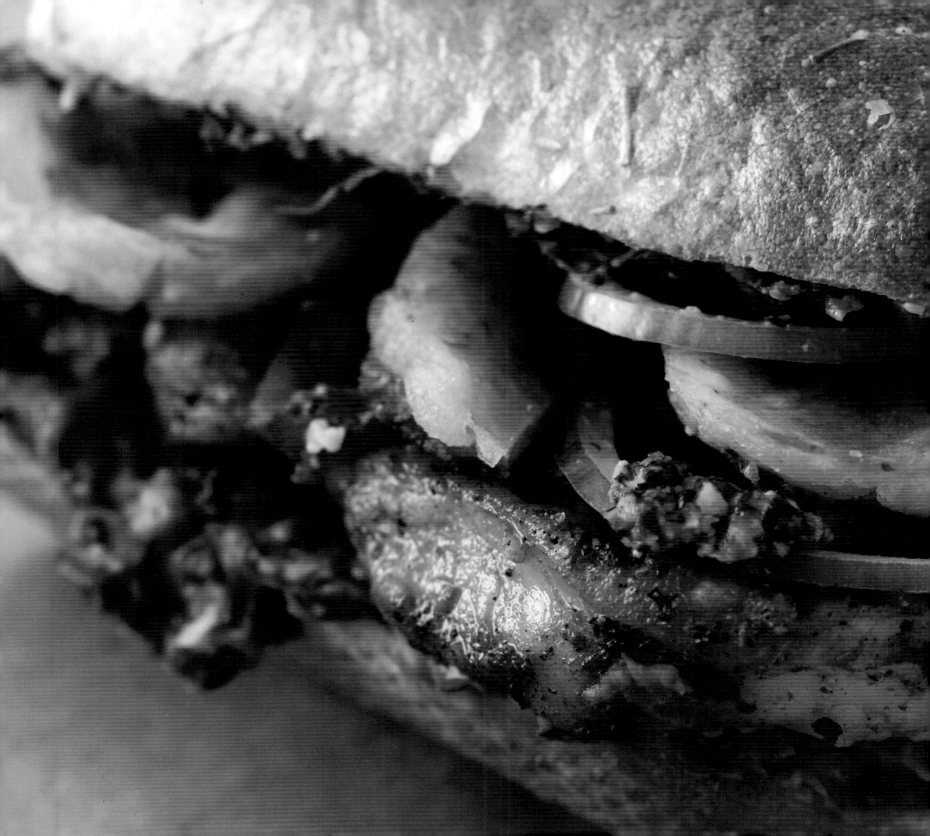

Cilantro Pesto:

1 cup   fresh cilantro leaves

1½ Tbsp.   pepitas

1   clove garlic, peeled

juice from ½ lime

1 oz.   crumbled cotija cheese

¼ tsp.   kosher salt, plus extra

¼ tsp.   freshly cracked black pepper, plus extra

2 Tbsp.   canola oil

Fried Plantains:

1   ripe plantain, peeled, ends removed and cut in ¼-inch thick slices on a diagonal

2 Tbsp.   canola or peanut oil

kosher salt

For assembly:

4   hoagie rolls (or rolls of choice), sliced in half, sandwich style

2   roasted poblano peppers (seeds and stem removed), julienned (see page 239)

thinly sliced red onion

Process all pesto ingredients *except* canola oil in a food processor until pulverized. While pesto is processing, drizzle in oil. Adjust seasonings to taste with more kosher salt and freshly cracked black pepper. If you like a tart pesto, add a bit more lime juice as well.

FRIED PLANTAINS

Heat oil in a large sauté pan over medium to medium-high heat for about 2 to 3 minutes or until pan and oil are hot.

While pan is heating, season both sides of plantain slices with kosher salt.

Sauté plantain slices in heated oil until golden—4 to 6 minutes. Flip and sauté until other side is golden as well—4 to 6 minutes. Remove from heat and drain on a paper towel.

ASSEMBLY

To assemble sandwiches, smear refried black beans on the inside of the bottom half of each hoagie roll. For each sandwich, place one achiote-marinated grilled pork chop on top of the refried beans. Next add a layer of julienned roasted poblano peppers, then fried plantains, and finally a few rings of thinly sliced red onion. Smear a thick layer of cilantro pesto over the inside of the top half of each hoagie roll. Place the top half of the rolls cilantro-side down onto the fillings to close each sandwich. Slice sandwiches in half and serve immediately.

Grilled Blue Cheese Burger

with Caramelized Onions, Mushrooms & Horseradish Mayo and Hand-Cut Truffle Fries

It's well-known that the best fries are first blanched in oil, and then drained before being fried at a higher temperature until golden and crisp. This technique is used in the fry recipe below, but to make them even more delicious they are tossed with truffle oil, Parmesan, and parsley before serving. If you have a spare truffle lying around, feel free to add some freshly shaved truffle too.

BLUE CHEESE BURGERS

Blue Cheese Burgers:

1⅓ lb.	ground buffalo, (if you do not like or cannot find buffalo, substitute ground beef)
	kosher salt
	freshly cracked black pepper

For Assembly:

4	sesame seed buns
	horseradish mayonnaise
	caramelized onions
	sautéed cremini mushrooms
4 oz.	crumbled blue cheese

Sautéed Cremini Mushrooms:

1½ tbsp	canola or olive oil
20–25	cremini mushrooms, sliced
1 tsp.	fresh thyme leaves
1 Tbsp.	freshly squeezed lemon juice
	kosher salt
	freshly cracked black pepper

Horseradish Mayonnaise:

See Page 234

Prepare grill to medium-high heat.

While the grill is heating, form ground buffalo into 4 evenly sized patties, ⅓-pound each. Liberally season both sides of each patty with kosher salt and freshly cracked black pepper.

Place the patties onto the hot grill. Grill over medium-high heat for about 5 minutes per side (10 minutes total) until just cooked through, flipping only once. (If you know and trust the butcher who grinds your meat, feel free to cook the burgers for less time for a more medium to medium rare burger.)

Remove from heat and assemble burgers. Place one patty on the bottom half of a sesame seed bun. Spread about 1 tbsp of horseradish mayonnaise on the cut-side of the top half of the bun. Sprinkle the patty with 1 ounce of crumbled blue cheese then top with caramelized onions and sautéed cremini mushrooms. Cover with the top bun. Repeat the dressing process with the rest of the burgers. Serve immediately with hot freshly-cooked truffle fries.

SAUTÉED CREMINI MUSHROOMS

Add oil to a large sauté pan and place over medium heat. Once the pan is hot and the oil is rippling from the heat, add the sliced mushrooms to the pan. Sprinkle with fresh thyme leaves, kosher salt, and freshly cracked black pepper. Toss to coat with oil and distribute the seasonings. Sauté, undisturbed for about 4 minutes to allow the mushrooms to caramelize. Stir and sauté for another 4 to 5 minutes until cooked through and well caramelized. Deglaze the pan with the lemon juice, stirring and scraping up any bits on the bottom. Adjust seasonings to taste with more kosher salt and freshly cracked black pepper.

Continued on Next Page

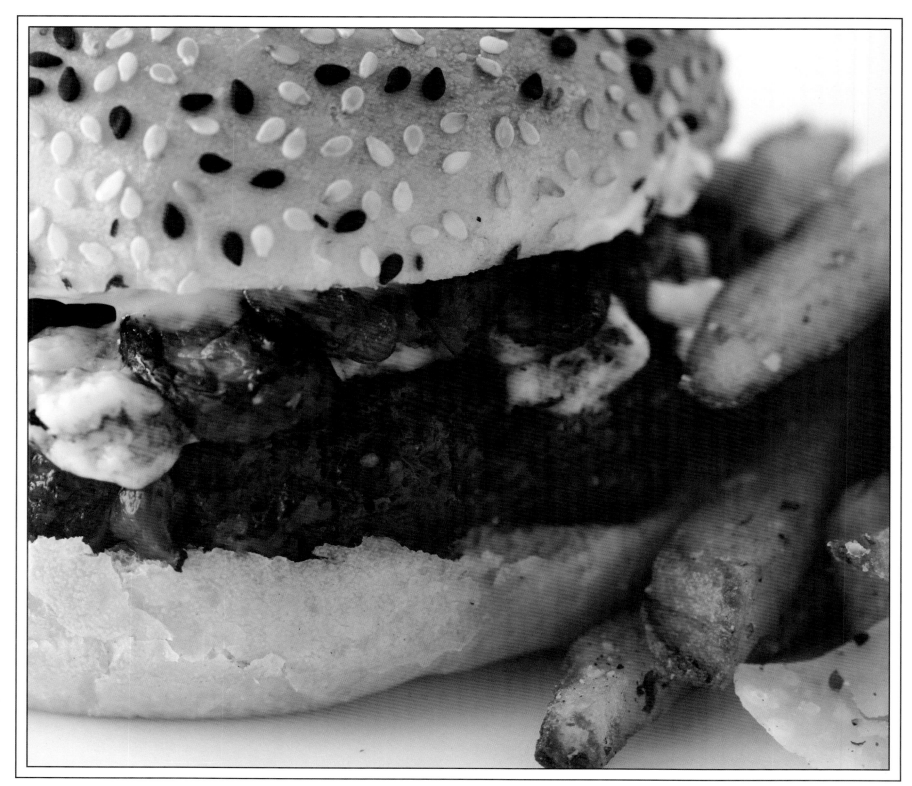

Caramelized Onions:

2 Tbsp.	canola oil
2	large yellow onions, peeled and sliced
	kosher salt
	freshly cracked black pepper

Truffled Parmesan Fries:

3	large russet potatoes
	peanut oil, for frying (enough to fill your deep fryer or halfway up a large pot)
	kosher salt
2–3 tsp.	truffle oil
	shaved Parmesan cheese
2 Tbsp.	fresh parsley, minced

Add oil to a large sauté pan and place over medium to medium-low heat. Once the pan is hot, add the onions. Toss to coat with oil. Slowly sauté onions, stirring frequently to prevent burning, until the onions have caramelized and are golden, sweet, and tender, about 30 to 45 minutes. Season onions to taste with kosher salt and freshly cracked black pepper. Caramelized onions can be made a few days in advance and heated just before ready for use.

TRUFFLED FRENCH FRIES

Peel russet potatoes. Slice potatoes into ⅓-inch thick slices then cut into ⅓-inch x ⅓-inch thick batons. Immediately place batons into a bowl and cover with 1-inch water. Add 2 cups of ice to the water and place in the fridge. Let the potatoes sit in the ice water for at least 30 minutes and up to 24 hours. This process helps remove some of the starch from the potatoes.

Heat the oil in a deep fryer to 280 degrees. Monitor the oil using a deep fryer thermometer.

Line a couple of sheet pans with paper towels and set aside.

Once the oil has come up to temperature, Drain the potato batons from the ice water. Pat completely dry with a kitchen towel or paper towels. Working in batches, blanch the batons in the oil for about 8 minutes per batch, stirring occasionally, until the fries are soft and turning translucent. During this step you do not want the potatoes to brown at all. If they begin to brown, your oil is too hot.

Remove the par-cooked fries from the oil and transfer to the lined sheet pans to drain. Repeat process with the rest of the potatoes. Once all the potatoes are par-cooked, let them drain on paper towels for at 30 minutes to 2 hours.

When ready to finish the fries, raise the heat of the oil to 350 to 360 degrees. Once the oil has come up to temperature, fry the french fries in batches for 1 to 2 minutes until golden brown and crispy. Let oil return to 350 to 360 degrees before frying the next batch. Remove from oil, drain on paper towels and sprinkle with kosher salt immediately. After about 30 seconds of draining, transfer the fries to a heat-safe bowl and drizzle with a small amount of truffle oil, a couple of pinches of shaved Parmesan cheese and chopped parsley. Toss to evenly distribute the oil, cheese and herbs. Taste and adjust seasoning with more salt if necessary. Serve immediately. (Because fries are best immediately after cooking, serve the batches as soon as they are finished rather than waiting for all of the batches to cook before serving.)

A NOTE ON DEEP FRYING

It is ideal to use a deep fryer because they heat the oil from all sides so the oil is more easily kept at an even temperature both at the top and bottom of the pot. If using a pot on the stove be very careful because the oil at the bottom of the pot will be significantly hotter than at the top of the pot. To help diffuse the heat, carefully stir the oil without splashing. Not only can oil cause very serious burns, it can also catch on fire if overheated or if spilled onto the heating element. (Again, this is a great reason to use a deep fryer rather than the stove.)

Marinade:

2 cups	buttermilk
3 Tbsp.	sugar
1 Tbsp.	kosher salt
2	cloves garlic, peeled and minced
1 Tbsp.	hot sauce
1 tsp.	freshly cracked black pepper

3–4	firm, unripe green tomatoes cut in ½-inch thick slices, ends removed
	peanut oil, for frying.

Crust:

1 cup	flour
1 cup	stone-ground corn meal
1 Tbsp.	kosher salt
1 tsp.	freshly cracked black pepper
1 tsp.	granulated garlic
½ tsp.	onion powder

Grilled Shrimp:

2–3 Tbsp.	canola oil
4	thin slices sopressata, cut in quarters
16	colossal shrimp, peeled and deveined
	kosher salt and freshly cracked black pepper

Salad:

2	navel oranges, supremed
3 cups	pea shoots
¼ cup	red onion, shaved
2 Tbsp.	Orange-Sage Vinaigrette (see page 236)
	kosher salt and freshly cracked black pepper

3 oz.	crumbled chevre, for assembly

Stir together marinade ingredients in a non-reactive bowl. Add tomatoes and marinate for 1 hour.

While tomatoes are marinating, whisk together all ingredients for crust in a large bowl to evenly distribute.

Heat 1 inch oil to 350 degrees in a large dutch oven or heavy-bottomed pot over medium-high heat.

While oil is heating, dredge buttermilk-marinated tomatoes in crust mixture to coat evenly. Place coated tomatoes onto a piece of parchment or wax paper until ready to fry.

Working in batches of four so you don't overcrowd the pan, add coated tomatoes to hot oil. Fry for about 4 minutes total or until golden brown, flipping halfway through cooking. Remove fried tomatoes from oil and place on paper towels to drain. Season lightly with kosher salt. Repeat this process with remaining tomatoes.

GRILLED SHRIMP & ORANGE-PEA SHOOT SALAD

Preheat oil in large sauté pan over medium-high heat for 3 minutes. Once oil is hot, add sopressata pieces and crisp until most of the fat has been rendered out—about 1 minute per side. Remove from pan and drain on a paper towel.

While sopressata is crisping, season shrimp with kosher salt and freshly cracked black pepper. Toss to coat.

Add shrimp to hot pan as soon as sopressata has been removed. Sear shrimp about 2 minutes per side— 4 minutes total—until caramelized and just cooked through, working in batches depending on the size of your sauté pan to prevent overcrowding. Remove from heat.

Toss salad ingredients with orange-sage vinaigrette in a mixing bowl. Season to taste with kosher salt and freshly cracked black pepper.

To assemble:

Place a small bed of pea shoot salad in the middle of the plate. Place 1 fried green tomato on top of pea shoot salad followed by 2 shrimp, a few of pieces of sopressata, and a few pea shoots. Stack another fried green tomato on top of the shrimp and sopressata. Stand two more shrimp upright on top of the second tomato and carefully place a couple more pieces of sopressata. Scatter some crumbled chevre and navel orange-pea shoot salad around the plate. Finish with a drizzle of vinaigrette. Repeat plating three more times with remaining ingredients.

Fried Green Tomato Napoleons

with Grilled Shrimp, Sopressata, and Orange-Sage Vinaigrette

It's no secret that I was raised in the South, and most of my professional cooking experience happened in the even deeper South. This dish is a nod to the fresh bright flavors of nouvelle Southern cuisine.

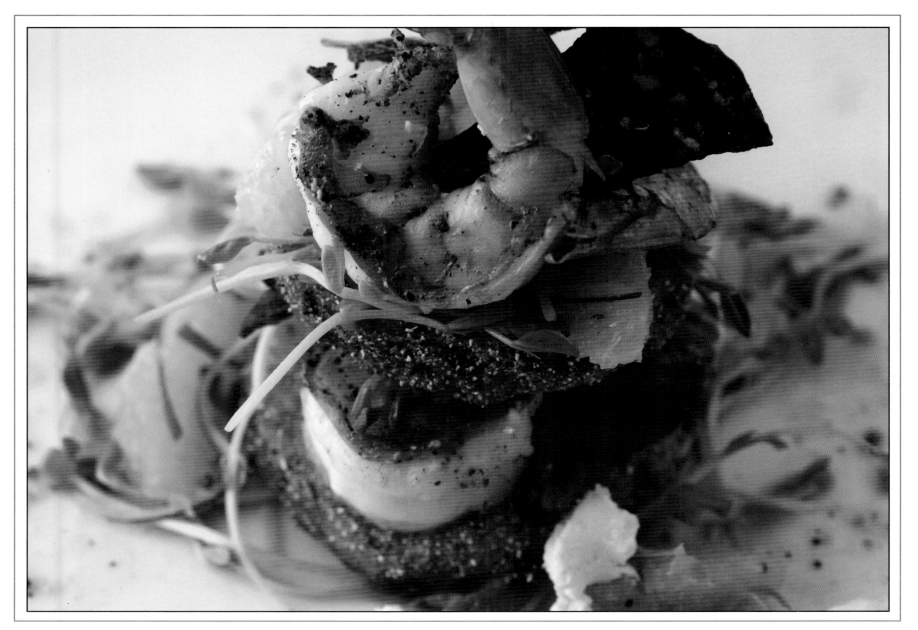

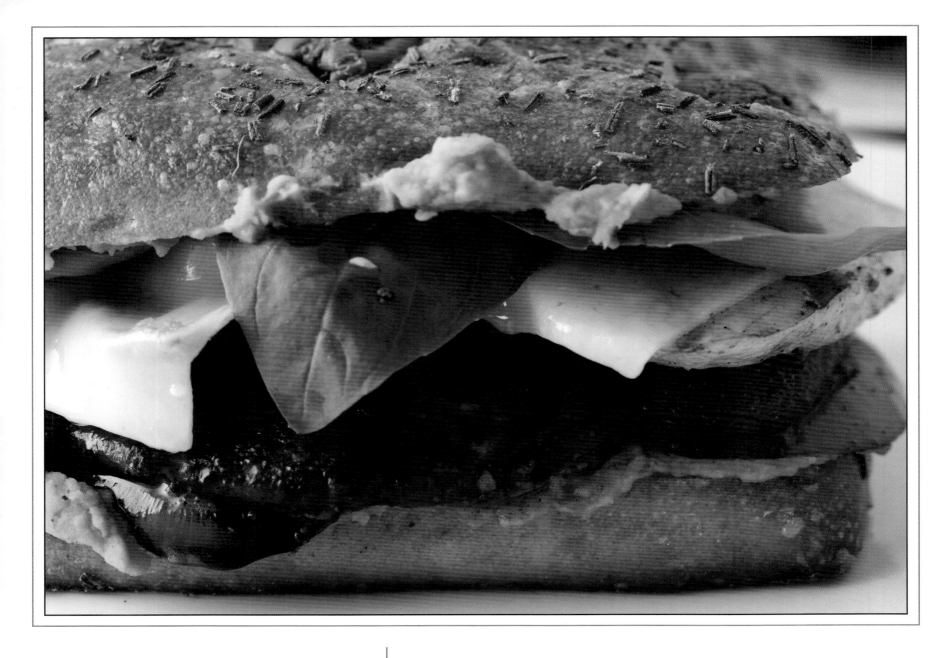

Marinated Grilled Veggie Sandwiches

with Truffled Sun-Dried Tomato Cannellini Hummus

Vegetarians and meat-eaters alike will love the bright bold flavors of this sandwich. To make it vegan friendly, simply leave off the cheese.

Marinade/Vinaigrette:

⅓ cup	red wine vinegar
1 tsp.	granulated garlic
1 tsp.	granulated onion
½ tsp.	dried oregano
1 tsp.	kosher salt
1 tsp.	freshly cracked black pepper
2 Tbsp.	Dijon mustard
⅓ cup	extra virgin olive oil

4	portabella mushroom caps, stems removed and "gills" carefully scraped out
2	small zucchini, stem ends removed and sliced ¼-inch thick on a diagonal
1	large yellow squash, stem ends removed and sliced ¼-inch thick on a diagonal
1	red onion, peeled and sliced into ½-inch rings
	kosher salt and freshly cracked black pepper

Hummus:

1	(14.5-oz.) can cannellini beans, drained and rinsed (or 1½ cups cooked cannellini beans)
½ cup	sun-dried tomatoes (packed in oil and drained)
	zest from 1 lemon
	juice from 1 to 2 lemons
1½ Tbsp.	white truffle oil
2 Tbsp.	extra virgin olive oil
	cloves from 1 bulb of roasted garlic (see page 240)
1 tsp.	kosher salt, plus extra
1 tsp.	freshly cracked black pepper, plus extra

Assembly

4	ciabatta rolls or rolls of choice, sliced in half, sandwich style
	sliced asiago cheese
	fresh basil leaves

GRILLED VEGGIE SANDWICH

In a mixing bowl, whisk together all marinade ingredients *except* oil. While whisking continuously, slowly drizzle in the oil to form an emulsified marinade/vinaigrette.

Pour marinade over prepared portabella mushroom caps in a resealable plastic bag. Make sure that all sides of mushrooms are touched by marinade. Seal the bag, removing as much air as possible to emulate a vacuum seal. Marinate mushrooms in refrigerator for 2 to 4 hours.

Prepare grill for medium-high heat.

Once grill is hot, remove mushrooms from marinade and place directly onto grill. Set remaining marinade aside. Sprinkle mushrooms lightly with kosher salt and freshly cracked black pepper. Grill for 4 to 5 minutes until nicely charred. Flip and grill another 4 to 5 minutes until cooked through.

Immediately after putting mushrooms on the grill, place sliced zucchini, yellow squash, and red onions into the bag with remaining marinade. Toss to coat. Let sit for 1 minute before placing veggies onto grill with portabella mushrooms. Sprinkle with kosher salt and pepper. Cook for 2 to 3 minutes until grill marks appear. Flip and grill for another 2 to 3 minutes until just cooked through.

TRUFFLED SUN-DRIED TOMATO CANNELLINI HUMMUS

Place all ingredients into a food processor or blender. Blend/process until smooth. If necessary, thin hummus out with a little bit of water. Adjust seasoning to taste with more lemon juice, kosher salt, and freshly cracked black pepper.

ASSEMBLY

Preheat oven to 400 degrees.

Heat buns in oven for 5 minutes. Remove from oven and layer 1 grilled portabella cap, several slices of zucchini and yellow squash, and several onion slices onto bottom halves of each roll. Top grilled veggies with sliced asiago cheese. Place in oven for 2 to 3 minutes or until cheese has melted.

While the cheese is melting, smear prepared hummus on top halves of each bun.

Remove sandwich bottoms from oven. Top melted cheese with fresh basil leaves. Close sandwiches by placing top half of each bun, hummus-side down, over filling. Serve immediately.

Homemade Mustard:

⅓ cup   mustard powder

1½ Tbsp.   brown mustard seeds

½ tsp.   kosher salt, plus extra

     small pinch ground allspice

¼ tsp.   granulated garlic

2 tsp.   honey

1 tsp.   truffle oil

1 Tbsp.   sherry vinegar

3 Tbsp.   water, plus extra

Artichoke-Pepper Relish:

½ cup   peppadew peppers

½ cup   pickled cherry peppers, stems removed

½ cup   pickled pearl onions (also called cocktail onions)

1 cup   marinated artichoke hearts, drained

Grilled Hot Dogs:

4   (¼ lb.) all-beef hot dogs

4   high-quality hot dog buns

     pea shoots or sprouts (optional)

     Artichoke-Pepper Relish

     Smoked Gouda, thinly sliced

     Sweet & Spicy Homemade Mustard

SWEET & SPICY HOMEMADE MUSTARD

Combine all ingredients for mustard in a mixing bowl and whisk into a paste. Let sit for 2 hours at room temperature. Thin paste to standard mustard consistency with extra water. Adjust seasoning to taste with kosher salt. Store, chilled, in a glass or plastic container until ready for use. (*Note: Mustard is hottest as soon as it's made. As it sits in the fridge for days the heat will subside. Mustard will last indefinitely when stored properly. Due to its highly acidic nature, do not store mustard in anything aluminum or covered with aluminum.*)

ARTICHOKE-PEPPER RELISH

Process ingredients in a food processor until mixture is the consistency of relish.

GRILLED HOT DOGS

Preheat broiler. Prepare grill for medium-high heat.

When grill is heated, grill hot dogs until cooked through and charred on all sides—2 to 3 minutes per side. If desired, warm buns on grill, about 1 to 2 minutes per side.

To assemble:

Place hot dog in bun. Sprinkle pea shoots on either side of the hot dog, follow with a liberal amount of relish. Cover the top of the hot dog with slices of Gouda. Repeat this process with the next three hot dogs. Place hot dogs upright on a baking sheet under the broiler. Broil for 1 to 2 minutes until the cheese begins to melt. Remove from oven and drizzle mustard over the top of the hot dogs. Serve immediately.

Look for a nearby grocery store that has an olive bar. Many of the items in the Artichoke-Pepper Relish can be purchased there in the portions that this recipe calls for, which is much nicer than having to buy large individual jars of each item. If you can't find peppadews, just double the amount of cherry peppers.

Grilled Hot Dogs

with Smoked Gouda, Sweet and Spicy Homemade
Mustard, and Artichoke-Pepper Relish

Hot dogs are the perfect summer food for any barbecue or get-together—quick and easy, yet oddly satisfying. When you make the mustard for this dish, resist the urge to taste it before it's had a chance to sit for two hours. The initial flavor of mustard powder combined with water is quite bitter and rather unappealing. Once the mustard has a chance to mellow slightly, you can taste it to adjust the seasoning levels.

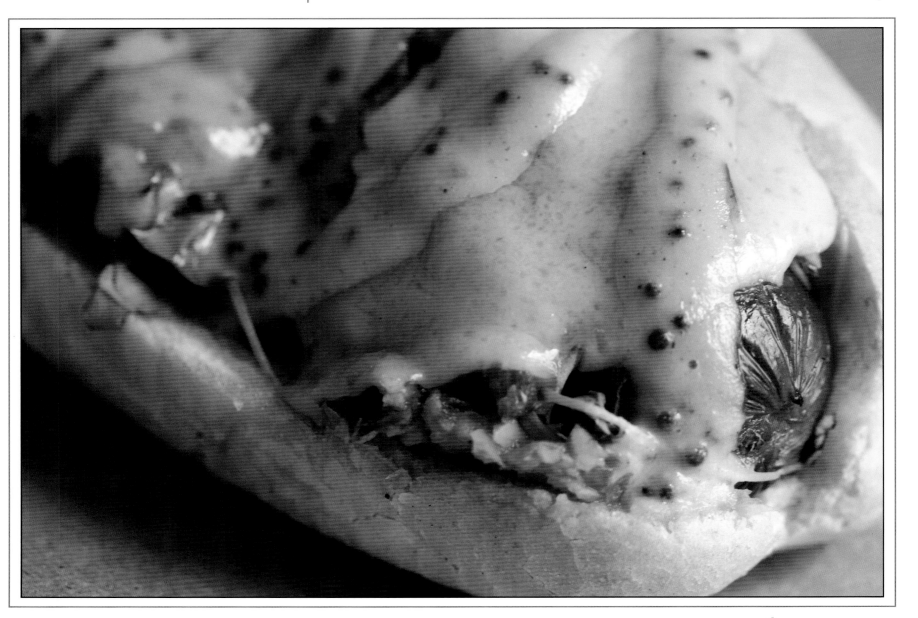

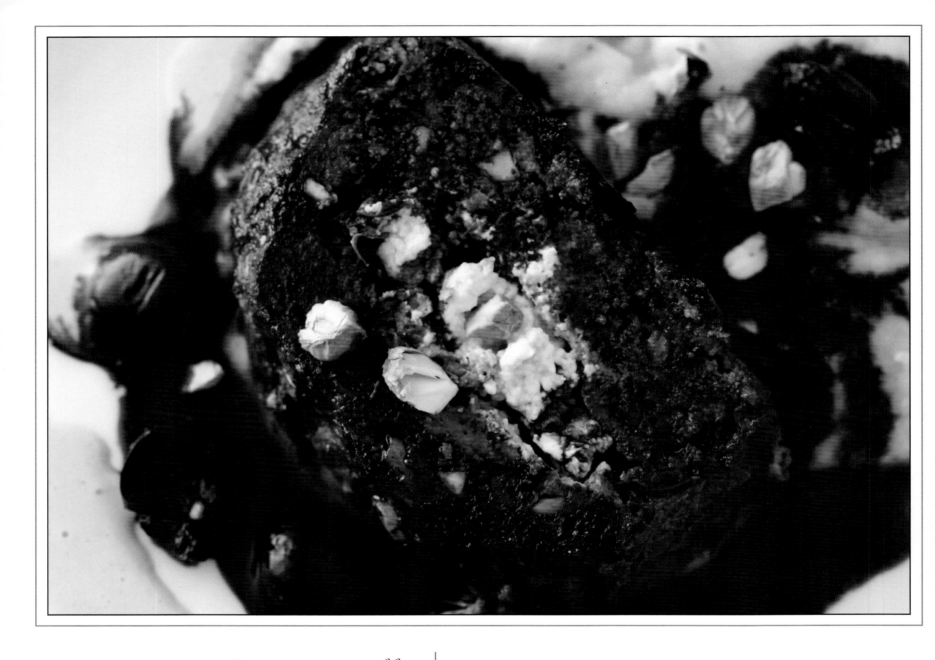

Sheep's Milk Feta Stuffed Lamb Kofta Meatloaf

with Roasted Garlic Turnip Puree and Bing Cherry-Red Wine Reduction

Bing cherries have a short harvesting season that peaks in mid June. While not a fundamental element of this dish, they add a delightful, sweet, fruity pop that complements the heavily-seasoned lamb meatloaf nicely. If Bing cherries aren't available, you can substitute any sweet ripe cherry.

LAMB KOFTA MEATLOAF

Meatloaf:

1¾ lb	ground lamb
3 Tbsp.	sumac
1 Tbsp.	ground cumin
1 Tbsp.	chili powder
1 tsp.	dried thyme
2 tsp.	kosher salt
1 tsp.	freshly ground black pepper
1 tsp.	granulated garlic
¼ cup	bread crumbs
¼ cup	dried sour cherries, roughly chopped
¼ cup	shelled pistachios, roughly chopped
⅔ cup	crumbled sheep's milk feta (can substitute with cow's milk feta)

Bing Cherry-Red Wine Reduction:

⅓ cup	balsamic vinegar
1 cup	dry red wine
15	Bing cherries, pitted and halved

Herbed Yogurt Sauce:

1 cup	Greek-style strained yogurt, not fat-free
	juice from ½ lemon
2 Tbsp.	water
½ tsp.	kosher salt, plus extra
½ cup	packed mint leaves
½ cup	packed parsley leaves
1	clove garlic

Roasted Garlic Turnip Puree

See Page 240

chopped salted pistachios, for garnishing

Preheat oven to 350 degrees.

In a large bowl, mix all ingredients for meatloaf *except* crumbled feta by hand until all seasonings have been worked into the lamb.

Form meat loaf. Line a sheet pan with parchment paper. Using about two-thirds of the ground lamb mixture, form a rectangular "boat" with an indentation in the middle and approximately 1-inch thick wall on all sides. Fill indentation with crumbled feta. Using remaining lamb mixture, press out a similar rectangle and place over the filling. Press together sides and top of meatloaf to form a completely sealed meatloaf.

Bake meatloaf at for 50 minutes. Remove from oven and let cool for 10 minutes before slicing.

BING CHERRY-RED WINE REDUCTION

Reduce balsamic vinegar and red wine by one third in a small saucepan over medium-high heat. Add cherries to reduction and reduce, again by one third. Remove from heat and let cool slightly before using.

HERBED YOGURT SAUCE

Blend all ingredients in blender until smooth. Adjust seasonings to taste with kosher salt.

ASSEMBLY

To plate, place a scoop of turnip puree in the middle of a plate. Lean a slice of meatloaf up against turnips. Drizzle cherry-red wine reduction over meatloaf and turnips. To garnish drizzle herbed yogurt around the outside of the plate and sprinkle dish with chopped pistachios.

Seared Mahi Tacos

on Fresh Corn Tortillas with Pico De Gallo, Red Cabbage, and White Sauce

There is something so inherently right about sautéing a piece of freshly caught fish, throwing it into a fresh corn tortilla and dousing it with salsa fresca, lime, and white sauce. While fish tacos are great with fried, grilled, or sautéed fish, we prefer the latter. This recipe calls for mahi mahi but really, any fresh fish that is available locally will do.

Corn Tortillas:

1¾ cups	instant masa harina, like Maseca
1 tsp.	kosher salt
1¼ cups	hot tap water

Special Equipment: tortilla press

Pico De Gallo:

½ lb	ripe tomatoes, cored & diced
½–1	jalapeño pepper, finely diced (vary amount depending on how spicy you like it. For even less spice, remove seeds and veins)
¼ cup	red onion, finely diced
2–3 Tbsp.	(packed) cilantro, roughly chopped
1	clove garlic, peeled and minced
	juice from ½ lime
	kosher salt and freshly cracked black pepper, to taste

Red Cabbage:

4 cups	red cabbage, finely shredded
	juice from ½ lime
	pinch of salt

FRESH CORN TORTILLAS

Preheat oven to its lowest setting, ideally under 200 degrees.

Whisk masa and salt in a mixing bowl to combine. Add hot tap water and stir until mixture comes together to form a dough similar in consistency to soft cookie dough. Knead dough in bowl, working it into a ball. Cover bowl with a slightly damp cloth and let set for 20 minutes.

While dough is resting, preheat a griddle or large sauté pan to medium-high heat. (*Note: Have a large piece of aluminum foil on hand. As the tortillas are finished you will use this to keep them warm.*)

Line a corn tortilla press with a plastic bag (a cut up plastic grocery bag works best). Pinch off about a 1½-inch piece of dough and roll into a ball in your hands. Place dough ball into center of lined tortilla press. Close press and press down on the handle as far as it will go. Open press and carefully peel tortilla away from plastic. Tortilla will easily crumble, so be gentle! Cook tortilla on preheated griddle for 60 to 90 seconds until tortilla starts to brown in spots. Flip tortilla and cook for another 60 or so seconds until tortilla begins to puff and brown in places. Wrap tortilla in aluminum foil and keep warm in oven. Repeat process with remaining dough. Tortillas are best eaten fresh and are typically not good the next day.

PICO DE GALLO

Combine all ingredients for pico de gallo in a mixing bowl. Season to taste with kosher salt and freshly cracked black pepper. Let sit, chilled, for 30 minutes before serving to allow flavors to marry.

RED CABBAGE

Toss cabbage with lime juice and a pinch of salt. Let set for 1 hour, tossing every 15 minutes or so. Cabbage will begin to soften and release water and color.

Continued on Next Page

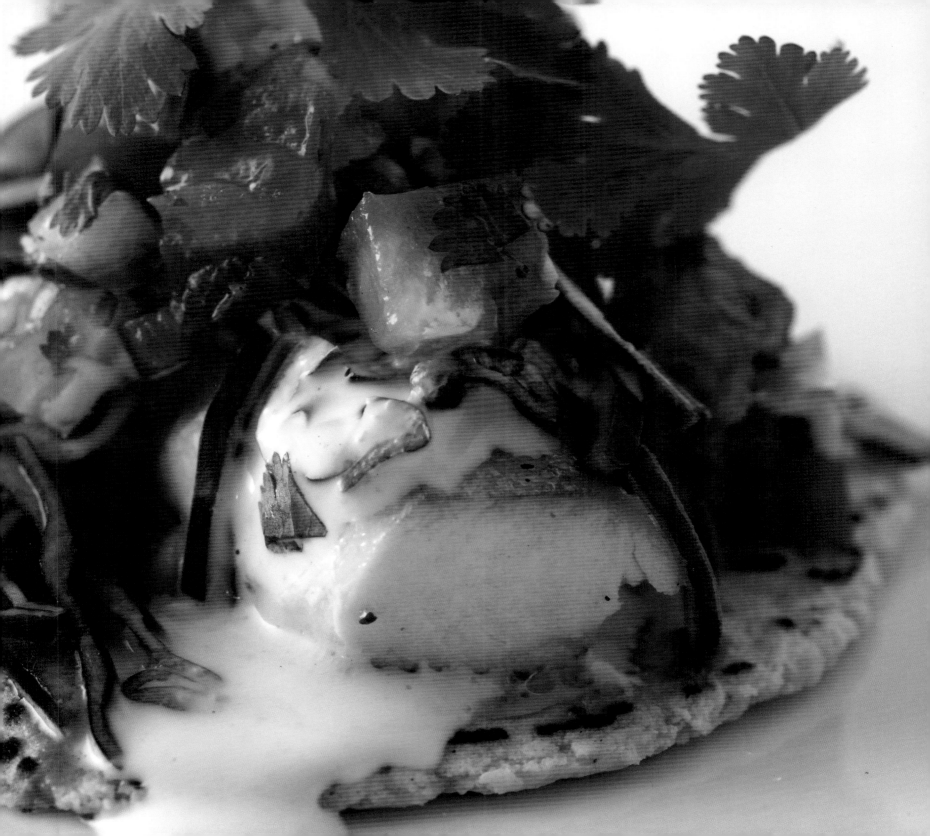

White Sauce:

¼ cup   mayonnaise

¼ cup   buttermilk

¼ tsp.   kosher salt

¼ tsp.   granulated garlic

Seared Mahi:

1½ lbs.   mahi mahi, cut in 1-inch thick slices

2–3 Tbsp. canola oil

kosher salt

freshly cracked black pepper

Whisk together all ingredients thoroughly. Chill in an airtight container in the refrigerator for at least 30 minutes. Stir before use.

SEARED MAHI

Preheat a large *non-stick* sauté pan over medium-high heat for 3 minutes.

While pan is heating, season fish liberally with kosher salt and freshly cracked black pepper. Toss to coat.

Add canola oil to heated pan. Once oil ripples with heat, but before it begins to smoke, add half of the fish to the pan. (*Note: Cooking the fish in two batches prevents overcrowding the pan.*) Sear fish over medium-high heat for 3 to 4 minutes until caramelized, flip, and continue cooking for another 3 to 4 minutes until just cooked through. Remove from pan and set aside. Repeat with second batch.

ASSEMBLY

To construct tacos, place 1 tortilla on a plate. Place a piece of mahi down the middle of tortilla. Add wilted cabbage on top of mahi and drizzle with white sauce. Spoon on pico de gallo. Serve with various hot sauces, Sriracha, lime wedges, and fresh cilantro leaves to garnish.

Rosemary-Garlic Roasted Rack of Lamb

with Sautéed Green Beans and Rosemary-Garlic Brown Butter Croutons

If it's too hot inside to use your oven, grilling the lamb is always an option . . . actually, it may taste even better than searing and roasting it. Either way, this is one of my personal all-time favorite meals.

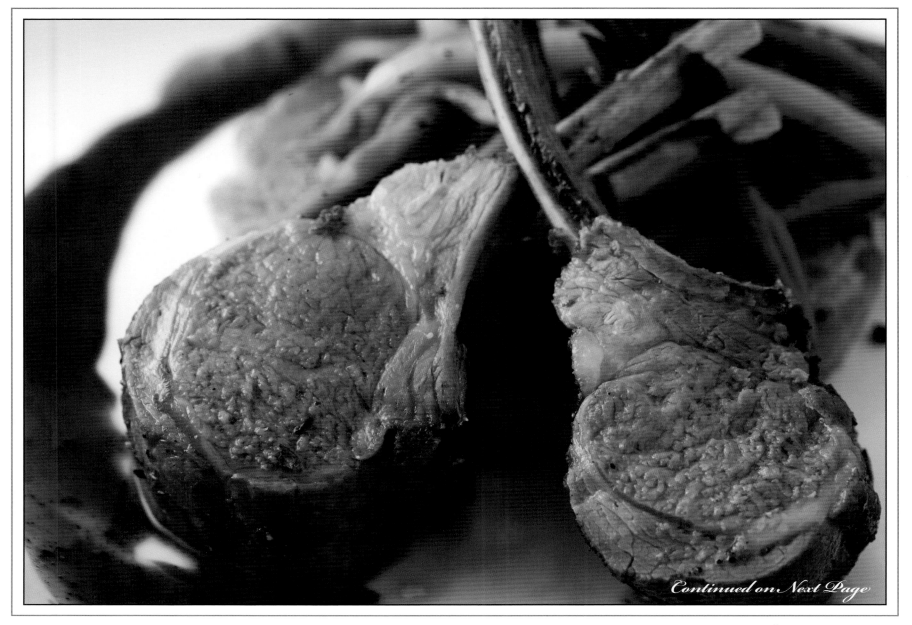

Continued on Next Page

Marinade:

- 3 sprigs rosemary, roughly chopped
- 5 cloves garlic, peeled, smashed and roughly chopped
- 1 tsp. kosher salt
- ½ cup extra virgin olive oil

Rack of Lamb:

- 2 frenched racks of lamb
- 1 Tbsp. canola or peanut oil
  kosher salt
  freshly cracked black pepper

Rosemary Garlic Brown Butter:

- 1 stick (8 Tbsp.) butter
- 1 (3-inch) sprig rosemary
- 2 large cloves garlic, peeled and smashed

Toss to combine all marinade ingredients in a gallon-size resealable plastic bag. Add racks of lamb and coat in marinade. Seal bag, removing as much air as possible to emulate a vacuum seal. Refrigerate and allow lamb to marinate, chilled, in herb-oil combination for at least 4 hours and up to 24 hours.

If roasting, preheat oven to 350 degrees. If grilling, preheat half of grill for medium-high heat and half for indirect cooking.

Remove lamb from herb oil; discard any pieces of rosemary or garlic that might have stuck to lamb; spices will burn during the browning process and give the lamb a bitter flavor. Season entire surface area of racks with kosher salt and freshly cracked black pepper.

Roasting instructions:

Preheat a large sauté pan over high heat for 3 minutes. Once the pan is hot, add canola oil. Working with one rack at a time, sear lamb on all sides (not including ends) until well browned, about 2 minutes per side. Place on a sheet pan, fat-side up. Once both racks have been seared, insert an internal thermometer into thickest part of one rack, not touching the bones. Roast lamb in preheated oven until lamb reaches an internal temperature of 130 degrees for medium-rare doneness—15 to 25 minutes, depending on thickness of racks. Remove from oven and cover loosely with aluminum foil. Let rest for at least 10 minutes before slicing. Temperature will continue rising as racks rest. Slice racks into pieces of 2 rib-bones each, serving 4 bones total per person.

Grilling instructions:

Place seasoned racks fat-side down onto preheated grill over direct heat. Sear for 4 minutes, then rotate a quarter turn (for hatch marks) and grill for another 4 minutes. Flip and grill the lamb for another 4 minutes, rotate a quarter turn and grill 4 more minutes. Insert an internal meat thermometer into thickest part of rack away from any bones. Move racks to side of grill preheated for indirect cooking. Close dome and cook lamb with indirect heat until internal temperature reaches 130 degrees for medium-rare doneness—5 to 15 minutes. Cooking times will vary depending on the width of lamb, so an internal thermometer is necessary to ensure perfectly cooked meat. Remove from grill and cover loosely with aluminum foil. Let rest for at least 10 minutes before slicing.

ROSEMARY GARLIC BROWN BUTTER

Place butter in a small saucepan over medium heat. Cook butter over medium heat, stirring or swishing occasionally until milk solids brown and butter turns amber—5 to 8 minutes. Do not burn or butter will taste bitter.

Remove from heat and submerge rosemary and garlic cloves completely in brown butter. (*Note: Be careful because the butter will splatter from the water content of the herbs when first added.*) Allow rosemary and garlic to infuse in brown butter for 5 minutes, then remove and discard.

BROWN BUTTER CROUTONS

Brown Butter Croutons:

    4   (1-inch thick) slices of day-old sourdough bread

        Rosemary Garlic Brown Butter

Sautéed Green Beans:

1½ lbs.   green beans, stem ends trimmed

   ½   red onion, peeled and thinly sliced

2 Tbsp.   rosemary garlic brown butter

        juice from half a lemon

        kosher salt and freshly cracked black pepper

Red Wine Demi-Glace Sauce:

        See Page 239

Brush all sides of sourdough bread liberally with Rosemary Garlic Brown Butter.

Preheat a large sauté pan over medium heat and add ½ tablespoon brown butter to pan to coat bottom.

Add bread to pan in a single layer, working in batches if necessary. Toast bread in butter until browned—3 to 5 minutes—and then flip and toast other side. Add more brown butter to pan as necessary. Once both sides have been browned, remove from heat. Repeat with remaining croutons and serve immediately.

SAUTÉED GREEN BEANS

Bring a large pot of salted water to a boil over high heat. Once boiling, add green beans. Boil for 4 minutes. Drain, and then run under cold water to cool. Set aside.

Heat 2 tablespoons brown butter in a large pan over medium heat until hot. Add sliced red onion and sauté for 1 minute, stirring occasionally. Add blanched green beans to pan. Sprinkle with kosher salt and freshly cracked black pepper. Sauté until crisp-tender, stirring occasionally, about 4 minutes. Squeeze lemon juice over green beans, stir, and remove from heat. Adjust seasoning to taste with kosher salt and freshly cracked black pepper.

ASSEMBLY

To assemble:

Place 1 brown butter crouton in the middle of a plate. Stack green beans on top of crouton and then lean 2 pieces (4 bones total) of rack of lamb up against the crouton and green beans. Drizzle red wine demi-glace sauce around the plate. If desired, garnish with a sprig of rosemary stuck straight into the crouton behind the lamb. Repeat plating process 3 more times for 4 servings.

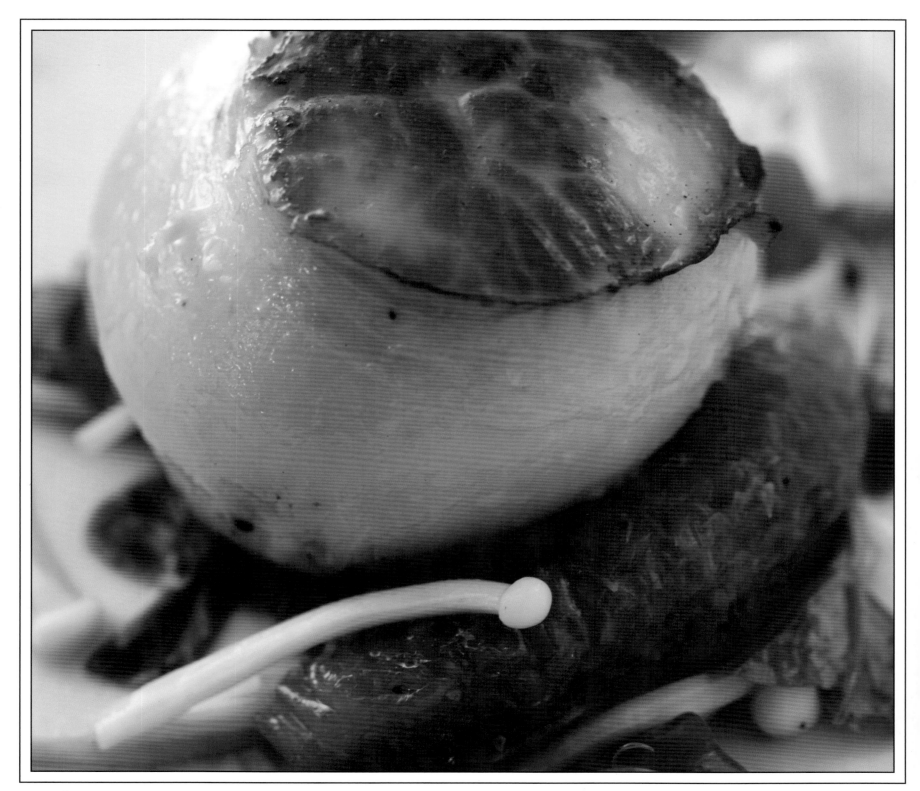

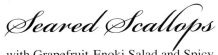

Seared Scallops

with Grapefruit-Enoki Salad and Spicy Mango Peanut Sauce

The spicy mango peanut sauce has a relatively bold flavor in comparison to the delicate sweetness of scallops, so be sure to use it sparingly in order to allow the flavor of the scallop to shine through.

Seared Scallops:

12	sea scallops, side muscles removed if still present
3 Tbsp.	canola or peanut oil
	kosher salt
	freshly cracked black pepper

Grapefruit-Enoki Salad:

2	ripe pink grapefruits
1½ cups	Enoki mushrooms, trimmed
3 cups	pea tendrils or sprouts
1 tsp.	Dijon mustard
1 Tbsp.	extra virgin olive oil
	kosher salt
	freshly cracked black pepper

Spicy Mango Peanut Sauce:

See Page 242

SEARED SCALLOPS

Preheat a large sauté pan over high heat for two minutes and add canola oil.

While pan is heating, liberally season the sea scallops with kosher salt and freshly cracked black pepper.

Once oil is very hot, but before it starts smoking, add 6 sea scallops to pan and sear over high heat, undisturbed, for 3 minutes until a golden brown crust has formed. Flip scallops and cook for another 3 minutes, undisturbed, until scallops have just turned opaque in the middle. Remove from pan and loosely cover with foil. Repeat searing process with remaining scallops. (*Note: Searing in two batches keeps from over-crowding the pan and allows for a hotter pan and a better crust.*)

GRAPEFRUIT-ENOKI SALAD

Cut grapefruit into supremes (see page 230) over a bowl to collect juice. Place supremes in a separate bowl from juice. Once all supremes have been cut, squeeze any excess juice from remaining membranes. Discard membranes.

Add Enoki mushrooms and pea tendrils to grapefruit supremes.

Set aside 3 tablespoons of grapefruit juice and drink or reserve excess juice for another purpose.

Whisk Dijon mustard and a pinch of kosher salt and freshly cracked black pepper into remaining 3 tablespoons juice. While continuously whisking, slowly drizzle in olive oil for an emulsified vinaigrette.

Add vinaigrette to supremes, Enoki, and pea tendrils. Toss and season to taste with kosher salt and freshly cracked black pepper.

ASSEMBLY

To serve, place three small piles of grapefruit salad in a row down a long rectangular plate. Top each pile of salad with one scallop. Spoon a small amount of sauce around outside of each pile, spreading sauce with the back of the spoon in a semi-circle swoop around the scallop. Repeat plating three more times for a total of four servings.

Seared Salmon

with Fresh Corn, Chorizo and Radish Salad and Avocado-Yogurt Sauce

The summer Alaskan salmon season runs from May through August. If you cannot find fresh Alaskan salmon for this dish, substitute Arctic Char or any other fresh sustainable fish available in your area.

Seared Salmon:

4 (6-oz.)	wild Alaskan salmon filets
3 Tbsp.	canola or peanut oil
	kosher salt
	freshly cracked black pepper

Corn and Radish Salad:

3	large ears sweet corn, shucked and cleaned
½ lbs.	fresh chorizo, browned and drained
4	large radishes, trimmed and cut in a small dice
3	green onions, thinly sliced
1 tsp.	fresh oregano, chopped
1 Tbsp.	red wine vinegar
1 Tbsp.	canola oil
1 tsp.	Dijon mustard
	kosher salt
	freshly cracked black pepper

Avocado-Yogurt Sauce:

See Page 228

SEARED SALMON

Preheat oil in a large, heavy-bottomed, nonstick sauté pan over medium-high heat until oil ripples and is nearly smoking—3 to 4 minutes.

While pan is heating, liberally season salmon filets on all sides with kosher salt and freshly cracked black pepper.

Once pan is hot, place salmon into the pan, flesh-side down. (*Note: Do not over-crowd the pan. If your pan is not large enough work in two batches or in two separate pans at the same time.*) Sear salmon for 4 to 5 minutes over medium-high heat until a golden crust forms and flesh releases from pan. Flip salmon and sear other side for another 4 to 5 minutes until golden and just cooked through. (*Note: The fish will release itself from the pan when it's ready to flip. So, if it sticks to the pan when you try to turn it, it's not ready! Also, assuming you are using high quality fresh fish, slightly underdone is completely acceptable and far more preferable than overdone fish.*) Remove from pan.

CORN & RADISH SALAD

Bring a large pot of water to a boil over high heat. Add ears of corn to the pot and turn off heat. Allow corn to sit in the hot water for 5 minutes, rotating the side of the ear that is submerged beneath water after 2½ minutes. Remove from pot and let cool.

Cut kernels from cobs. Discard cobs. Combine kernels with next 4 ingredients in a bowl and toss to evenly distribute.

In a separate small bowl, whisk together red wine vinegar, canola oil, and Dijon.

Pour vinegar mixture over corn salad and toss to evenly coat. Season to taste with kosher salt and freshly cracked black pepper.

ASSEMBLY

To plate, spoon a liberal dollop of avocado-yogurt sauce onto a plate. Using back of a spoon, spread sauce in a diagonal line across the plate. Place one seared salmon filet on top of sauce going in the opposite diagonal direction so that the sauce is visible from either side of the filet. Spoon corn salad over fish and around the plate.

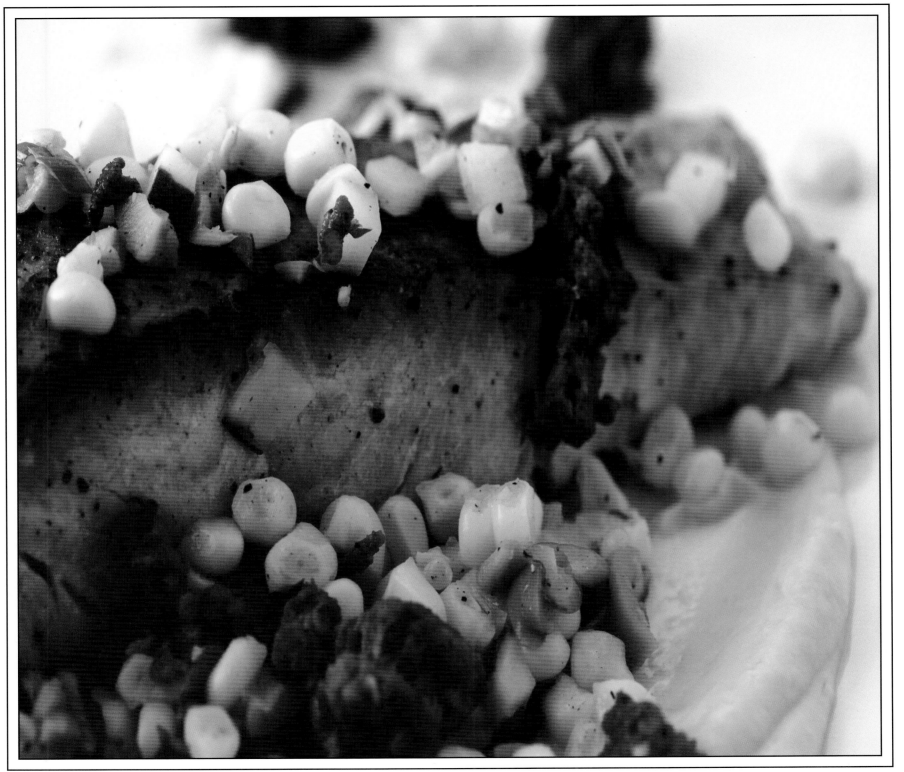

Rub:

1½ Tbsp.	kosher salt
2 Tbsp.	packed brown sugar
2 tsp.	freshly cracked black pepper
2 tsp.	Coleman's mustard powder
1½ tsp.	smoked paprika
1 tsp.	sweet paprika
½ tsp.	ground cayenne
¼ tsp.	ground cumin
½ tsp.	ground ginger
1 tsp.	granulated onion
1½ tsp.	granulated garlic

3	racks baby back ribs
4 oz.	hickory wood chips

Mop:

1½ cups	apple cider vinegar
1 Tbsp.	fresh ginger, peeled and minced
3	cloves garlic, peeled
1 Tbsp.	crushed red pepper
1 tsp.	freshly cracked black pepper
1 Tbsp.	kosher salt
4	anchovy filets
3 Tbsp.	(packed) brown sugar

Homemade Barbecue Sauce

See Page 234

In a bowl, whisk together all ingredients for rub until well mixed. Set aside.

Evenly coat all sides of prepared ribs with rub. Place ribs onto a sheet pan and wrap tightly in plastic wrap or, if you have one, place into a jumbo-sized resealable bag. Seal bag, removing as much air as possible to emulate a vacuum seal. Let ribs sit in the rub, refrigerated, for 6 to 12 hours. Remove ribs from the fridge 1 hour before you are ready to start smoking them and let come to room temperature.

Blend all ingredients for mop in a blender until very smooth. Refrigerate in an airtight container for at least 4 hours or up to 4 days before use.

When ready to cook ribs, prepare a gas grill or smoker for 225 degree indirect heat. If you have one, feel free to use a rib rack. If using a smoker, add hickory chips directly to fire. If using a gas grill, add hickory chips to a foil container poked with large holes and place directly over flames. Place ribs onto grill or rib rack in an area with no direct heat beneath them.

Close lid and let smoke for 3½ to 5 hours, depending on size of ribs, or until tender. Baste ribs with mop every 30 to 40 minutes. If ribs are not in a rib rack, flip them with each basting. *(Note: Make sure to maintain a temperature of 225 degrees inside dome of the grill at all times. While it's hard to maintain an exact temperature, it's important that the heat does not fall below 200 degrees or rise above 250 degrees, so keep a watchful eye on the temperature throughout the entire smoking process.)*

To check ribs for doneness, lift them up using tongs and wiggle them gently. If outside bark starts to crack and meat pulls away slightly, ribs are tender and ready to eat. Baste all sides of ribs with homemade barbecue sauce. Grill ribs over direct heat until barbecue sauce has caramelized—3 to 4 minutes—and then flip and caramelize other side.

Remove from heat and let cool for 5 to 10 minutes before slicing. Cut into individual ribs or serve in half or quarter rack portions with extra barbecue sauce on the side.

To prepare ribs, place rack of ribs flesh-side down onto a cutting board or flat surface. To remove the thin membrane on the back of the ribs, start with the first rib at the short end of the rack and work your fingers or paring knife underneath the membrane. Wiggle your finger or knife back and forth until you can fully grasp the membrane. Using your hand, carefully pull back the membrane to remove it from the entire rack. If you're careful, you'll be able to remove the membrane quickly and in one piece. However, if the membrane *does* break, simply work your fingers or knife back under the membrane and continue pulling. While it is edible, removing the membrane is an important step in ensuring tender ribs.

Sweet and Tangy Hickory Smoked Baby Back Ribs

with Homemade Barbecue Sauce

Similar to fried chicken, I can be happy chowing down on a feast of ribs alone. For this main course, I am not including any side dish recipes although baked beans, coleslaw, or other traditional barbecue sides make great accompaniments.

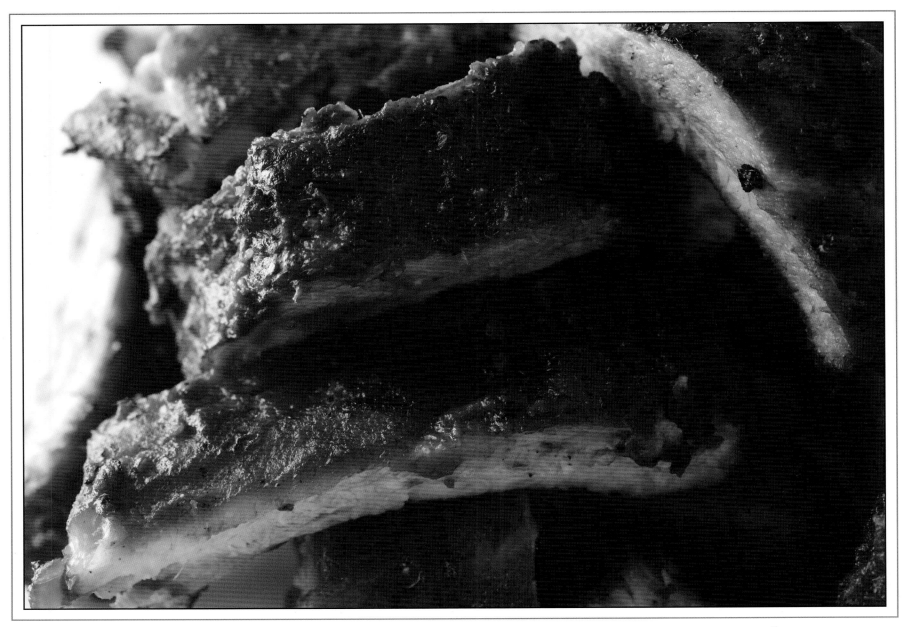

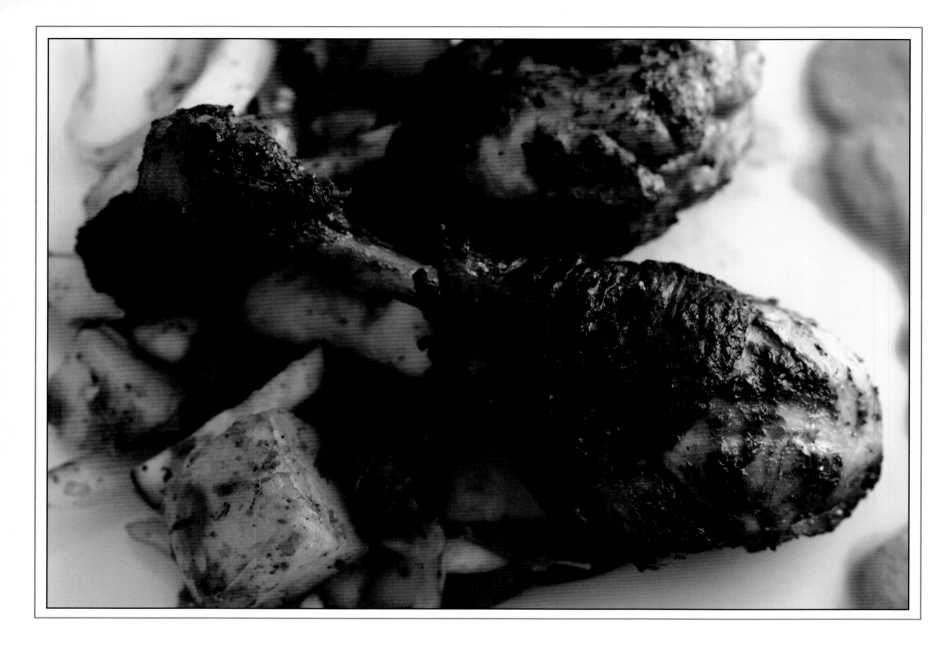

Tandoori Marinated Grilled Chicken

with Indian-Spiced Sautéed Veggies and Cilantro Chutney

Feel free to use your favorite type of chicken for this recipe, adjusting the cooking time accordingly. We love drumsticks due to the high ratio of skin to meat, as well as their built in handle.

Marinade:

1 cup	plain yogurt, NOT non-fat
	juice from 1 lime
1½ tsp.	kosher salt, plus extra
1 tsp.	ground cumin
¼ tsp.	fenugreek, ground
1 tsp.	achiote paste
½ tsp.	turmeric
½ tsp.	ground coriander
½ tsp.	brown mustard seeds
1	serrano chile, stem removed
2	cloves garlic, peeled
1 Tbsp.	ginger, peeled and roughly chopped
1	small shallot, peeled and roughly chopped

8–10	chicken drumsticks (or any chicken part desired)

Indian-Spiced Sautéed Vegetables:

3	Yukon Gold potatoes
3 Tbsp.	canola or ghee or peanut oil
½	yellow onion, sliced
1	red bell pepper (stem and seeds removed), julienne
1	large zucchini, stem ends trimmed and sliced in ¼-inch thick half-moons
2	cloves garlic, minced
1 tsp.	ginger, peeled and minced
½–1	serrano chile, minced (vary depending on spice preference)
½ tsp.	ground cumin
¼ tsp.	ground fenugreek
¼ tsp.	brown mustard seeds
¼ tsp.	turmeric
½ tsp.	achiote (ground annato; optional)
	kosher salt
	freshly cracked black pepper

Yogurt-Cilantro Chutney

See Page 244

TANDOORI CHICKEN

Whisk together all ingredients for marinade until well combined. Place chicken into a resealable plastic bag with marinade, tossing to coat. Seal bag, removing as much air as possible to emulate a vacuum seal. Marinate chicken, refrigerated, for at least 4 hours and up to 24 hours.

Prepare grill for medium-high heat. Once grill is hot, remove chicken from marinade. Lightly season chicken on all sides with kosher salt. Grill chicken over direct medium-high heat turning a quarter turn every 5 to 6 minutes until completely cooked through (about 20 to 24 minutes) or until internal temperature of chicken reaches 175 degrees. Remove from grill and let cool for 5 minutes before serving.

INDIAN-SPICED SAUTÉED VEGETABLES

Cover potatoes in a small pot with approximately 1 inch of cold water. Bring water to a boil over high heat and boil until potatoes are mostly cooked through and tender when pierced with a knife—8 to 10 minutes. (*Note: Do not overcook the potatoes, or the skin will begin to come away from the flesh.*)

Drain potatoes and let cool until able to handle. Cut potatoes into about 1-inch pieces

Preheat a large sauté pan with 2 tablespoons ghee over medium-high heat. Once the pan has preheated and the ghee is hot, add potato, onions, and peppers to pan. Season liberally with salt and pepper and stir. Sauté for 4 to 5 minutes, stirring occasionally, until veggies start to brown a little. Add zucchini and sauté for another 2 minutes, stirring occasionally. Add remaining ingredients and sauté for 1 to 2 more minutes, stirring frequently. Do not let garlic burn— if it begins to brown, remove pan from heat. Adjust seasoning to taste with more kosher salt and freshly cracked black pepper.

ASSEMBLY

To assemble:

Spoon some veggies into the middle of a plate, top with grilled chicken, and then drizzle chutney around the plate. Garnish with fresh cilantro leaves, if desired.

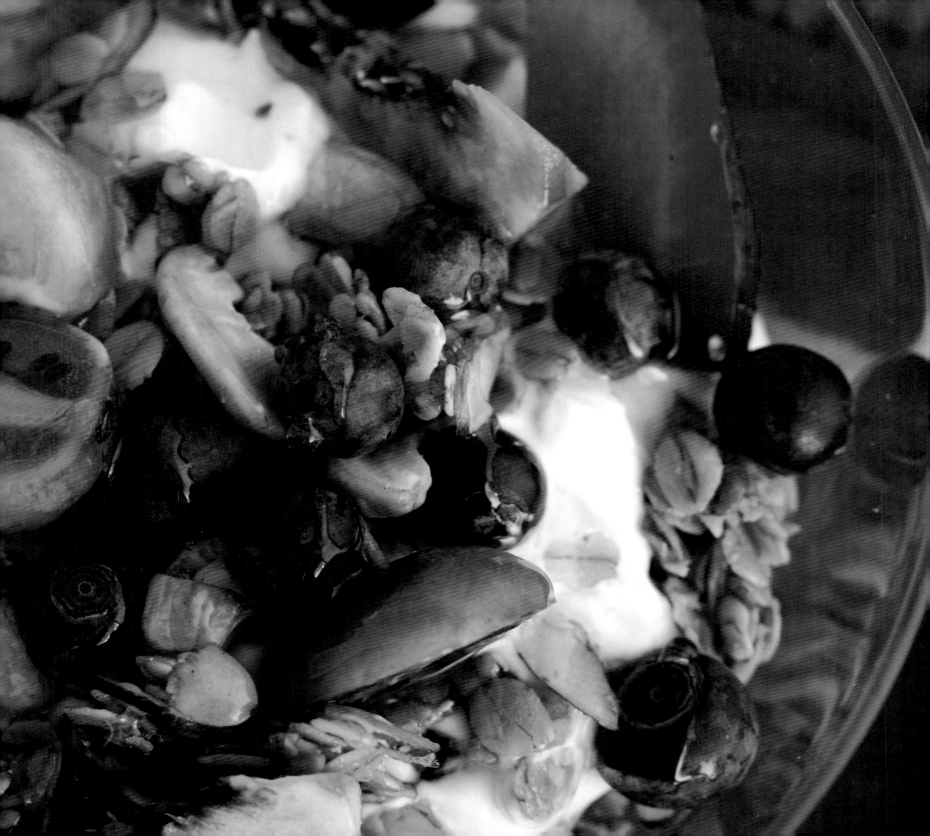

Honeyed Cashew and Almond Granola

Summer Fruit and Greek Yogurt Breakfast Parfaits

Granola is extremely easy to make, and a parfait made with fruit, granola, and yogurt is the perfect breakfast for a hot summer morning.

Granola:

½ cup	honey
¼ tsp.	cinnamon
1 tsp.	pure vanilla extract
½ tsp.	kosher salt
½ cup	canola oil or melted butter
3 cups	rolled oats (also called old-fashioned oats)
1 cup	raw almond slices
1 cup	raw cashews
1 cup	sweetened flaked coconut flakes (optional)

Fruit Granola Yogurt Bowls:

1 recipe	Almond and Cashew Granola
4 cups	plain low-fat Greek-style strained yogurt
8–12	strawberries, hulled and cut in half, lengthwise
1 pint	raspberries
1 pint	blueberries
2 ripe	peaches, peeled, pitted and sliced
8	baby kiwi fruit, cut in half lengthwise (optional)
	good honey

GRANOLA

Preheat oven to 350 degrees. Line a sheet pan with parchment paper.

In large mixing bowl, stir together first 5 ingredients. Add oats and nuts to honey mixture and stir to coat thoroughly.

Spread granola out onto parchment-lined sheet pan in a single layer.

Bake at 350 degrees, stirring every 5 minutes or so until golden brown, about 30 minutes. The deeper the golden color, the crispier the granola will be, but do not allow oats and nuts to burn, or the granola will be bitter.

Remove from oven and place pan on a wire rack to cool for 1 hour. Once cooled completely, break granola up into small chunks and toss with coconut flakes. Granola will stay good stored in an airtight container, refrigerated, for over a month.

FRUIT GRANOLA YOGURT BOWLS

In a bowl, layer ¼ cup granola, 1 cup yogurt, ⅓ cup granola, and one-fourth of each fruit. Drizzle with honey. Repeat the plating process three more times with remaining ingredients for a total of 4 parfaits. Serve immediately.

Crust:

¾ cup	flour
1 tsp.	sugar
¼ tsp.	salt
4 Tbsp.	(½ stick) butter, very cold, and cut in cubes
4 oz.	cream cheese, very cold, and cut in cubes

Filling:

5 ripe	peaches or nectarines, peeled and pitted, cut in eighths
5 cups	ripe blackberries
	juice from ½ lemon
¼ tsp.	salt
½ cup	sugar, plus extra if your fruit is tart
¼ tsp.	ground cinnamon
¼ cup	cornstarch

Crumb Topping:

½ cup	sugar
½ cup	flour
¼ tsp.	salt
¼ tsp.	cinnamon
6 Tbsp.	butter, very cold and cut in cubes
½ cup	quick cooking oats

CRUST

Add flour, sugar, and salt to a food processor. Pulse to mix. Add butter and cream cheese and process until ingredients come together in a ball and form a dough. Transfer dough to a lightly floured board and shape into a compressed disk. Wrap dough tightly in plastic wrap and place in the fridge. Chill for at least 1 hour and up to 2 days.

Preheat oven to 350 degrees with a rack in center position.

Roll chilled pie crust out on a lightly floured surface into an approximately 12-inch round circle. If dough starts to get warm, move it to a lightly floured surface where it can lay flat in the refrigerator and chill for 15 minutes. Once circle has been formed, carefully transfer dough onto a 9-inch pie pan and fit it flush against the pan, with approximately 1 inch of dough hanging over the edge of the pan. Fold overhanging pieces under and pinch, causing edges to stand up. Form a scalloped edge by using the thumb and forefinger of one hand to loosely press the outside edge of the crust inward while pressing outward from the opposite side using a finger of your other hand and working around the edge of the crust. Return pie shell to refrigerator to chill while finishing pie.

FILLING

Gently mix all filling ingredients in a large mixing bowl until evenly disbursed and coated with sugar and cornstarch, taking care not to smash the fruit. If your fruit is particularly tart, add extra sugar to balance flavor. Let sit for 20 to 25 minutes, stirring occasionally.

CRUMB TOPPING AND BAKING

While the fruit is sitting, make the crumb topping.

In a food processor, pulse-blend sugar, flour, salt, and cinnamon. Add butter to processor and pulse until mixture has pea-sized crumbs. Transfer to a bowl. Add oats and mash together with other ingredients until mostly incorporated into crumb topping, working quickly so the butter doesn't melt. Chill crumb topping until ready to use, at least 10 minutes.

Pour fruit into chilled pie crust, using a rubber spatula to scrape any residual juices lingering on the sides of the bowl into the pie pan. Sprinkle handfuls of crumb topping over fruit to form an even top-layer. Bake pie at 350 degrees on a foil-lined baking sheet for 1 hour or until crumb topping is golden and filling bubbles. (*Note: Placing the pie on a foil-lined baking sheet will catch any fruit juices that may spill over during baking.*)

Remove from oven and cool on a wire rack for at least 45 minutes before cutting. Serve with lightly sweetened whipped cream or vanilla ice cream.

Blackberry-Nectarine Crumb Pie

There are very few fruits that can beat a tree-ripened, freshly picked peach or nectarine at the height of summer. Feel free to use whatever stone fruit is freshest in this pie—peaches, nectarines, apricots, even plums or cherries. Locally grown and freshly harvested fruits picked at peak season always taste the best.

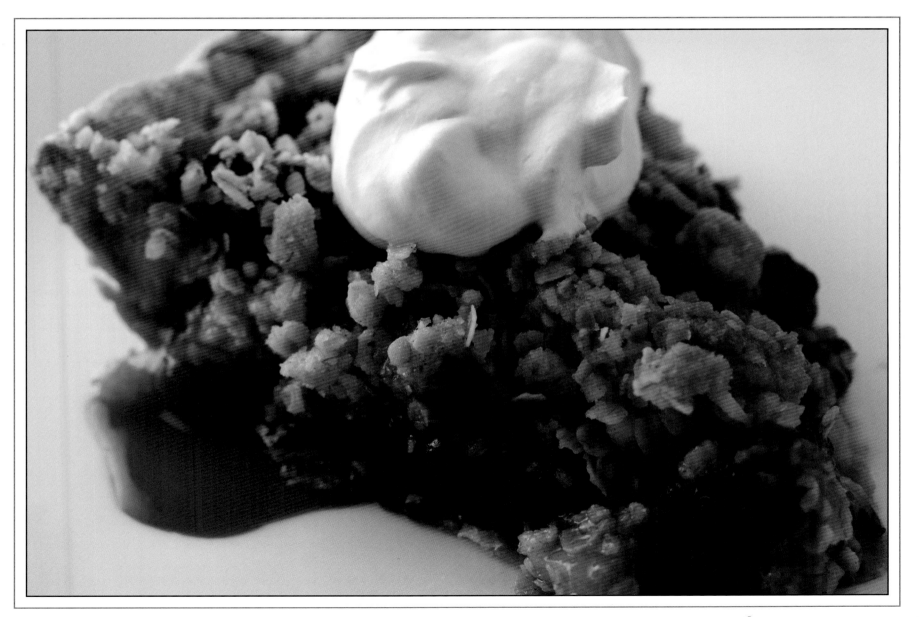

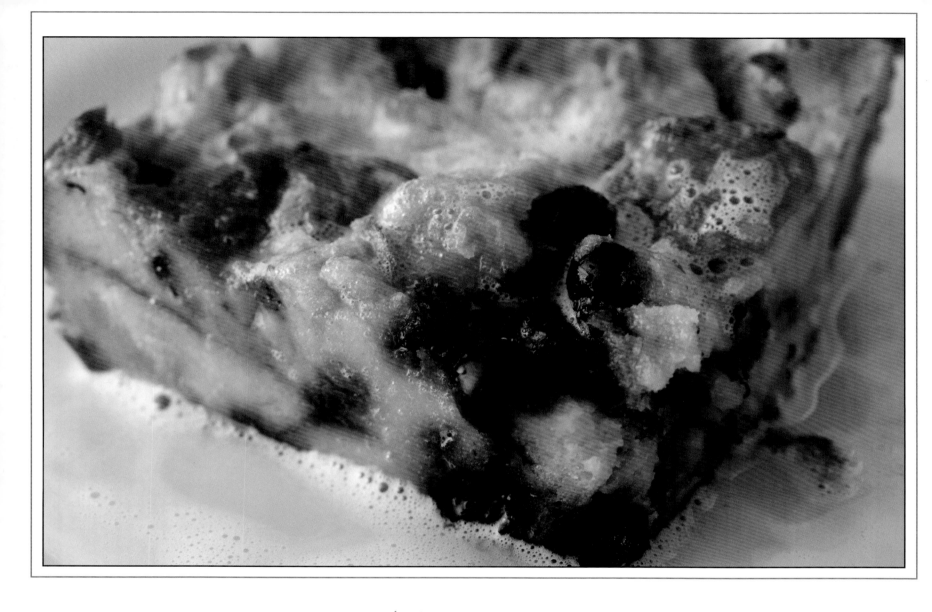

White Chocolate-Blueberry Bread Pudding

with White Chocolate-Frangelico Sauce

In the U.S., the French bread sold in most grocery stores is fluffy and not particularly crusty. This is the type of French bread that I think works best for this recipe. If you don't want to wait until the bread is a day old to make the bread pudding, simply cut the bread into cubes and dry it out in a 300 degree oven for 30 to 40 minutes, stirring occasionally so the bread cubes do not toast. Once the moisture has been extracted from the bread, let it cool to room temperature before proceeding with the recipe.

Bread Pudding:

½ cup	heavy cream
1 cup	good-quality white chocolate chips
1½ cups	whole milk
¾ cup	granulated sugar
5	eggs
½ tsp.	salt
1 tsp.	pure vanilla extract
½ tsp.	pure almond or hazelnut extract
1 lb.	loaf of day-old french bread (not a baguette), cut into 1 inch cubes
1½ cups	ripe blueberries
½ cup	white chocolate chips (separate from those listed above)
1 Tbsp.	butter, diced into small pieces

White Chocolate Frangelico Sauce:

1	egg yolk
⅓ cup	heavy cream
2 Tbsp.	sugar
¼ tsp.	salt
2 oz.	white chocolate
1.5 oz.	Frangelico hazelnut liqueur

Preheat oven to 350 degrees. Butter or grease an 8x11.5x2-inch glass or ceramic baking dish. Set aside.

Pour heavy cream into a small saucepan and place over medium-high heat. Heat cream until almost boiling, stirring occasionally to prevent cream from burning.

Place 1 cup white chocolate chips into large heat-safe mixing bowl. Pour almost-boiling cream over white chocolate chips. Let chocolate sit in hot cream for 1 minute, and then whisk until chocolate has completely dissolved into cream. Add whole milk, granulated sugar, eggs, salt, and vanilla and almond extracts to white chocolate-cream mixture. Whisk until all ingredients are fully incorporated and eggs are completely beat into liquid.

Add bread cubes to liquid mixture tossing to coat thoroughly. Let bread sit in mixture for 30 to 40 minutes until most of the liquid has been absorbed and bread is very mushy. Stir bread 2 or 3 times to ensure that all surfaces absorb liquid equally.

Stir in blueberries and ½ cup white chocolate chips into bread pudding mixture until evenly disbursed. Pour pudding into buttered baking dish in an even layer. Sprinkle diced butter pieces over pudding.

Bake bread pudding at 350 degrees for 55 to 65 minutes or until top is golden and pudding has set.

Remove from heat and let cool for at least 20 minutes before serving. Serve warm or cold with white chocolate Frangelico sauce.

WHITE CHOCOLATE FRANGELICO SAUCE

Bring 2 inches of water to a boil in a medium-sized saucepan or bottom pan of a double boiler. Whisk together egg yolk, heavy cream, sugar, and salt in a heat-proof metal mixing bowl or top pan of a double boiler until smooth. Place bowl or double boiler top with the cream mixture over the boiling water. Whisk constantly until mixture thickens slightly and sugar dissolves completely. Do not allow sauce to reach a simmer, or egg will curdle. Once thickened, add white chocolate to sauce. Stir until white chocolate has melted. Remove from heat and add Frangelico. Stir until completely incorporated and strain through a fine mesh sieve. Use immediately. To store, allow sauce to cool to room temperature and then store in an airtight container in the refrigerator for up to 1 week.

Fluffy Mango Cheesecake

with Mango-Macadamia Nut Toffee Sauce

If you don't think you'll use all of the toffee sauce the day it's made, try sprinkling the mango that the sauce calls for on top as a garnish rather than stirring it in with the macadamia nuts.

FLUFFY MANGO CHEESECAKE

Crust:

1½ cups	vanilla wafer cookie crumbs (about ½ box)
1 cup	macadamia nuts, minced or pulsed in a food processor
¼ cup	sugar
½ cup	(1 stick) butter, melted

Filling:

3	mangoes, peeled and pitted
3 (8-oz.)	packages cream cheese, full fat only
1 cup + 2 Tbsp.	granulated sugar
4	eggs
1 tsp.	good vanilla extract
¼ tsp.	salt

Mango-Macadamia Toffee Sauce:

2 Tbsp.	butter
½ cup	packed brown sugar
½ cup	heavy cream
½ tsp.	kosher salt
½ cup	macadamia nuts, roughly chopped
1	mango, peeled, pitted, and diced

Preheat oven to 350 degrees with a rack placed in the center. Wrap the outside of a deep 9-inch springform pan with several layers of aluminum foil. (*Note: The cheesecake is cooked in a water bath and the foil wrap will help prevent any water from seeping into the pan during cooking just in case the seal on the pan isn't tight enough.*)

Stir together crust ingredients in a mixing bowl until well-mixed and thoroughly moistened by butter.

Pour crust mixture into springform pan. Using a straight-sided cup, press crumbs down into an even layer across the bottom of the pan and up the sides to form the cookie-nut crust. Set aside.

Boil a large kettle of water for later use as a water bath.

Puree peeled and pitted mangos in a blender until very smooth and set aside.

Using either a stand mixer and whisk attachment or a large mixing bowl and hand-beaters, beat cream cheese until fluffy. Add sugar and beat again until fluffy. Add eggs one at a time, beating until fully incorporated, scraping down sides as necessary before next addition. Finally add mango puree, vanilla, and salt. Beat until smooth.

Place foil-wrapped springform pan in a large, flat-bottomed roasting pan. Pour filling into prepared crust. Pour enough boiling water into roasting pan—taking care not to get any water in the cheesecake itself—so that water comes about halfway up the outside of the springform pan. Carefully place in oven and bake for about 1 hour until cheesecake has just set. Cheesecake will still be jiggly but should not be at all liquidy. Remove cheesecake from water bath and aluminum foil. Place springform pan on a wire rack to cool. Cool cheesecake for 1 hour at room temperature before transferring it to refrigerator. Chill, refrigerated, for at least 12 hours before serving. Cheesecake may be made up to two days in advance. To serve, place an individual slice of cheesecake into the middle of a serving plate and spoon Mango-Macadamia Nut Toffee Sauce (see below) over the slice.

MANGO-MACADAMIA TOFFEE SAUCE

Melt butter in a small saucepan over medium-high heat. Add brown sugar, heavy cream, and salt to melted butter and stir until brown sugar has dissolved into liquid. Place a candy thermometer into sauce and boil until sauce reaches 225 degrees. Remove sauce from heat and stir in macadamia nuts and diced mango. Cool for at least 30 minutes before serving.

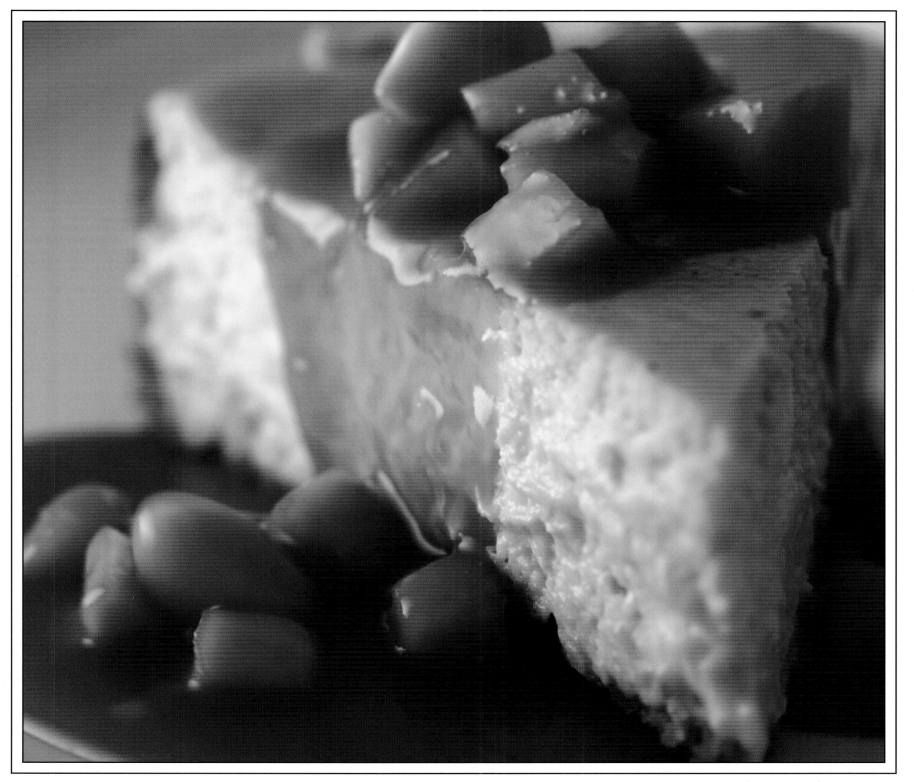

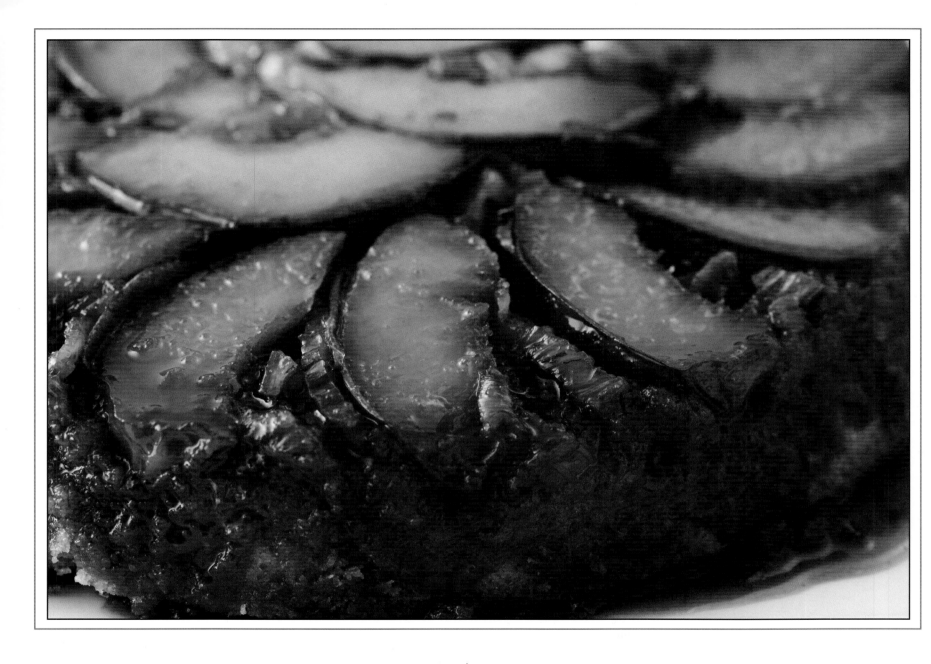

Nectarine and Candied Fennel Upside-Down Cake

Don't be scared by the addition of fennel in the topping for this cake. It adds a delightful texture as well as a mild fennel flavor that marries beautifully with the nectarines, separating it from other run-of-the-mill upside-down cakes.

Nectarine-Candied Fennel Topping:

½ + 5 Tbsp. butter

1 bulb fennel, trimmed and diced

2 tsp. brown sugar

¾ cup (packed) dark brown sugar

¼ tsp. kosher salt

⅛ tsp. ground cardamom

3 ripe nectarines, pitted and cut into 8 slices per nectarine

Upside-Down Cake:

1¾ cup cake flour

¼ tsp. salt

1½ tsp. baking powder

¼ tsp. ground cardamom

½ cup (1 stick) of butter, at room temperature

⅔ cup granulated sugar

2 eggs

1½ tsp. quality vanilla extract

⅔ cup whole milk

Preheat oven to 350 degrees.

Preheat a sauté pan over medium heat for two minutes. Add ½ tablespoon butter. Once butter has melted, sauté fennel over medium heat—stirring occasionally—for 6 minutes. Stir in 2 teaspoons brown sugar and a small pinch of kosher salt to fennel. Continue cooking for another 3 minutes, stirring frequently. Remove fennel from sauté pan and set aside.

Return sauté pan to medium heat. Melt 5 tablespoons butter and then add brown sugar, kosher salt and ground cardamom. Stir. Cook until sugar has dissolved into butter—stirring frequently—for 3 to 4 minutes. Pour brown sugar mixture into an ungreased 9-inch cake pan and spread to evenly coat the bottom of the pan.

Place nectarine slices into brown sugar mixture in concentric circles. Sprinkle sautéed fennel over nectarine, taking care to get it into the brown sugar cracks between nectarine slices. Set aside.

UPSIDE-DOWN CAKE

In a mixing bowl, sift together cake flour, salt, baking powder, and ground cardamom.

In a separate mixing bowl or the bowl of a stand mixer with a whisk attachment, beat butter and sugar until fluffy and well-blended, scraping down the sides with a rubber spatula. Add eggs, one at a time, beating after each addition until completely incorporated; scrape down the sides of the bowl as necessary. Add vanilla and then beat until incorporated.

Add a third of the flour mixture to butter-sugar-egg mixture. Beat until just barely incorporated. Using a rubber spatula, scrape down the walls of the bowl, then add ⅓ cup milk. Beat until just incorporated. Repeat this process by adding another third of flour, remaining milk and ending with remaining flour, beating after each addition until just incorporated. (*Note: It's very important not to overbeat the batter as that will lead to a tough cake instead of a tender, crumbly one.*)

Pour cake batter evenly over nectarines in the cake pan. Place cake pan onto a foil-lined baking sheet to catch any sugar that may bubble over while baking. Bake cake on the center rack of a 350 degree oven for 50 to 55 minutes, or until a toothpick inserted into the middle of the cake comes out clean (a couple of crumbs are okay, but NO batter should be present).

Cool cake on a wire rack for 15 minutes and then run a knife around the edges to loosen. Place a plate over the pan, and then invert the cake onto the plate. Gently lift the cake pan to reveal the upside-down cake. Using a rubber spatula, scrape any remaining brown sugar syrup out of the bottom of the pan and onto the cake. This cake is best served fresh from the oven, but if necessary, it can be made it up to 1 day in advance and stored chilled once removed from the pan. Bring to room temperature before serving.

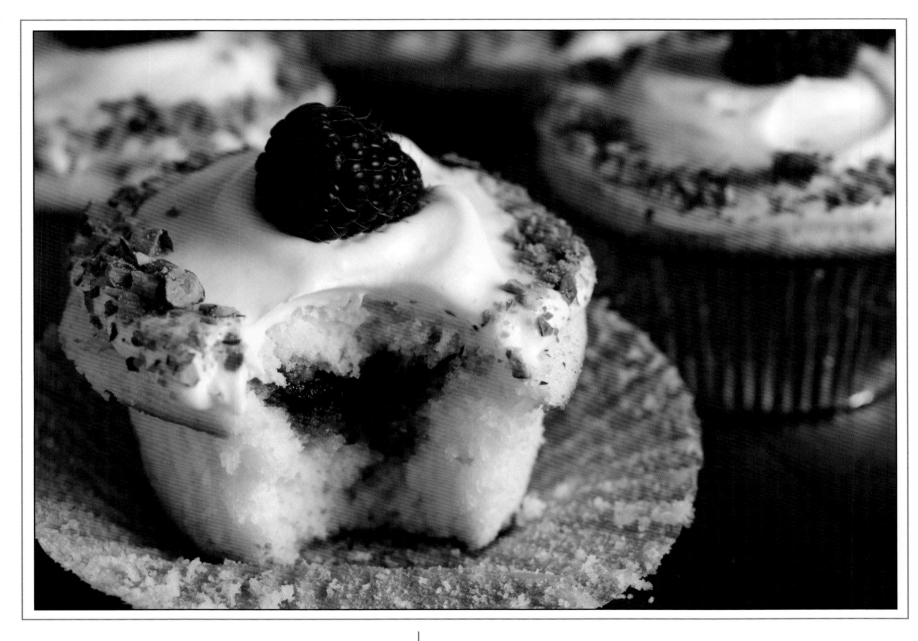

Almondy White Cupcakes

Filled with Raspberry Jam and Frosted with Whipped White Chocolate Ganache

The texture of whipped white chocolate ganache is so silky and fluffy and the flavor is so delicious that I have a hard time resisting the urge to eat it by the spoonful before I've had a chance to decorate the cupcakes. Fortunately the recipe makes a little more ganache than necessary, so spoon away!

ALMONDY WHITE CUPCAKES

Cupcakes:

3 cups	cake flour
1 Tbsp.	baking powder
¾ tsp.	kosher salt
1 cup	buttermilk
1 tsp.	pure vanilla extract
2 tsp.	pure almond extract
1 cup	(2 sticks) butter, at room temperature
1½ cups	granulated sugar
½ tsp.	lemon zest, grated
6	egg whites, kept separated

Raspberry Jam:

See Page 239

Whipped White Chocolate Ganache:

See Page 244

Preheat oven to 350 degrees with a rack positioned in the middle. Line two (12-count) muffin tins with cupcake liners. (Recipe makes about 24 cupcakes total.)

Sift together cake flour, baking powder, and salt. Set aside.

Whisk together buttermilk, vanilla, and almond extract.

Using either a stand mixer with whisk attachment or a mixing bowl and hand-beaters, beat butter until fluffy. Add granulated sugar and lemon zest to butter and beat until well-incorporated and fluffy. Add egg whites to butter mixture one at a time, beating until fully incorporated and fluffy before adding next egg white.

Once egg whites have been added, add a third of the flour mixture. Beat until just barely incorporated. Using a rubber spatula, scrape down the walls of the bowl and add half of the milk mixture. Beat until just incorporated. Alternate additions of a third of the flour, half of the milk mixture, and the remaining third of the flour mixture until all ingredients have just been incorporated. (*Note: It's very important not to over-beat the batter as that will lead to tough, dense cupcakes rather than tender, crumbly ones.*)

Fill prepared muffin tins evenly with batter about two-thirds full. Bake cupcakes at 350 degrees on the middle rack for 18 to 20 minutes until a toothpick inserted into the middle of a cupcake comes out clean. If your oven is large enough to bake both tins at the same time on the middle rack, do so; otherwise, bake cupcakes in two batches. Remove from oven and place on a wire rack to cool completely—about 1 hour.

ASSEMBLY

(*Note: Work with cupcakes one at a time so you don't confuse which top goes with which cupcake.*) Using a paring knife, cut out a cone from the top of the cupcake, leaving a about a ¼-inch border on all sides and cutting about halfway into the cupcake. (Picture cutting the lid off of a pumpkin when creating a jack-o'-lantern.) Remove the cone-shaped lid and cut off ¼-inch of cone tip that used to be in the middle of the cupcake. Using a ½-teaspoon measuring spoon, scoop out about ½ teaspoon of cake from the middle of the cupcake. Spoon in 1 tablespoon raspberry jam. Replace the cupcake's cone-shaped lid to conceal the jam in the middle of the cake and restore the cupcake to normal. Repeat the process with remaining cupcakes.

Frost each cupcake with 1 or 2 tablespoons of the whipped white chocolate ganache. spreading it evenly over the top of the cupcakes. Sprinkle chopped almonds over the outside ¼-inch rim of frosting all the way around the cupcake. Place a ripe raspberry directly in the center of each cupcake. Cupcakes can be kept at room temperature for up to 12 hours. Store chilled for up to 2 days. Let cupcakes return to room temperature before serving.

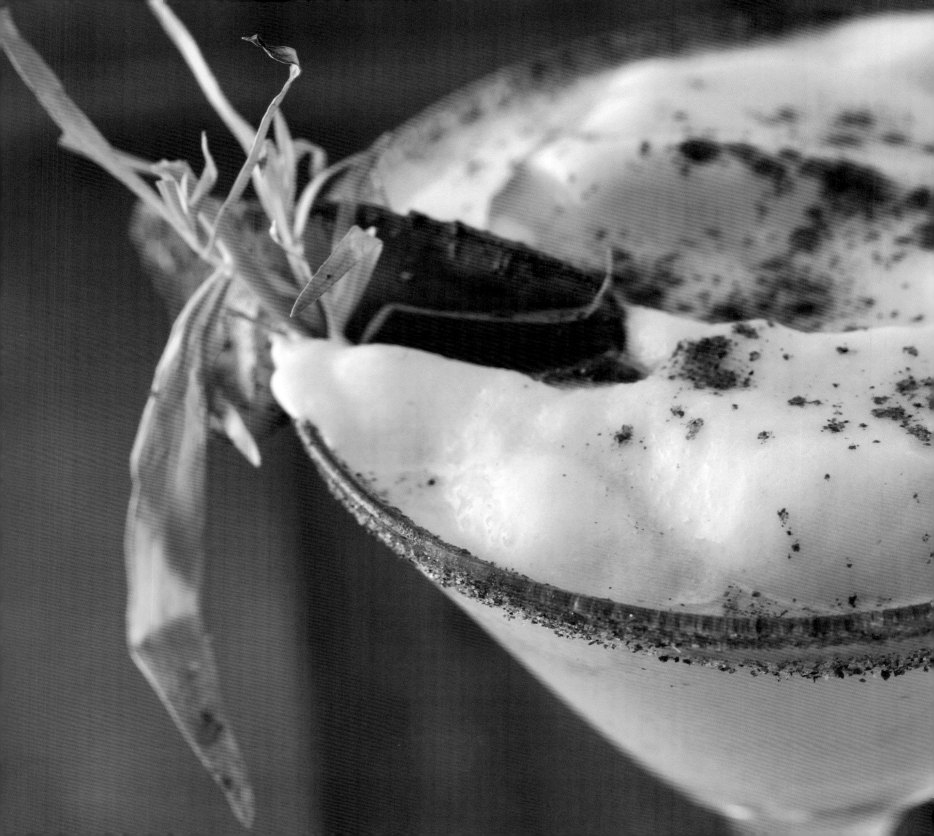

Mango, Pineapple, and Tarragon Daiquiri

with a Sweet and Salty Chili Rim

I don't particularly like cloyingly sweet mixed drinks. So in this recipe, I only call for a single tablespoon of simple syrup. Taste the first daiquiri you make, and if you prefer a sweeter beverage, simply add more syrup until the flavor works for you.

Rich Simple Syrup:

1 cup	sugar
½ cup	water

For dipping the rims:

2 Tbsp.	kosher salt
3 Tbsp.	granulated sugar
1 Tbsp.	chili powder
	lime wedges

For each drink:

½	ripe mango, peeled and diced
1 cup	fresh ripe pineapple, diced
1½ tsp.	fresh tarragon leaves
1 Tbsp.	Rich Simple Syrup
2 oz.	rum
1¼ cups	ice

Garnish:

	dried chili mango
	fresh tarragon

RICH SIMPLE SYRUP

Stir sugar into water in a small saucepan over medium-high heat until sugar has dissolved completely. Bring to a simmer and cook for about 3 minutes until syrup has thickened slightly. Remove from heat and let cool completely before refrigerating.

Rich, simple syrup, a bar staple, is simply a syrup made with a 2:1 sugar to water ratio. Knowing this you can make as much or as little as you like. Store syrup in an airtight container in the refrigerator for up to 1 month.

DAIQUIRI

Whisk together all rim ingredients in a bowl big enough to fit the rim of a glass. Set aside.

Blend all ingredients for the drink in a blender until smooth.

Using a lime wedge, moisten the rim of your serving glass. Dip moistened rim into chile powder mixture, rocking glass back and forth until rim is fully coated. Pour daiquiri into glass, taking care not to mess up the rim. Garnish with fresh tarragon sprigs and dried chili mango.

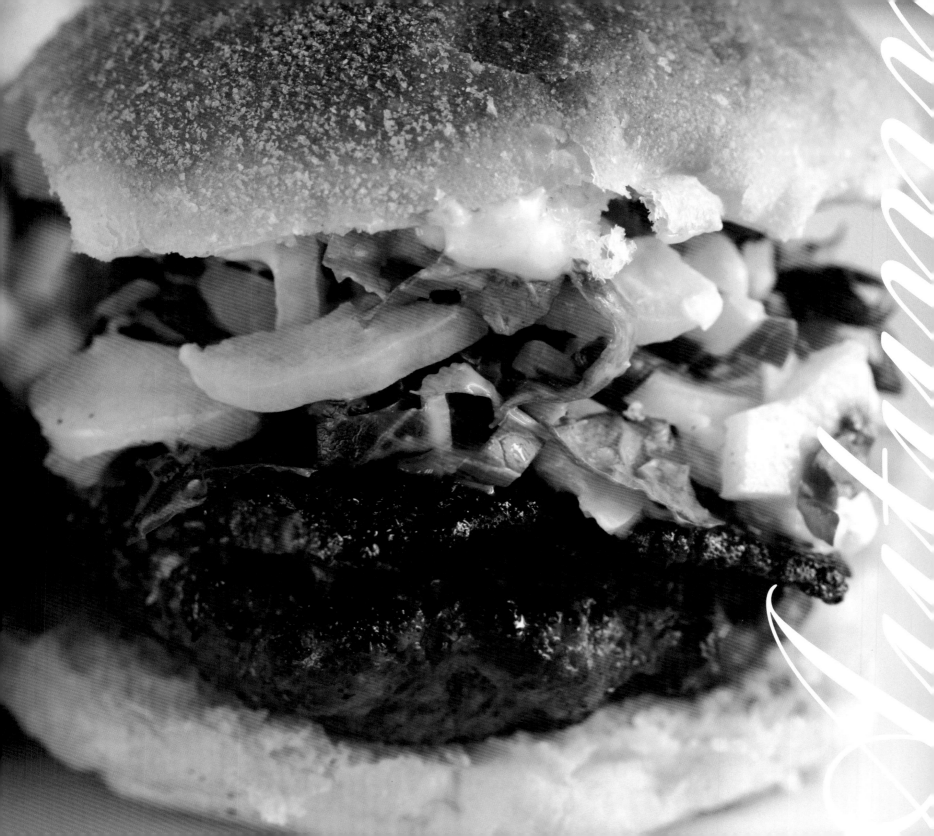

Openers

Main

Breakfast

Dessert

Drinks

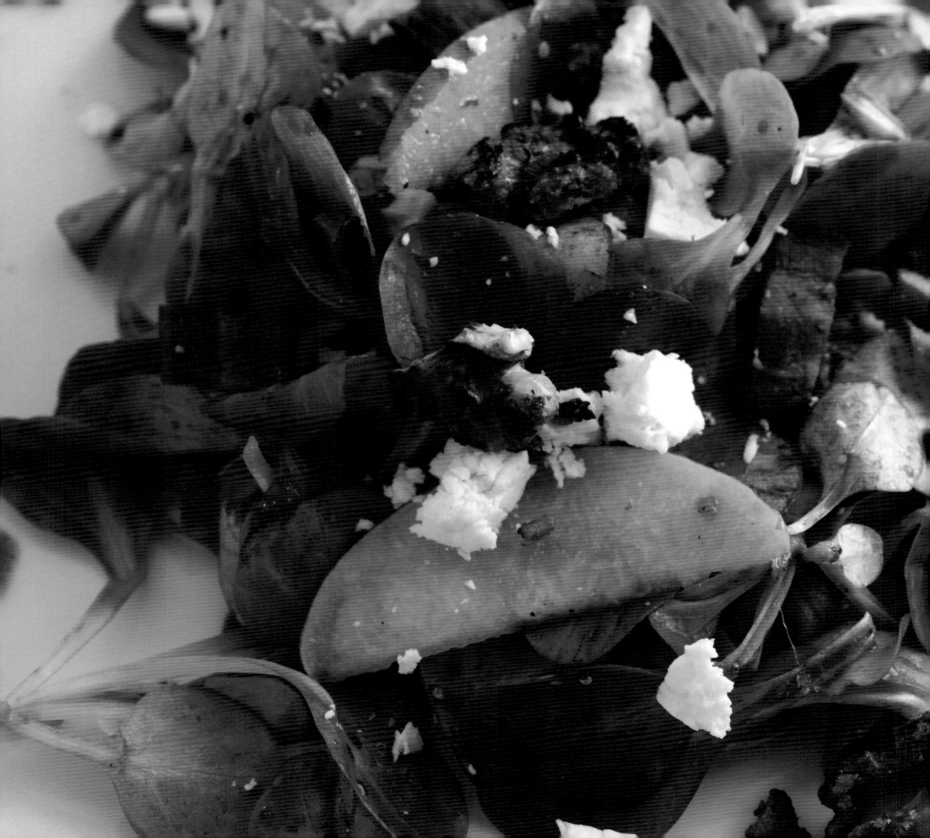

Asian Pear, Mache, Feta, &
Bacon Salad

with Coarse-Grain Mustard & Molasses Vinaigrette

The vinaigrette for this salad is slightly sweetened by brown sugar and a touch of molasses. The mild flavor of the molasses plays really well with the Asian pear and peppery walnuts in the salad.

Vinaigrette:

1½ Tbsp.	coarse grain mustard
½ tsp.	molasses
¼ tsp.	(packed) brown sugar
2 Tbsp.	red wine vinegar
¼ tsp.	freshly cracked black pepper
	pinch kosher salt
3 Tbsp.	olive oil

Salad

1 Asian pear, core removed, sliced thin	
5–6 cups	mache, can substitute any greens
½ cup	feta, crumbled
4	slices cooked bacon, crumbled

Peppery Candied Walnuts:

1 cup	walnuts
2 Tbsp.	light corn syrup
1 Tbsp.	(packed) brown sugar
¾ tsp.	salt
½ tsp.	freshly cracked black pepper
⅛ tsp.	red pepper flakes

SALAD

In a large mixing bowl, whisk together all ingredients for the vinaigrette *except* olive oil until thoroughly combined. While continuing to whisk constantly, slowly drizzle in olive oil to form an emulsified vinaigrette. Adjust seasoning to taste with kosher salt and freshly cracked black pepper. Reserve 1½ tablespoons of dressing for garnish.

Add mache and sliced pear to vinaigrette and toss to coat. Divide salad evenly among four plates. Sprinkle each salad with crumbled feta, bacon, and candied walnuts (see below). To garnish, drizzle a teaspoon of reserved vinaigrette around the perimeter of the plate.

PEPPERY CANDIED WALNUTS

Preheat oven to 350 degrees and spray a baking sheet with cooking spray.

Mix together all candied walnut ingredients in a bowl until walnuts are evenly coated. Pour walnuts onto prepared baking sheet and scatter into a single layer. Bake at 350 degrees for 10 to 15 minutes until nuts turn a deep golden. Stir every 5 minutes to prevent nuts from burning.

Remove from oven. Cool nuts completely on the pan. Store in an airtight container at room temperature.

Crab-Stuffed Okra Wrapped in Prosciutto

Crab-stuffed okra are an elegant hors d'oeuvres that can be stuffed and wrapped in prosciutto ahead of time and then thrown into the oven just before guests arrive for an early fall dinner party.

STUFFED OKRA

15	large whole okra pods
2 oz.	chevre, at room temperature
1 oz.	cream cheese, at room temperature
½ cup	cooked crab meat
8	slices prosciutto, cut in half widthwise

Preheat oven to 450 degrees and lightly grease a sheet pan.

Cut okra in half lengthwise. Using either your fingers (if you don't mind getting a little slimy) or a small spoon, carefully scrape out seeds from each okra half, leaving exterior completely intact. (*Note: Be sure to keep okra halves together as you go to prevent a hassle when stuffing.*)

In a mixing bowl, cream together chevre and cream cheese until fluffy. Mix crab and cheeses until completely shredded and incorporated into a homogeneous mixture.

Spread a teaspoon of crab mixture into a hollowed-out okra half. Replace matching okra half to conceal stuffing. Wrap tightly in prosciutto. Repeat process of filling and wrapping with remaining pods and crab mixture. The stuffed okra can be refrigerated for up to 8 hours before baking.

Arrange stuffed okra on prepared baking sheet. Bake at 450 degrees for 20 to 25 minutes until prosciutto is crispy and okra is cooked through. Flip okra halfway through cooking. Serve hot.

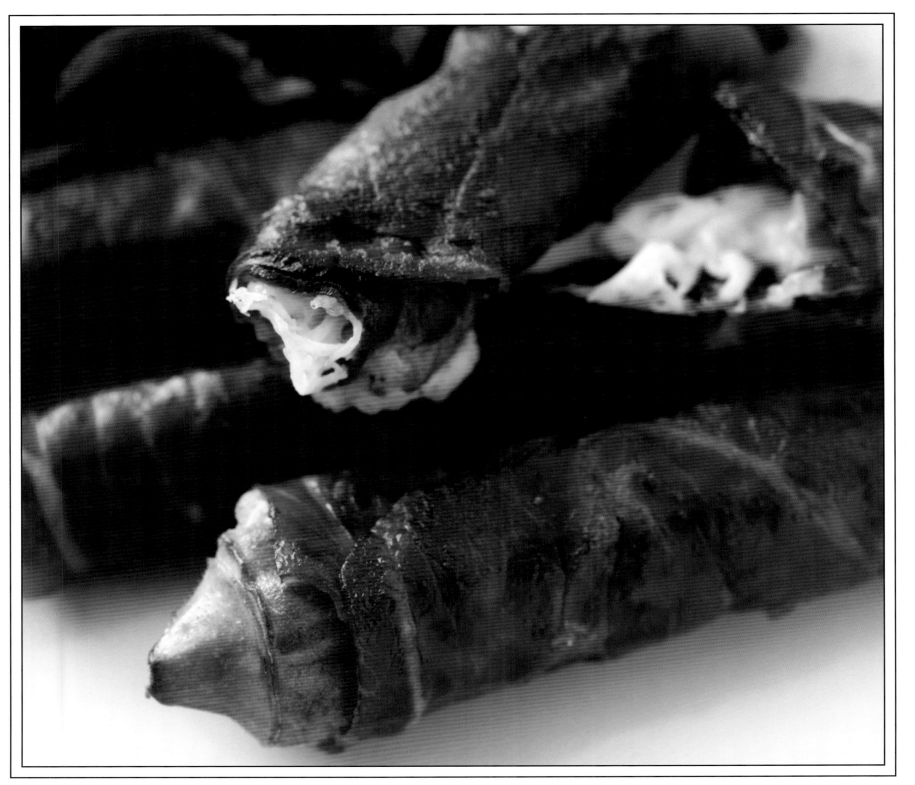

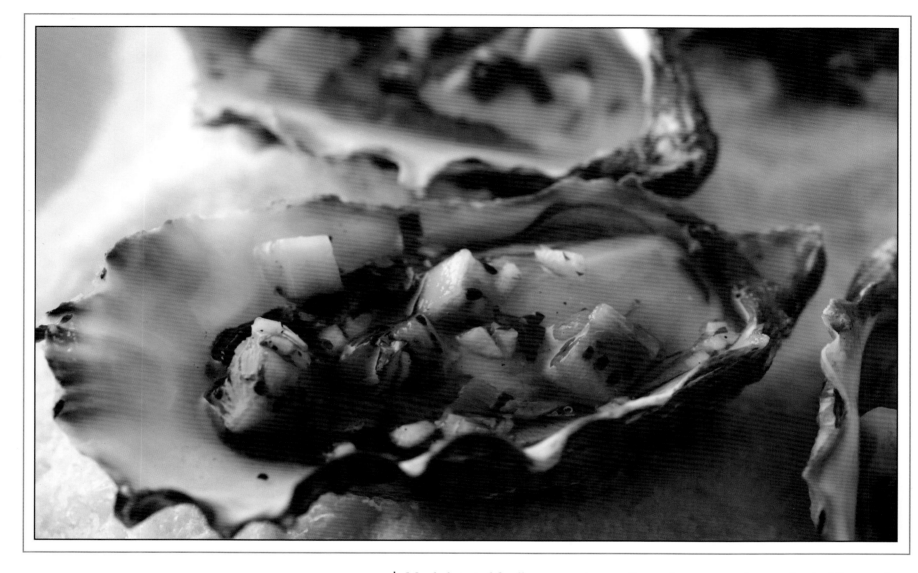

Oysters on the Half Shell

with Kiwi-Ginger Mignonette

My dad started feeding me oysters pretty much as soon as I popped out of the womb, and to this day they are one of my favorite ways to start a meal. I was raised on the old folklore that you should never consume oysters in months without Rs in them, namely May through August. During those summer months, the water is the warmest and provides the best environment for toxins and algae to grow. Nowadays, most of the oysters that you find in U.S. restaurants and markets are grown and harvested in water that is kept cool enough to prevent the growth of such toxins, so the oysters are pretty much as safe during the summer months as they are during the rest of the year. That being said, oysters spawn during the summer, and the quality of reproducing oysters is sub par when compared to those harvested in other months. Even though they are safe, I still prefer eating oysters in the months with Rs in them.

Ginger Mignonette:

1 Tbsp.	white wine vinegar
½ tsp.	finely minced or grated ginger
1 tsp.	finely chopped shallot
½ tsp.	sugar
¼ tsp.	freshly cracked black pepper
1 tsp.	finely chopped fresh parsley

1	kiwi fruit, peeled and cut in a small dice
12	raw oysters on the half shell, shucked immediately before use

In a small bowl, combine all ingredients for mignonette. Set aside for at least 30 minutes to allow flavors to marry.

Place raw oysters on a bed of crushed ice, or if serving immediately, rock salt. (*Note: The ice or salt will keep the oysters from spilling their liquor and the mignonette sauce.*)

To each oyster, add a few pieces of diced kiwi and ¼ teaspoon or so of mignonette sauce. Serve immediately.

ON SHUCKING OYSTERS

Do not attempt to shuck an oyster with an actual knife as a beginner. Oyster knives are thick, dull, and super strong—made with the sole purpose of breaking into oyster rocks. If you attempt to shuck an oyster with a knife, it is likely that all you will end up doing is ruining the blade and cutting yourself in the process.

Before beginning, make sure that the outsides of the oysters have been scrubbed clean of any sand or grit. All oysters have a completely flat side and a curved, cupped side. Begin by holding the oyster in a thick towel on a firm surface, the cupped side of the oyster facing down. The oyster is filled with precious liquor, and by opening it with the cupped side down, you will be able to preserve this liquor.

Slip the tip of the knife directly into the hinge at the back of the oyster. Wiggle the knife around like you are working a lock, twisting a little until you feel the hinge pop and give way. Once the hinge has been broken, run the oyster knife along the top of the shell to separate, being careful not to pop the belly of the oyster. Popping the belly is the worst thing you can do to an oyster! Remove the top shell, making sure to keep the oyster flat so as to not spill any of the liquor. Gently slide the oyster knife beneath the oyster and run it along the bottom to detach the oyster from the shell. Once you get the hang of it you'll, find that oyster shucking is relatively easy—all it requires is a little finesse.

Rosemary and Sea Salt Soft Pretzels

with Mustard Stout Cheese Dip

I grew up eating the most delicious soft pretzels from the Amish market in Annapolis, Maryland, and these are as close as I've come at being able to reproduce them. The addition of rosemary, sea salt, and black pepper may not be traditional, but it sure is delicious.

SOFT PRETZELS

Dough:

1	packet dry active yeast
1 tsp.	granulated sugar
1¼ cup	warm water, about 105 to 110 degrees
3¼ cups	flour
1 tsp.	kosher salt
½ cup	powdered sugar, sifted

Dipping Mix:

5 cups	water
1 cup	baking soda

Topping:

fresh rosemary, minced

coarse sea salt

freshly cracked black pepper

brown mustard seeds

melted butter, for brushing

Mustard Stout Cheese Dip:

See Page 236

Preheat oven to 425 degrees. Line two sheet pans with parchment paper and set aside. Oil a large bowl and set aside.

Add yeast and granulated sugar to warm water. Stir. Set aside for about 5 minutes. The yeast should become active and start bubbling or frothing. If after 5 or 10 minutes the yeast appears inactive, start again with fresh ingredients.

While yeast is activating, add remaining dough ingredients into a large mixing bowl and stir. Add activated yeast and water to dry ingredients. Stir until dough comes together. If kneading by hand, turn dough out onto a lightly floured surface and knead for 10 minutes until elastic and smooth. If using a stand mixer, use the dough hook and knead at medium speed for 5 to 7 minutes until elastic and smooth.

Transfer dough to oiled bowl. Flip dough to coat both sides in oil. Cover with oiled plastic wrap and a kitchen towel, and then place in a warm, draft-free spot. (*Note: I prefer to place the bowl near the preheating oven.*) Let dough rise for approximately 1 hour or until doubled in size.

In a 9x13-inch baking dish (or other equally wide dish), whisk together 5 cups water and 1 cup baking soda for dipping. (*Note: Most of the baking soda will*

not stay dissolved in the water, so right before dipping pretzels, whisk the mixture again.)

Divide dough into 8 even pieces. Roll out 1 piece into a 3-foot thin rope. Twist rope once or twice by swinging it in a jump-rope fashion. Twist rope into pretzel shape, pinching dough together where the ends intersect the dough. Holding the pretzel where the ends are connected to the dough, completely submerge the pretzel into the baking soda-water mixture. Place dipped pretzel onto prepared sheet pan, making sure that the holes in the pretzel are as wide as possible without the dough tearing or breaking the seal.

Repeat process three more times with three more pieces of dough, spacing pretzels as far apart as possible on the baking sheet. Sprinkle pretzels with minced rosemary, sea salt, black pepper, and mustard seeds. Bake at 425 degrees until golden brown—8 to 10 minutes—rotating the pan half way through baking for even browning. Remove from oven, brush with melted butter, and let cool for 10 minutes before serving.

While the first pan of pretzels is baking, prepare the second pan by following the process described above. As soon as the first batch of pretzels comes out of the oven, put the second batch in. Bake following above directions. Serve with Mustard Stout Cheese dip.

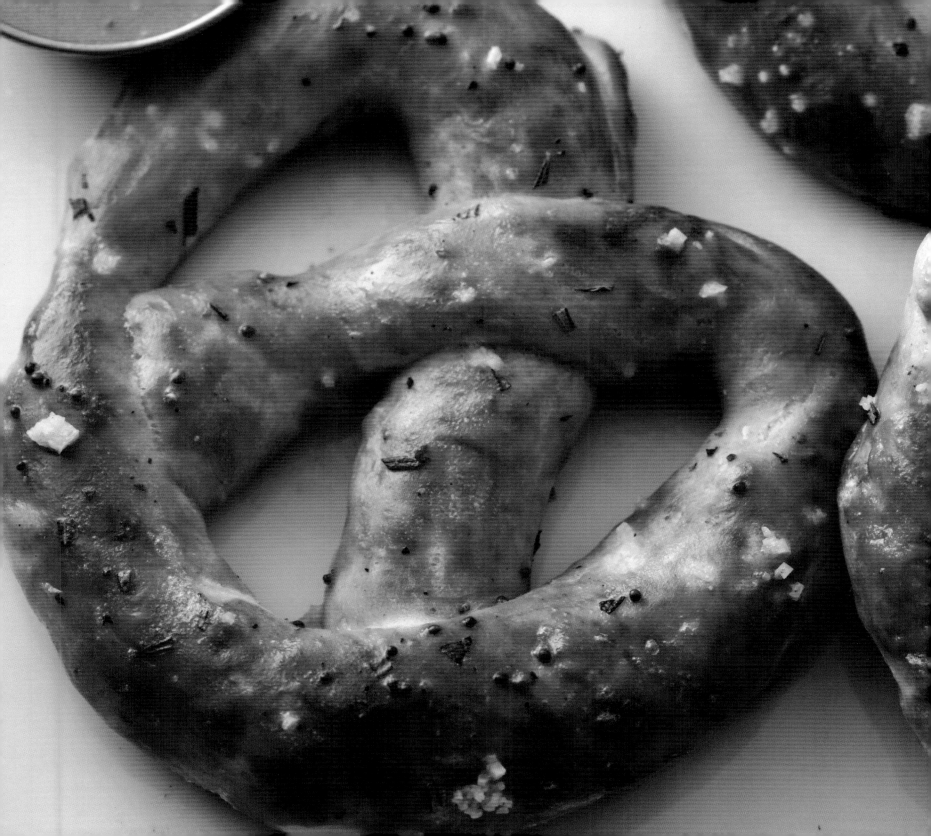

White Bean, Kale, and Sweet Potato Soup

with Chorizo

Spending the last 5 years in San Diego—20 miles from the Mexico border—has certainly influenced the flavors that I use in many of my dishes. Unintentionally, many of my dishes end up with a Mexican flare. Such is the case with this soup. Chorizo, cumin, achiote paste, and poblano chiles give this sweet potato and kale soup a distinctly south-of-the-border feel.

Stock:

1	ham hock
1	bay leaf
1	carrot, roughly chopped
1	stalk celery, roughly chopped
2	cloves garlic, smashed
1	yellow onion, quartered
1 tsp.	whole black peppercorns

Soup:

1 lb.	chorizo
1 Tbsp.	canola oil
1	yellow onion, peeled and diced
2	poblano chiles, stem and seeds removed and diced
5	cloves garlic, minced
1 tsp.	ground cumin
1 tsp.	ground chili powder
1½ tsp.	achiote paste
½ tsp.	freshly cracked black pepper, plus extra
2 tsp.	kosher salt, plus extra
2 cups	dried great northern beans
1	large sweet potato, peeled and diced
1	bunch kale, stems removed and roughly chopped

STOCK

Combine all stock ingredients in a large pot with 13 to 14 cups of water. Bring stock to a boil over high heat and then reduce heat to medium-low and simmer for 3 hours. Strain stock, reserving ham hock. Stock can be made up to 3 days in advance and stored in the refrigerator until ready for use.

SOUP

Preheat a large pot over medium-high heat. Once pan is heated, add chorizo. Brown chorizo until cooked through. Remove from pan and place on paper towels to drain.

Return pot to stove and reduce heat to medium. Heat canola oil in the pot for 1 minute. Once oil is hot, stir in diced onion and poblano chiles. Sauté veggies for about 10 minutes over medium heat, stirring occasionally, until onions are translucent and chiles are soft. Add garlic, cumin, chili powder, achiote paste, black pepper, and kosher salt and stir. Sauté for 1 more minute until garlic and spices release their aromas. Add dried beans and sauté for another 2 minutes, stirring frequently. Add drained stock and reserved ham hock and raise heat to medium-high. Bring soup to a boil. Reduce heat to medium-low, add reserved chorizo, and simmer for 2 hours, stirring occasionally until beans are almost tender. Add sweet potatoes and kale. Simmer for another 1 to 1½ hours until beans are tender and sweet potato is very soft. If soup needs more liquid during cooking process, add 1 cup at a time until desired consistency is achieved. Adjust seasoning levels as desired with more kosher salt and freshly cracked black pepper. (*Note: As with most soups or stews, this one tastes best on the second day.*)

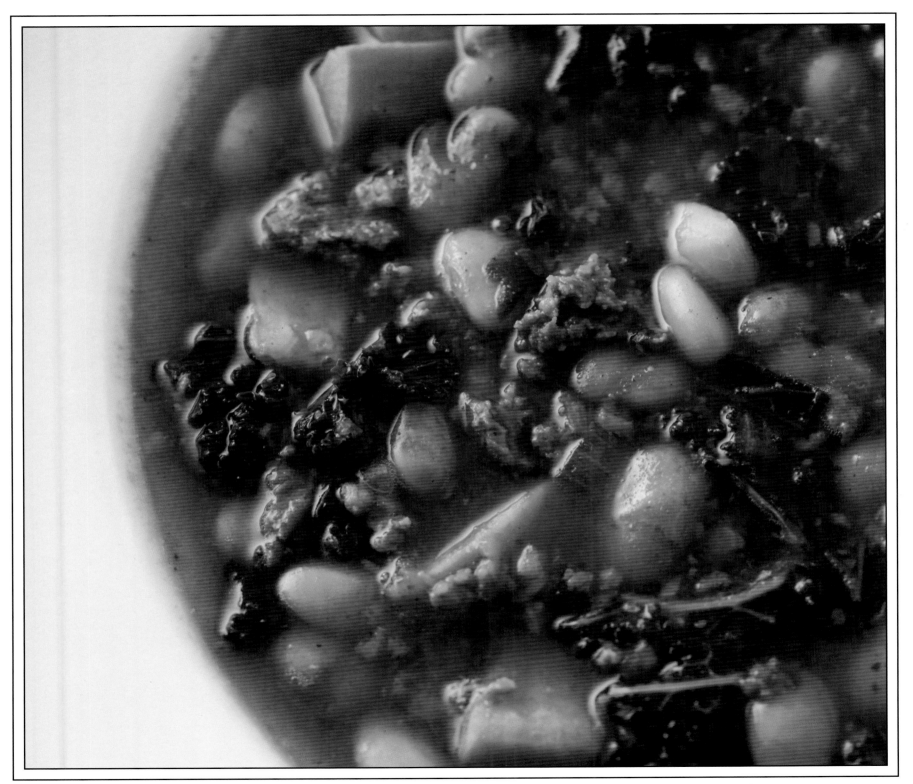

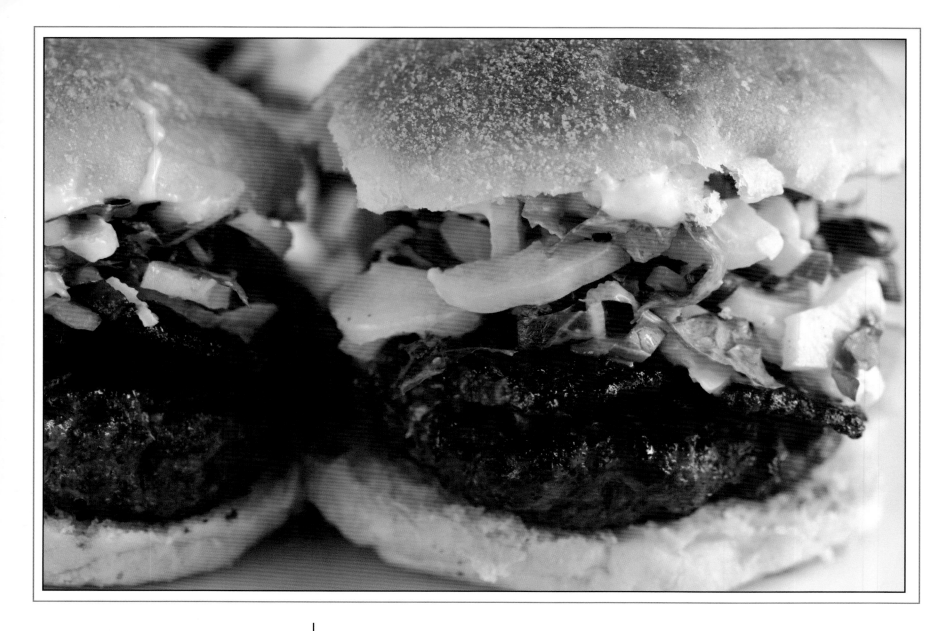

Asian Sliders

with Sambal-Glazed Bacon and Bok Choy Slaw

Most wasabi powders and pastes on the market actually contain *zero* true wasabi. Generally these products are just dyed horseradish. Regardless of authenticity, any wasabi paste or powder will work for this recipe. If you buy the powdered form, mix 1 part wasabi powder with 1 part water and let sit for about 15 minutes to form a slightly dry wasabi paste. It's important to let it sit so the enzymes in the powder have time to activate.

Sliders

1⅓ lb.	ground beef
	kosher salt
	freshly cracked black pepper
	Sambal-Glazed Bacon
	Wasabi Lemongrass Mayonnaise
	Wasabi Bok Choy slaw
8	slider buns

Sambal-Glazed Bacon:

1½ Tbsp.	Sambal Oelek
2 tsp.	(packed) brown sugar
6	thick-cut slices bacon (the thicker the better), cut into thirds lengthwise

Wasabi Bok Choy Slaw

1 tsp.	wasabi paste
1½ tsp.	Sambal Oelek
1½ Tbsp.	mayonnaise
1½ Tbsp.	rice wine vinegar
1 tsp.	(packed) brown sugar
1	head bok choy (*not* baby), rinsed and shredded
	kosher salt
	freshly cracked black pepper

Wasabi Lemongrass Mayonnaise:

1½ tsp.	minced lemongrass, tough outer layers removed
4 tsp.	wasabi paste
4 Tbsp.	mayonnaise
¼ tsp.	freshly cracked black pepper

Preheat grill to medium-high heat.

While grill is heating, form ground beef into 8 small patties, about 2½ inches in diameter. Liberally season both sides of patties with kosher salt and freshly cracked black pepper.

Grill over medium-high heat for 8 to 10 minutes total, flipping halfway through cooking, until just cooked through. Remove from grill.

Assemble sliders by layering each bottom half of the bun with a burger, followed by Sambal-glazed Bacon and Wasabi Bok Choy Slaw. Spread Wasabi Lemongrass Mayonnaise on top buns and place on top of the Wasabi Bok Choy Slaw to close the sandwiches.

SAMBAL-GLAZED BACON

Preheat oven to 400 degrees.

Place bacon slices onto a baking sheet in a single layer with 1 inch between each slice. Bake for 10 minutes.

While bacon is baking, whisk together sambal and brown sugar.

Remove pan from oven. Flip bacon over and then, using a pastry brush, evenly coat each slice of bacon with sambal–brown sugar mixture. Return pan to oven and continue baking until crisp, about 5 more minutes. Cooking times will vary depending on thickness of bacon. Remove from oven. Place bacon, glazed-side up, on a paper towel to drain.

WASABI BOK CHOY SLAW

In a small bowl, whisk together first 5 ingredients.

Pour wasabi dressing over shredded bok choy in a large mixing bowl. Toss to coat and season to taste with kosher salt and freshly cracked black pepper. Let salad marinate for 20 to 30 minutes before serving. Salad will wilt and release water. If desired, adjust seasoning to taste with kosher salt and freshly cracked black pepper.

WASABI-LEMONGRASS MAYONNAISE

Whisk together all ingredients until thoroughly incorporated. Chill until ready for use.

Ginger-Sumac Roasted Turkey Breast

with Brown Butter Vinaigrette and Roasted Brussels Sprouts

Roasted Brussels sprouts are one of my all-time favorite veggies. Before you call me crazy, try out this recipe and make sure to dip at least one of the roasted sprouts into the brown butter vinaigrette.

ROASTED TURKEY BREAST

Rub:

1 Tbsp.	minced or pureed ginger
2	cloves garlic, minced
1 Tbsp.	ground sumac, plus extra
1 tsp.	kosher salt
½ tsp.	freshly cracked black pepper

1	turkey breast split, bone-in, and skin on
2 Tbsp.	butter at room temperature
	kosher salt
	freshly cracked black pepper

Mash all rub ingredients together to form a paste.

Gently work your fingers under turkey skin and coat turkey breast with rub, massaging it in and making certain to focus on the area beneath the skin. Do not use rub on the skin but on the meat directly.

Seal turkey breast inside a large resealable plastic bag, removing as much air as possible in trying to emulate a vacuum seal. Let turkey breast chill in rub for 4 to 24 hours.

Preheat oven to 425 degrees.

Place turkey breast rib-side down onto a baking sheet lined with aluminum foil. Coat entire surface of turkey breast with room temperature butter, both under and over skin. Season skin with a sprinkle of kosher salt, freshly cracked black pepper, and sumac. Insert meat thermometer into thickest part of breast, away from any bones.

Roast turkey breast at 425 degrees for 50 to 55 minutes or until thermometer reaches 165 degrees. Cooking time will vary depending on the size of the turkey breast. For best results, rely on a digital meat thermometer with an alarm that you can set to go off when the temperature reaches 165.

Remove from oven and let rest for at least 10 minutes before slicing.

To plate, place a pile of roasted Brussels sprouts in the middle of a plate. Lean slices of turkey breast up against sprouts. To finish, drizzle plate with brown butter vinaigrette.

Continued on Next Page

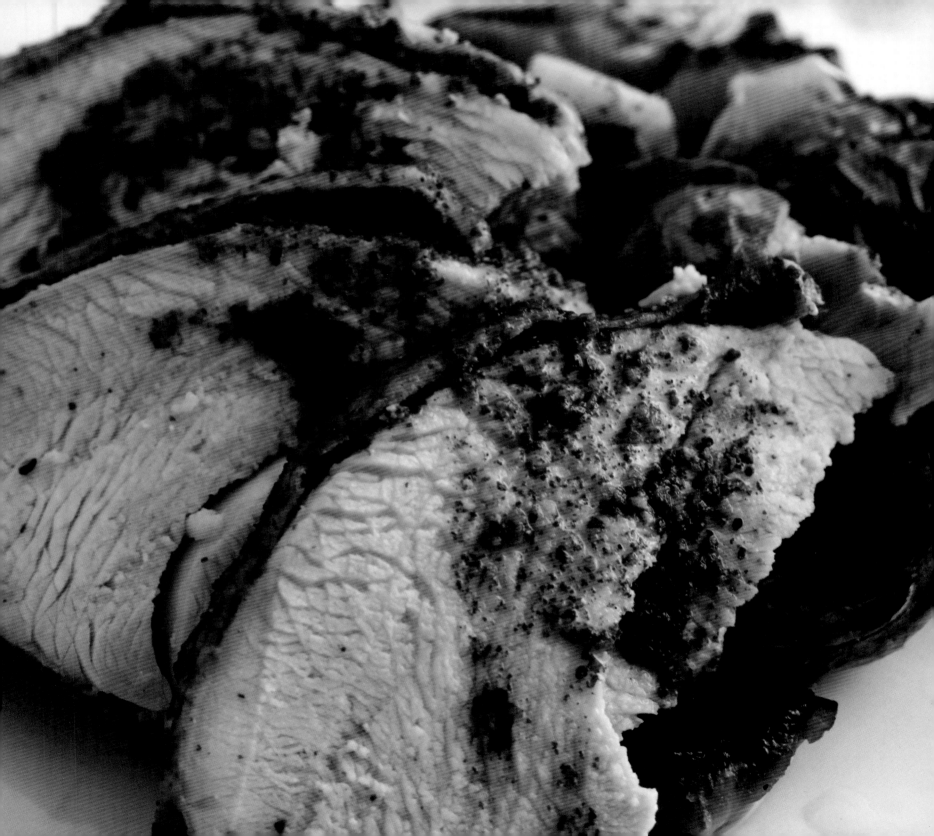

Roasted Brussels Sprouts

2 lbs.	Brussels sprouts
1 Tbsp.	butter, melted
1 Tbsp.	canola oil
	kosher salt
	freshly cracked black pepper

Ginger Sumac Brown Butter Vinaigrette:

4 Tbsp.	salted butter
1½ tsp.	ginger, minced
1	large clove garlic, peeled and minced
2 tsp.	ground sumac
2 Tbsp.	red wine vinegar
¼ tsp.	kosher salt, plus extra
	freshly cracked black pepper

Preheat oven to 425 degrees with a rack positioned in the upper third of the oven.

Trim off the very tip of the stem end of each Brussels sprout and remove any discolored or bruised outer leaves. Cut sprouts in half lengthwise. Drizzle melted butter and canola oil over prepared sprouts in a mixing bowl. Toss to coat evenly. Sprinkle sprouts liberally with kosher salt and freshly cracked black pepper. Toss again.

Arrange seasoned Brussels sprouts cut-side down onto a sheet pan. Roast sprouts at 425 degrees on the upper rack for 30 to 45 minutes—shaking pan every 15 minutes to prevent burning—until cut sides of sprouts are well caramelized, top leaves are crispy and brown in places, and sprouts' centers are tender. Serve immediately.

GINGER SUMAC BROWN BUTTER VINAIGRETTE

Cook butter in a small saucepan over medium heat, stirring occasionally, for 3 to 6 minutes until milk solids foam up, subside, and butter turns a nutty brown.

Reduce heat to low and add ginger, garlic, and sumac to the pan. Whisk constantly and cook for about 30 seconds. While whisking constantly, drizzle in red wine vinegar, kosher salt, and a pinch of freshly cracked black pepper. Taste and adjust seasoning as desire with more kosher salt and freshly cracked black pepper. Serve immediately. Vinaigrette will not stay emulsified and will need to be whisked before each use.

Horseradish Crusted Chicken Breast

with Parsnip-Potato Hash & Cider Gastrique

Gastrique is the formal term for a sauce that is made from a reduction of vinegar, sugar, and often times fruit. The potency of the vinegar in the gastrique will vary depending on how long the vinegar reduces. The vinegar in this dish's gastrique doesn't reduce for very long, resulting in a stronger vinegar flavor. As with all strong flavors, use sparingly at first, and if you like how it complements the dish, add more.

Horseradish Crust

1 cup	panko bread crumbs
2 Tbsp.	prepared horseradish
1 tsp.	kosher salt
1 tsp.	freshly cracked black pepper
1 tsp.	fresh thyme, minced
⅓ cup	green onions, minced
1 tsp.	fresh sage, minced
2 Tbsp.	extra virgin olive oil

4	boneless skinless chicken breasts
	extra virgin olive oil, for coating
	kosher salt
	freshly cracked black pepper

	micro greens or sunflower sprouts, for garnish

Cider Horseradish Gastrique

¼ cup	sugar
½ tsp.	kosher salt
1 Tbsp.	water
¼ cup + 2 Tbsp.	cider vinegar
¼ tsp.	crushed red pepper
2 tsp.	prepared horseradish

HORSERADISH CRUSTED CHICKEN BREAST

Preheat oven to 450 degrees.

Arrange panko in a thin even layer on a sheet pan. Toast bread crumbs in preheated oven until golden—5 to 10 minutes—tossing a couple of times. Remove from oven and let cool about 10 minutes.

Using your fingers, mix together toasted panko and remaining crust ingredients in a mixing bowl until oil and horseradish have been evenly distributed throughout the panko.

Toss chicken with olive oil and season all sides with kosher salt and freshly cracked black pepper.

Place seasoned breasts onto a sheet pan. Distribute bread crumb mixture evenly over each chicken breast, pressing to help crust stick.

Bake chicken at 450 degrees for 14 to 18 minutes until cooked through to an internal temperature of 165 degrees. Cooking times will vary depending upon thickness of breasts. Remove from oven and let set 5 minutes.

To plate, spoon one-fourth of the hash in the middle of a serving plate. Place a horseradish-crusted chicken breast on top of the hash. Garnish plate with a drizzle of gastrique and a pinch of micro-greens or sunflower sprouts.

CIDER-HORSERADISH GASTRIQUE

Add water, salt, and sugar to a 1-quart saucepan over medium heat. Stir until sugar has dissolved into the water. Cook sugar *without stirring* until it reaches a golden brown amber color, swirling pan to prevent burning. (*Note: Have a pastry brush and water nearby during the cooking process to brush down any sugar that may crystallize on the sides of the pan.*) Once sugar has turned amber, remove from heat and carefully add cider vinegar. The molten sugar will bubble viciously, so be very careful. Return pan to heat once bubbling subsides. Add crushed red pepper and horseradish to pan. Stir to dissolve caramelized sugar into vinegar. Cook another 2 to 3 minutes until smooth. Remove from heat and let cool 10 minutes. Strain.

Continued on Next Page

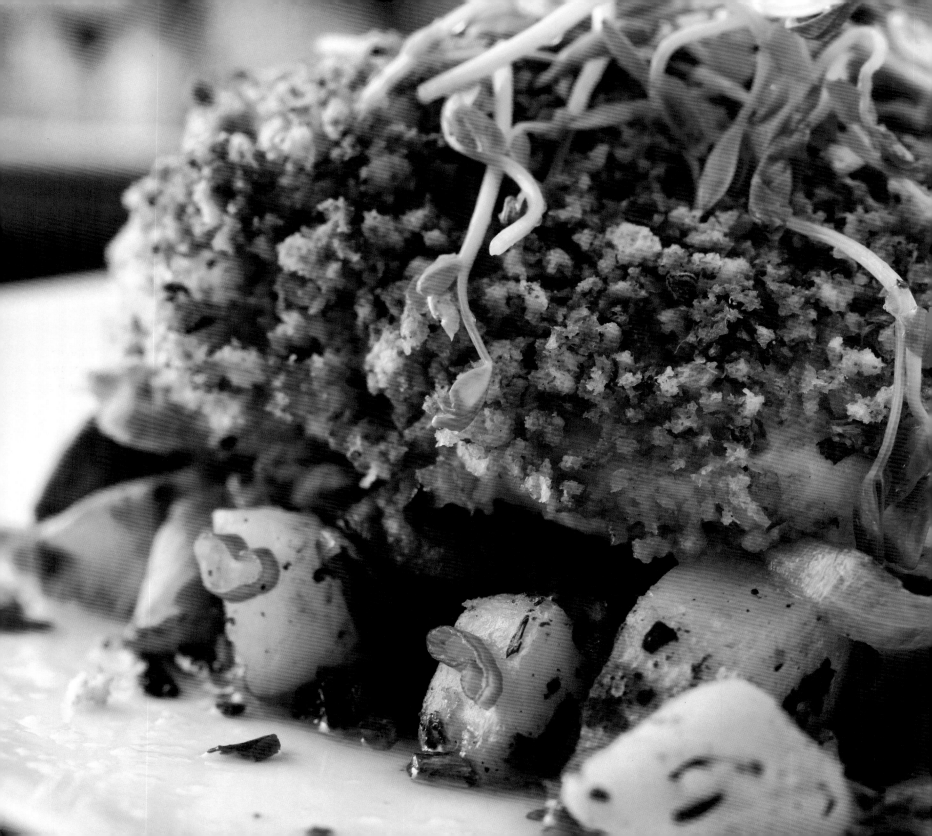

Parsnip-Potato Hash

1 Tbsp.	bacon fat
12	button mushrooms, thickly sliced
1	medium yellow onion, sliced
	kosher salt
	freshly cracked black pepper
1 Tbsp.	canola oil
1 tsp.	fresh sage, minced
1 tsp.	fresh thyme, minced
⅓ cup	green onions, thinly sliced

Boil a medium-sized pot of water over high heat. Once boiling, season water liberally with salt and add peeled, diced parsnips and potatoes. Boil 3 to 4 minutes until parboiled to a crisp-tender state. Drain and set aside until needed.

While water comes to a boil, preheat a large sauté pan over medium heat for about 5 minutes. Add bacon fat to heated pan. Once fat is hot, add mushrooms. Sauté for 7 minutes, stirring occasionally. Add onion to mushrooms and sprinkle with kosher salt and freshly cracked black pepper. Sauté for another 7 minutes, stirring occasionally.

Add parboiled parsnips and potatoes, as well as canola oil, sage, and thyme to mushrooms and onions. Season liberally with kosher salt and freshly cracked black pepper. Toss to evenly distribute ingredients and to coat veggies in oil. Sauté for 25 to 30 minutes, tossing occasionally, until hash is caramelized and potatoes and parsnips are cooked through. Adjust seasoning to taste with more kosher salt and freshly cracked black pepper. Remove from heat and add green onions. Toss to distribute. Serve immediately.

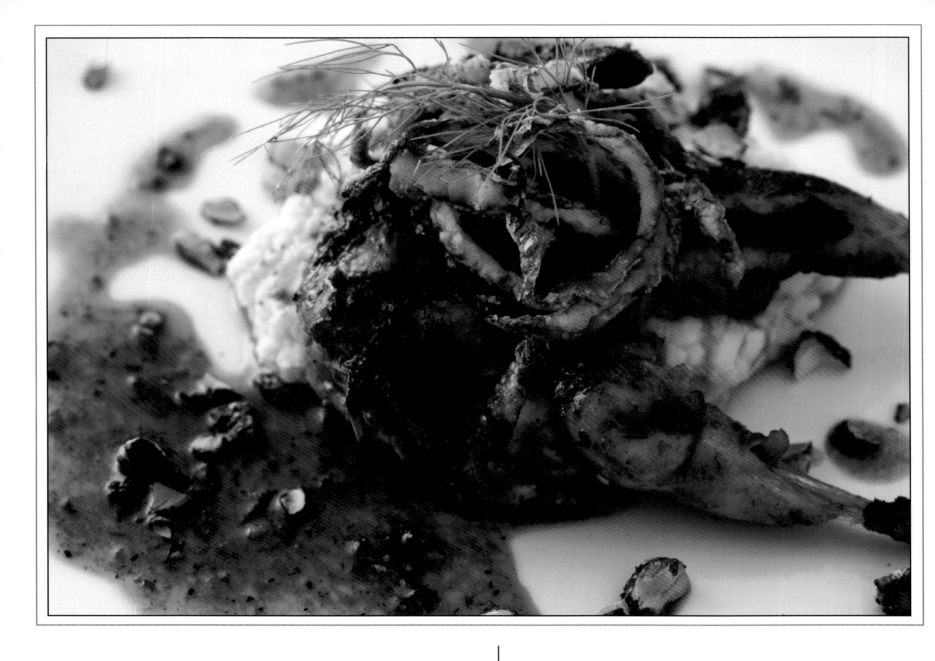

Harissa-Marinated Grilled Quail

with Celery Root Puree

Deboning quail is very tedious, time consuming work that is easier left to the professionals. Most of the time, if you can find quail from your local butcher, he will likely already offer them deboned or be willing to do it for you.

Marinade:

3 Tbsp.	Harissa, store-bought or homemade (see page 234)
1 Tbsp.	Dijon mustard
1 Tbsp.	honey
½ tsp.	freshly cracked black pepper
2 Tbsp.	extra virgin olive oil

4	semi-boneless quails
	kosher salt
	freshly cracked black pepper

Celery Root Puree:

1½ lbs.	celery root (celeriac), peeled and cut in 2-inch cubes
½ cup	whole milk, plus extra if necessary
2 Tbsp.	butter
	kosher salt and
	freshly cracked black pepper

Fried Fennel:

1 cup	fennel, sliced ⅛-inch thick (best done with a mandoline)
½ cup	flour
½ tsp.	kosher salt, plus extra for seasoning
½ tsp.	ground cumin
1 cup	peanut oil for frying

Pomegranate Harissa Vinaigrette:

See Page 238

Spiced Pomegranate Pistachios:

See Page 242

Whisk together marinade ingredients and pour over quail in a 1-gallon resealable plastic bag. Rub marinade into birds, making sure that all areas are evenly covered. Seal bag, removing as much air as possible, emulating a vacuum seal for best results. Refrigerate. Marinate quail, chilled, for 3 to 6 hours.

Prepare grill for high direct heat. Remove quail from marinade and sprinkle all sides with kosher salt and freshly cracked black pepper. Grill quail directly over high heat for about 3 minutes per side—6 minutes total—or until just cooked through. (*Note: Overcooking will result in an extremely dry bird, so be careful!*) Remove from heat and let rest for 5 minutes before serving.

To plate, place a scoop of celery root puree in the middle of a plate. Lay one whole grilled quail over celery root. Pile fried fennel on top of quail and drizzle vinaigrette around the plate. Finish with a sprinkle of chopped spiced pomegranate pistachios. Repeat plating 3 more times for a total of four servings.

CELERY ROOT PUREE

Cover celery root in a pot with 1 inch water. Season water liberally with salt. Bring to boil over high heat. Boil celery root until very tender, about 15 minutes.

While celery root is boiling, add milk and butter to a food processor or blender.

Once celery root is tender, strain and then add to milk and butter. Process until very smooth. If puree is too thick, thin it out with more milk, adding a tablespoon at a time until you've reached the consistency of mashed potatoes. Adjust seasonings to taste with kosher salt and freshly cracked black pepper.

FRIED FENNEL

Heat oil in a 2-quart heavy-bottomed pot to 350 degrees.

Whisk together flour, kosher salt, and cumin in a separate bowl.

Added fennel slices to flour mixture and toss to coat. Shake off excess flour and carefully add to preheated oil.

Fry fennel for 2 to 4 minutes, stirring occasionally, until fennel turns golden brown. Using a slotted spoon or spider, remove fennel from oil and drain on a paper towel. Sprinkle immediately with a pinch of kosher salt.

Seared Mahi Mahi

with Fennel-Grape Salad and Sweet Potato Gratin

At the very top of the stalk of fennel, there are soft, emerald green fronds that look a lot like dill. Similar to dill, these fronds can be used as an herb. Rather than discarding the fronds with the stalks, save them and use them as an herb in salads or to garnish a dish.

Seared Mahi Filets:

	kosher salt
	freshly cracked white or black pepper
4 (6-oz.)	mahi filets
3 Tbsp.	canola, peanut, or safflower oil

Fennel-Grape Salad:

1	bulb fennel, trimmed and sliced ⅛-inch thick
2 cups	seedless red grapes, cut in half lengthwise
2 Tbsp.	flat-leaf parsley, minced
2 Tbsp.	fennel fronds, minced
⅓ cup	pine nuts, toasted (see page 243)
	kosher salt
	freshly cracked black pepper

Vinaigrette:

3 Tbsp.	white wine vinegar
1 Tbsp.	Dijon mustard
1	large garlic clove, minced (or 2 small cloves)
½ tsp.	kosher salt
½ tsp.	freshly cracked black pepper
6 Tbsp.	canola or safflower oil

Sweet Potato, Fennel, and Anchovy Gratin:

See Page 242

SEARED MAHI FILETS

Preheat a large sauté pan over medium-high heat for 4 minutes.

While pan is heating, season all sides of filets liberally with kosher salt and freshly cracked pepper.

Add oil to the pan. Swirl pan to evenly coat the bottom of the pan in oil. Sear mahi filets over medium-high heat until golden—3 to 4 minutes. Flip and sear for another 3 to 4 minutes until second side is golden as well and mahi is just cooked through. If necessary, cook in two batches to prevent overcrowding. (*Note: When cooking fish—or any meat—the flesh will release itself from the pan when it's ready to flip. If you try to flip the fish and it sticks to the pan, it's not ready to flip yet. Let it cook longer until it easily releases from the surface.*)

To assemble, place a square of sweet potato gratin in the middle of the plate. Lean a seared mahi filet up against the gratin. Spoon grape-fennel salad over the fish and around the plate. Garnish the plate with a drizzle of reserved white wine vinaigrette. Repeat plating for a total of 4 servings.

FENNEL-GRAPE SALAD

In a mixing bowl, whisk together all vinaigrette ingredients *except* oil. While continuing to whisk vigorously, slowly drizzle in oil to form an emulsified vinaigrette. Adjust seasonings to taste with kosher salt and freshly cracked black pepper.

Reserve half of the vinaigrette for plating.

Place remaining ingredients for salad and vinaigrette into a bowl. Toss to combine and evenly coat all ingredients with dressing. Adjust seasonings with kosher salt and freshly cracked black pepper as desired. Let salad chill for 20 minute to 1 hour before serving.

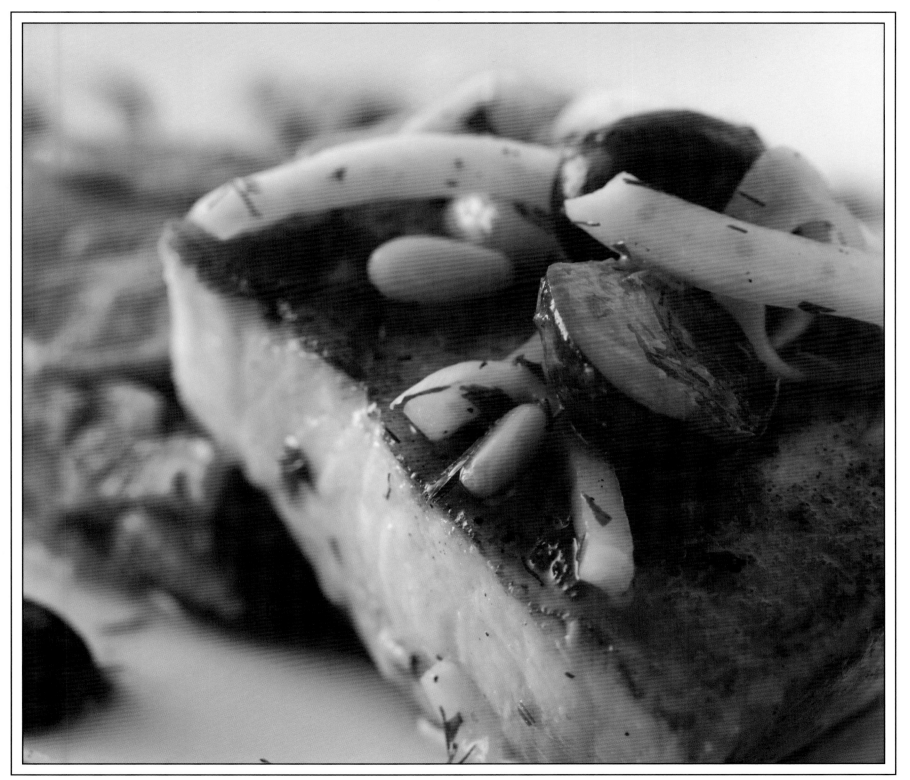

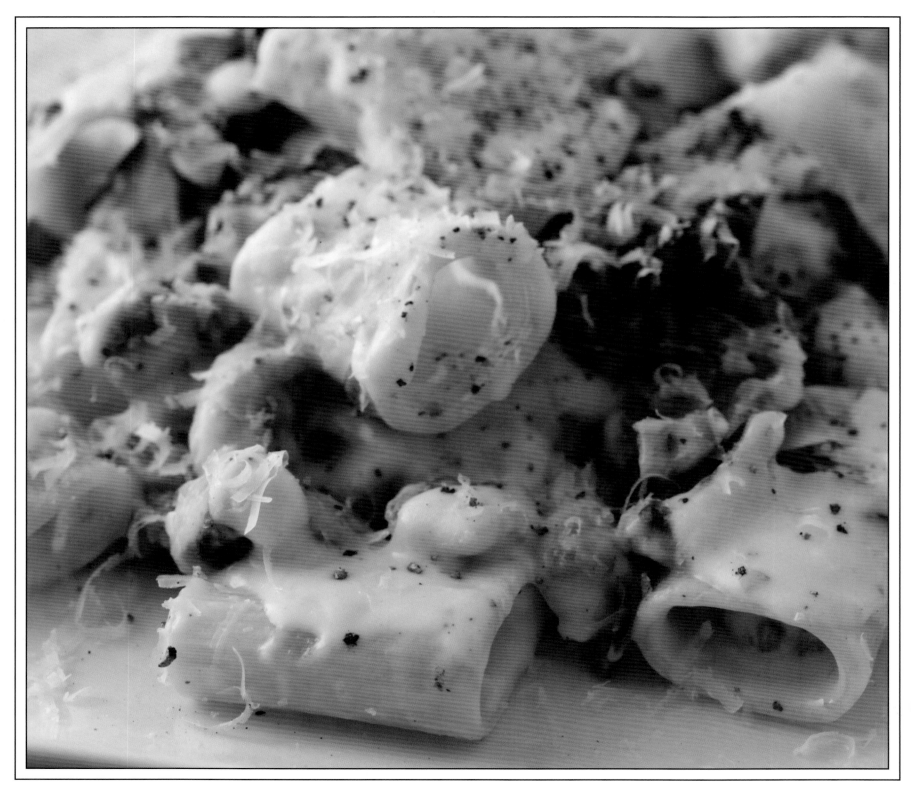

Paccheri Pasta

with Walnuts, Roasted Carrots, Swiss Chard, and Sage-Mornay Sauce

The addition of toasted walnuts adds the crunch that would otherwise be missing from this dish, and the carrots bring the sweet caramelized flavor. Both elements stand up nicely to the hearty Sage Mornay Sauce.

PACCHERI PASTA

40	baby carrots, cut in half
1 Tbsp.	canola oil
10 oz.	dried paccheri pasta, or any other large tube-shaped pasta
1 Tbsp.	butter
2	bunches Swiss chard, thick stems removed and roughly chopped
1 cup	walnut halves, toasted (see page 243)
	kosher salt
	freshly cracked black pepper
	Sage-Mornay Sauce
	Parmesan cheese, freshly grated, for garnishing

Sage-Mornay Sauce:

2½ Tbsp.	butter
1	clove garlic, minced
2½ Tbsp.	flour
2½ cups	whole milk, at room temperature
1 Tbsp.	fresh sage, minced
1 tsp.	lemon zest, minced or finely grated
2 oz.	Parmesan cheese, freshly grated
2 oz.	Gruyère, shredded
	kosher salt
	freshly cracked black pepper

Preheat oven to 425 degrees.

Place carrots on a baking sheet. Drizzle with oil and season with kosher salt and freshly cracked black pepper. Toss to coat. Bake carrots at 425 for 40 minutes, stirring every 15 minutes so all sides can caramelize. Remove from oven.

While carrots are roasting, bring a large pot of liberally salted water to boil over high heat. About 10 minutes before carrots should be done roasting, cook pasta to al dente according package directions and Drain.

While pasta is cooking, preheat a large sauté pan over medium-high heat for 2 minutes. Melt butter in preheated pan. Once butter has melted, add Swiss chard. Sprinkle with kosher salt and freshly cracked black pepper. Sauté Swiss chard, stirring frequently, until just wilted. Remove from heat and drain off liquid.

After draining pasta, return it to the pot. Pour Sage-Mornay sauce over pasta. Add sautéed Swiss chard, roasted carrots, and toasted walnuts to pasta and sauce. Toss to coat and thoroughly mix ingredients, being careful not to break pasta tubes.

To plate, divide pasta evenly among four plates. Garnish with freshly grated Parmesan cheese and cracked black pepper.

SAGE-MORNAY SAUCE

Melt butter in a saucepan over medium heat. and then add garlic. Sauté, stirring occasionally for 60 seconds. Whisk in flour. Cook, whisking continuously, for 2 minutes. While continuing to whisk, slowly pour in milk until fully incorporated and smooth. Stir in sage and lemon zest. Cook sauce over medium heat until thickened, 10 to 15 minutes, stirring occasionally.

Once thick, whisk in Parmesan and Gruyère cheese. Season to taste with kosher salt and freshly cracked black pepper. Keep warm over low heat until ready to serve, stirring occasionally.

½ Tbsp.   canola oil

1½ lbs.   smoked Linguiça, diced

6 Tbsp.   butter or duck fat

6 Tbsp.   flour

1   large yellow onion, peeled and diced

1   large red bell pepper (stems and seeds removed), diced

1   jalapeño pepper, diced

3   stalks celery, diced

4   cloves garlic, minced

¼ tsp.   dried oregano

¼ tsp.   dried basil

¼ tsp.   dried thyme

1   bay leaf

½ tsp.   ground cayenne

2   (14.5-oz.) cans diced tomatoes with green chiles, like Rotel

10 cups   duck stock, plus extra as needed

shredded duck meat from two ducks

1   (20-oz.) bag frozen okra

kosher salt

freshly cracked black pepper

Duck Stock:

See Page 232

Preheat oil in a large stock pot and place over medium-high heat for 3 to 4 minutes. Cook Linguiça in preheated oil for about 8 minutes, stirring occasionally, until all sides have a chance to brown. Remove sausage from pot and set aside. Drain off all rendered fat.

Melt butter in the same stock pot over medium-high heat. Add flour to melted butter to form a roux. Cook roux over medium-high heat, stirring constantly, until it turns the color of milk chocolate. Do not leave roux unattended, or it will burn. If roux burns, wash out stock pot thoroughly and start over with more butter and flour. (*Note: It's unconventional to cook roux over a high temperature, but with constant stirring and supervision you can accurately gauge the color of the roux and cut the cooking time down from 45 minutes to about 15 minutes.*)

As soon as the roux is color of milk chocolate, add diced onions, bell pepper, jalapeño, and celery and reduce heat to medium. Sauté aromatics in the roux for about 10 minutes, stirring occasionally, until onion is translucent and veggies are soft. Add garlic, dried oregano, basil, and thyme and stir. Sauté for another 60 seconds or so until garlic releases its aroma.

Add canned tomatoes, bay leaf, and cayenne to pot and stir. Stir in browned sausage and 10 cups of duck stock. Raise heat to medium-high and bring to a boil. As soon as gumbo begins to boil, reduce heat to medium-low to low. Simmer for 1 hour, stirring occasionally and skimming off any fat that rises to the surface. Add shredded duck meat and frozen okra to the pot. Stir. Simmer gumbo for another 1½ to 2 hours, stirring and skimming occasionally, until okra is stewed down to a similar state as remaining veggies. If gumbo gets too thick while simmering, simply add a little more stock. Taste and adjust seasonings with kosher salt and freshly cracked black pepper. (*Note: I don't suggest seasoning the gumbo in the beginning because as the gumbo reduces, the seasoning levels change.*) Let gumbo cool to almost room temperature and refrigerate overnight. (*Note: Like all stews, gumbo is best eaten the day after it's made so that the flavors have a chance to meld and develop more fully.*)

If desired, scrape off any fat that has risen to the surface and hardened during the chilling process before reheating. Reheat gumbo over medium heat until simmering, stirring occasionally. Serve over cooked white rice.

Duck and Linguiça Gumbo

This recipes makes a huge pot of gumbo. Fortunately, gumbo freezes well. If you have more than you need, pop it in the freezer, and it will be there on nights when you don't feel like cooking dinner. Just make fresh rice to serve with the reheated gumbo. If you can't find Linguiça, substitute any smoked sausage. If duck isn't your thing, feel free to substitute chicken.

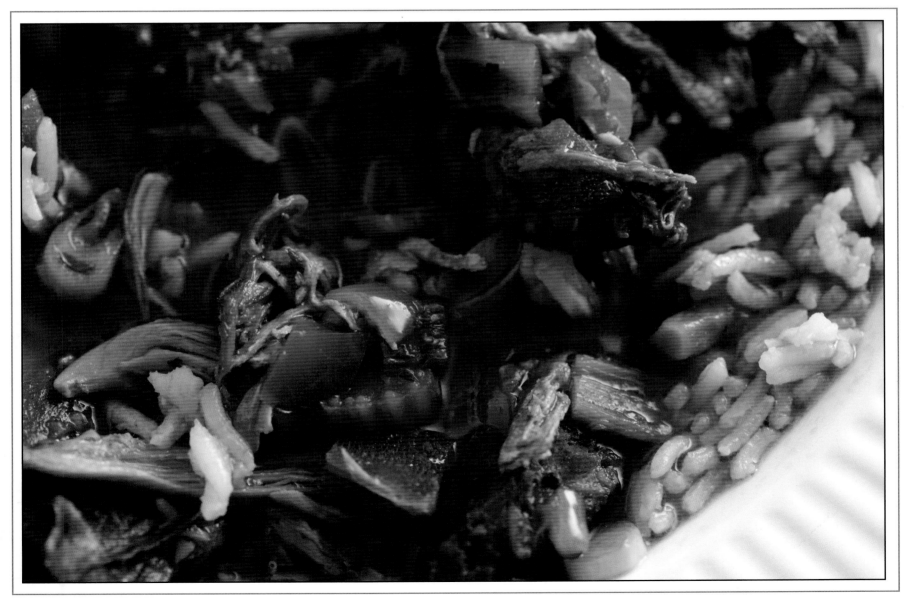

Pollo Asado Mexican Pizza

with Roasted Jalapeños and Cotija on a Cornmeal Crust

The pollo asado in this dish is one of our favorite quick fixes for dinner. It goes great on pizza, in tacos, or wherever else you can imagine using it. Whether you're making this pizza because you have leftover pollo asado from another meal or are making the chicken specifically for this pizza, I promise you won't be disappointed. Because of the cornmeal, the dough is really loose. You won't be tossing it into a nice shape so much as using your hands to pull the dough into a rough circle.

Mexican Pizza:

1 recipe	Cornmeal Pizza Crust (see page 229)
1 recipe	Ancho Chile Pizza Sauce (see page 277)
8 oz.	part-skim low-moisture mozzarella, shredded
½ recipe	Pollo Asado (see below)
3 oz,	cotija cheese, crumbled
½	small red onion, peeled and sliced
3	roasted red jalapeños, seeds and stem removed, julienned (can substitute roasted red peppers for less heat; see page 239)
	Cilantro Ranch Dressing (see page 175)
	fresh cilantro leaves

Pollo Asado Marinade:

½ cup	freshly squeezed lime juice
½ cup	freshly squeezed orange juice
1 Tbsp.	apple cider vinegar
1 Tbsp.	kosher salt
1½ tsp.	freshly cracked black pepper
1 tsp.	dried Mexican oregano (substitute regular oregano, if necessary)
⅛ tsp.	ground cinnamon
⅛ tsp.	ground cloves
6	large cloves garlic, minced mashed into paste or processed through press
2 lbs.	boneless skinless chicken thighs
2 Tbsp.	canola oil, for coating

MEXICAN PIZZA

Preheat oven to 500 degrees or as hot as your oven will go. (*Note: You're oven can't be too hot.*)

Spread pizza sauce evenly over prepared pizza crust, leaving only about a ½ inch of crust dry around the edges. Sprinkle dough with a layer of mozzarella cheese, followed by layers of pollo asado, red onions, and roasted red jalapeño peppers. To finish off, sprinkle pizza with crumbled cotija.

Bake pizza in hot oven for 10 to 12 minutes until crust is golden and cheese is bubbly. Remove from oven, drizzle with cilantro ranch dressing, and scatter cilantro leaves over pizza. Cool for 5 minutes. Cut in slices and enjoy. Recipe makes two pizzas.

POLLO ASADO

Whisk together marinade ingredients and pour over chicken thighs in a gallon-sized resealable plastic bag. Toss to coat completely. Seal bag, removing as much air as possible to emulate a vacuum seal. Marinate chicken in refrigerator for at least 4 hours and up to 24 hours.

Prepare grill for medium-high heat. Remove chicken from marinade and toss with canola oil. Grill chicken over direct heat for 5 to 6 minutes per side— 10 to 12 minutes total—until cooked through, moving as necessary to avoid any major flare-ups.(*Note: Thicker thighs may require additional cooking time.*) Remove from heat and let rest at least 5 minutes before chopping.

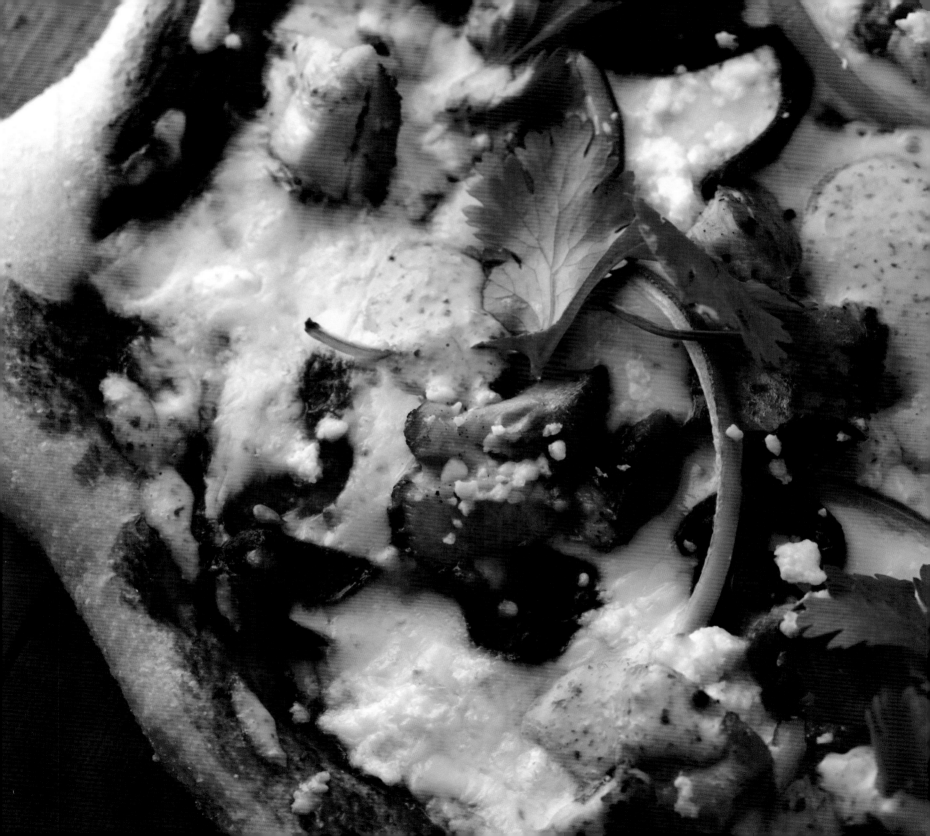

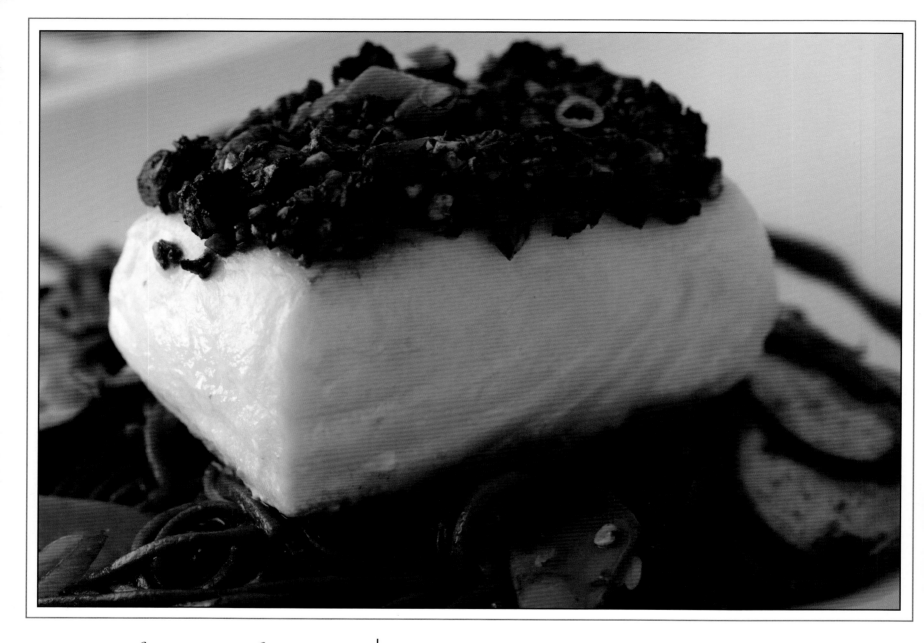

Pistachio-Wasabi Crusted Alaskan Halibut

with Soba Noodle Stir-Fry

If you can't find tamarind paste or tamarind pods in your local grocery store, look for it in either an Asian or Latin market. If you still have no luck, substitute molasses for the tamarind paste. The flavors are somewhat similar, and the amount called for is so small you probably won't be able to tell the difference.

Pistachio Wasabi Crust:

1 tsp.	wasabi paste
2 tsp.	dark soy sauce
1 tsp.	lime juice
⅔ cup	shelled unsalted pistachios, roughly chopped

4	(4-oz.) pieces Alaskan halibut
	kosher salt

Sauce:

½ tsp.	tamarind paste
1 tsp.	Dijon or Chinese mustard
2 tsp.	dark soy sauce
1 tsp.	regular soy sauce
1 Tbsp.	Chinese black vinegar
1 tsp.	Sambal Oelek (or less if you don't like spicy flavors)
1 Tbsp.	lime juice
1 Tbsp.	water

Soba Noodle Stir-Fry:

1 Tbsp.	canola oil
2	small zucchini, stem ends removed and thinly sliced
1	red bell pepper, stem and seeds removed, julienned
1½ cups	snow peas, ends trimmed slightly and cut in half lengthwise
½	yellow onion, sliced (optional)
8 oz.	dry soba noodles, cooked according to package directions
¼ cup	fresh cilantro leaves, roughly chopped
2	green onions, thinly sliced, divided

Preheat oven to 450 degrees.

Whisk together first three ingredients for crust in a small bowl. Add pistachios and toss to coat.

Sprinkle halibut lightly with kosher salt on all sides. Arrange halibut pieces on a sheet pan and top with equal amounts of pistachio crust mixture.

Bake at 450 degrees for 10 to 13 minutes—depending on thickness of halibut—until *just* cooked through; do not overcook. (*Note: On average, a 1-inch thick filet will be done in 8 to 10 minutes; however, most Alaskan halibut filets are thicker than 1 inch.*)

To plate, place one fourth soba noodle stir-fry onto the middle of a plate. Top with a piece of pistachio-crusted halibut. Garnish plate with a sprinkle of thinly sliced green onions. Repeat plating 3 more times for a total of 4 dishes.

SOBA NOODLE STIR-FRY

Whisk together all ingredients for sauce and set aside.

Preheat a large sauté pan over high heat for 4 minutes and add canola oil. Once oil ripples with heat—which will likely happen immediately if your pan has preheated long enough—add zucchini, red bell pepper, and snow peas. Sauté veggies over high heat, stirring constantly, for 2 to 3 minutes until crisp-tender. Add cooked soba noodles and sauce to pan. Toss to coat all ingredients with sauce. Sauté, tossing frequently for another 2 minutes. Remove from heat and add cilantro and green onion. Toss to incorporate. Adjust seasonings to taste with more kosher salt or soy sauce. Serve immediately.

Shepherd's Pie

with Potato-Turnip Topping

Although you may frequently see shepherd's pie recipes that call for beef, technically speaking, this dish must be made with lamb to actually be called a shepherd's pie. The same dish made with beef is called a cottage pie.

SHEPHERD'S PIE

Filling:

1 Tbsp.	canola or safflower oil
1½ lbs.	ground lamb (substitute buffalo or beef, if desired)
½ tsp.	kosher salt, plus extra
½ tsp.	freshly cracked black pepper, plus extra
1	yellow onion, peeled and diced
2	large parsnips, peeled and diced
2	large carrots, peeled and diced
4	cloves garlic, peeled and minced
2 Tbsp.	fresh rosemary, minced
2 Tbsp.	flat-leaf parsley, minced
2 Tbsp.	flour
1	(8-oz.) can tomato paste
½	bottle dry red wine
2 cups	beef or lamb broth
1	bay leaf
1 Tbsp.	sweet paprika

Topping:

1	large turnip, peeled right before use and cut in 1½-inch cubes
3	large russet potatoes, peeled right before use and cut in 1½-inch cubes
4 Tbsp.	butter, diced
2 oz.	cream cheese, diced
⅓ cup	whole milk, plus extra
	kosher salt
	freshly cracked black pepper
	chives, finely chopped, for garnishing

Preheat a large pot over medium-high heat for 3 minutes. Add canola oil to the pot. Once oil ripples from the heat, but before it begins to smoke, add lamb. Sprinkle with kosher salt and freshly cracked black pepper. Brown, stirring occasionally and break up the hunks of ground lamb. Once lamb is browned and cooked through, remove from pot and set aside.

Drain off all but 1 tablespoon oil from the pan and return to stove. Reduce heat to medium and sauté onion, parsnips, and carrots over medium heat, stirring occasionally, for about 10 minutes or until onions are translucent. Add garlic, rosemary, and parsley to the pot and cook for another minute, stirring continuously. Sprinkle with flour and stir to combine. Cook for another 60 seconds. Add remaining filling ingredients, browned lamb, and sautéed vegetables. Stir to combine. Raise heat to medium-high and bring to a boil. Reduce heat to low to medium-low and simmer until most of the liquid has been absorbed, about 1 to 1½ hours, stirring occasionally. Adjust seasonings to taste with kosher salt and freshly cracked black pepper.

While filling simmers, cover cubed potatoes in a pot with 1 inch water liberally seasoned with kosher salt. Boil over high heat for 2 minutes and add turnips. Boil for another 6 to 8 minutes or until the potatoes and turnips are very tender. Drain well. Using a stand mixer with whisk attachment, beat potatoes, turnips, butter, cream cheese, and milk until smooth, scraping down sides as necessary. If you don't have a stand mixer, mash veggies through a potato ricer and mix with butter, cream cheese, and milk until creamy. Adjust seasoning of mashed potato mixture with kosher salt and freshly cracked black pepper to taste.

Preheat broiler.

Once filling has finished cooking, pour into a large glass or ceramic casserole dish large enough that the filling only goes a little over halfway up the sides of the dish. Spread mashed potatoes and turnips evenly over filling. Using a spatula, swirl potatoes to create peaks.

Broil shepherd's pie until peaks of potato topping have browned, about 5 minutes. (*Note: Keep an eye on the shepherd's pie! Things under the broiler can go from brown to burnt quickly.*)

Remove from heat and let sit for 5 minutes before serving. Sprinkle with chopped chives to garnish. Serve hot.

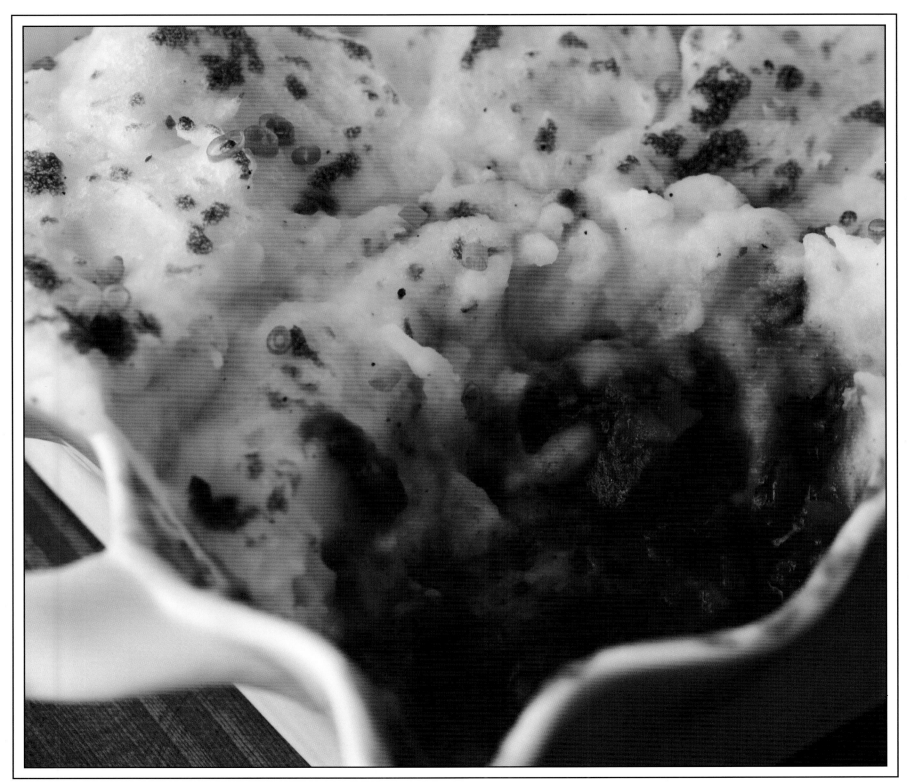

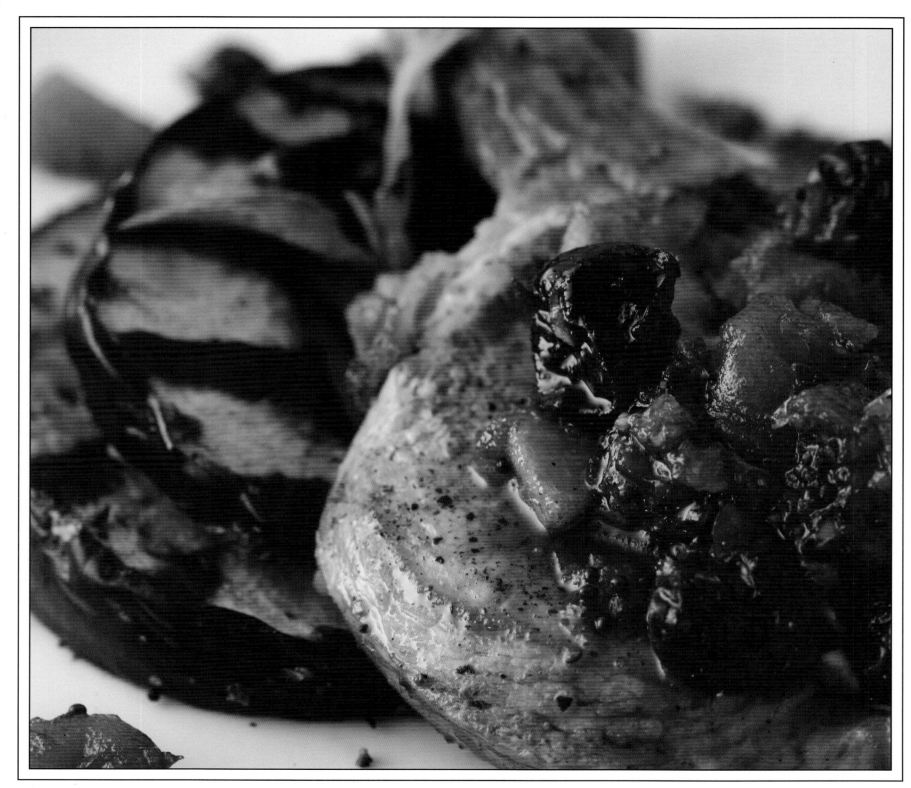

Pork Loin Chops

with Sliced Acorn Squash and Apple & Tart Cherry Chutney

During the fall you can still find some perfect days for grilling. We've included both outdoor grilling and indoor cooking instructions for this dish if you live in a place where it gets cold early in the year. Regardless of the weather, the flavors in this dish are undeniably fall.

PORK LOIN CHOPS:

2 Tbsp.	canola oil
4	(1-inch thick) pork loin rib chops
	kosher salt
	freshly cracked black pepper

Acorn Squash:

1	acorn squash, cut in half lengthwise, seeds scooped out
1½ Tbsp.	extra virgin olive oil
4	fresh sage leaves, chopped
3	cloves garlic, peeled and minced
	kosher salt
	freshly cracked black pepper

Apple & Tart Cherry Chutney:

See Page 227

PORK LOIN CHOPS

To sear chops: Heat oil in a large sauté pan over medium-high heat until oil ripples from the heat. While oil is heating, liberally season all sides of chops with kosher salt and freshly cracked black pepper. Working in batches if necessary to avoid overcrowding, sear chops for 4 to 5 minutes until well caramelized. Flip and sear for another 4 to 5 minutes, or until an internal thermometer reads 140 to 143 degrees, for medium doneness. Remove from heat and let rest for at least 5 minutes before serving.

To grill chops: Prepare grill for medium-high heat. Season chops liberally with kosher salt and freshly cracked black pepper on all sides. Once grill is very hot, brush chops with oil. Grill over direct heat for 6 to 7 minutes per side, a total of 12 to 14 minutes or until an internal thermometer reads 140 to 143 degrees, for medium doneness. Let rest for at least 5 minutes before serving.

ACORN SQUASH

Carefully cut acorn squash halves into ⅓-inch thick slices, similar to how you would slice a cantaloupe.

Toss squash slices with oil and sprinkle with sage leaves and garlic. Season liberally with kosher salt and freshly cracked black pepper, tossing evenly to coat.

In the oven: Preheat oven to 400 degrees. Arrange acorn squash slices flat on a sheet pan in a single layer.

Bake for 15 minutes until bottom side is golden. Flip slices and bake for another 10 to 15 minutes until cooked through.

On the grill: Prepare grill for medium heat. Grill seasoned acorn squash slices in a single layer over medium heat for about 10 minutes or until nicely charred. Flip and grill for another 10 minutes. Move squash to indirect heat and grill, covered, for another 5 to 10 minutes until slices are tender and cooked through.

ASSEMBLY

Pile several acorn squash slices in the middle of a plate. Lean a pork chop against acorn squash, with rib bone up in the air. Spoon chutney over pork and around the plate. If desired, garnish with fresh sage. Repeat plating 3 more times with remaining ingredients.

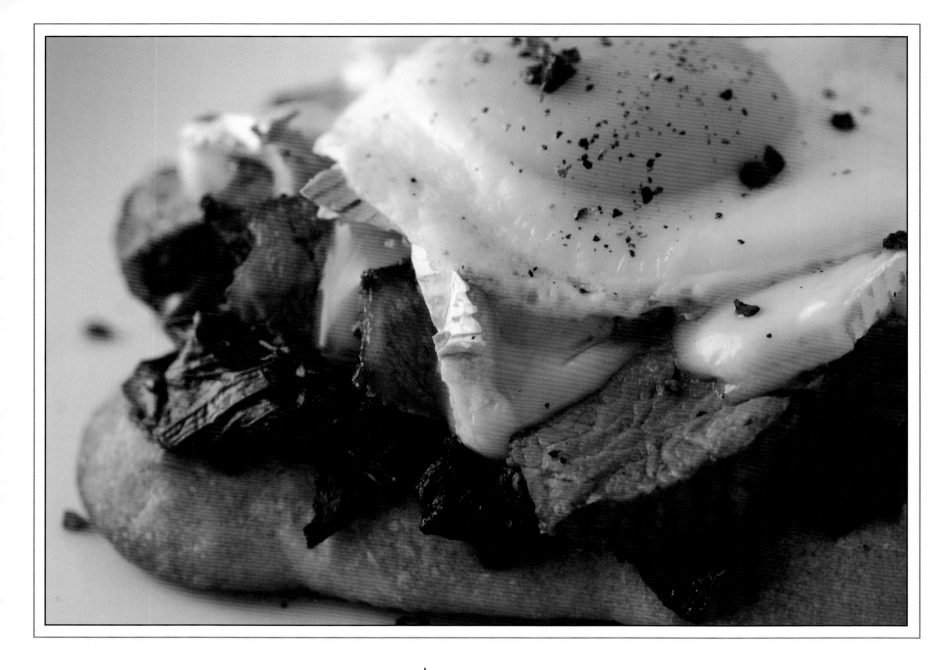

Open-Faced Steak and Egg Sandwiches

with Caramelized Onion-Tomato Jam

Dandelion greens by themselves tend to be quite bitter, but in this dish they are the perfect complement for the sweet, tangy caramelized onion-tomato jam and the rich, savory steak, eggs, and Brie.

Steak:

2　(10-oz.) New York Strip steaks, trimmed of external fat

　　canola oil

　　kosher salt

　　freshly cracked black pepper

Greens:

½ Tbsp.　butter

1　clove garlic, peeled and minced

2　bunches dandelion greens, roughly chopped

　　kosher salt

　　freshly cracked black pepper

Eggs:

4　large eggs

1–2 Tbsp.　butter

For assembly:

4　ciabatta buns, individual sandwich-sized, sliced in half lengthwise

　　Caramelized Onion-Tomato Jam

4–5 oz.　triple cream Brie, at room temperature, sliced

　　smoked sea salt

　　freshly cracked black pepper

Caramelized Onion-Tomato Jam:

1 Tbsp.　butter or bacon fat

1　yellow onion, peeled and sliced

¾ tsp.　freshly cracked black pepper, plus extra

½ tsp.　kosher salt, plus extra

1　(14.5-oz). can diced tomatoes

⅓ cup　balsamic vinegar

⅓ cup　dry red wine

¼ cup　granulated sugar

Preheat oven to 350 degrees and prepare grill for medium-high heat.

Drizzle steaks with oil and toss to coat. Season steaks on all sides liberally with kosher salt and freshly cracked black pepper. Grill over medium-high heat for 8 to 10 minutes for medium-rare to medium doneness, flipping once, halfway through. Remove from heat and let rest for 10 minutes.

Melt ½ tablespoon butter in a sauté pan over medium heat. Sauté garlic in melted butter for 1 minute. Add dandelion greens to garlic and season with a pinch of kosher salt and freshly cracked black pepper. Sauté greens until just wilted, about 2 to 3 minutes, stirring occasionally. Remove from heat.

Warm ciabatta buns in preheated oven for 5 to 6 minutes.

While bread is warming, cook eggs. Melt 1 tablespoon butter in a nonstick sauté pan over medium to medium-low heat. Once butter has melted and the pan is heated, add 1 or 2 eggs to pan if your pan is large enough for eggs to cook without touching. Cook eggs sunny-side up until whites are cooked through but yolks are still runny, about 3 to 4 minutes. Remove from pan and repeat cooking process with remaining eggs.

Slice steaks thinly against the grain just before assembly.

To assemble sandwiches, spread a layer of Caramelized Onion-Tomato Jam (see below) over the bottom half of each ciabatta bun. Add an even layer of sautéed greens and a layer of sliced steak. Top steak with several slices of Brie and top with 1 egg sunny-side up. Sprinkle with smoked sea salt and freshly cracked black pepper. Serve sandwiches open-faced with knife and fork but serve the top bun alongside for soaking up any of the yolk that may run onto the plate.

CARAMELIZED ONION-TOMATO JAM

Melt butter in a sauté pan over medium heat. Once butter has melted and the pan is hot, add onion and black pepper. Sauté onion, stirring occasionally, until caramelized, about 30 minutes. (*Note: Do not let the onion burn or the jam will be bitter. If necessary, reduce heat to prevent burning.*)

Stir in remaining ingredients. Simmer until liquid has almost all cooked off—30 to 45 minutes—stirring occasionally. Adjust seasoning to taste with more kosher salt and freshly cracked black pepper. Jam can store for up to two weeks refrigerated. Best when used at room temperature or warmed.

Dough:

4 Tbsp.	butter, melted
¼ cup	granulated sugar
½ tsp.	salt
1 cup	canned pumpkin puree or roasted pie pumpkin puree
1	egg beaten
1	packet active dry yeast
1 Tbsp.	sugar
½ cup	lukewarm water, 105–110 degrees
3¾ cups	flour, plus extra
	oil, for greasing the bowl

Filling:

⅔ cup	brown sugar
1 Tbsp.	ground cinnamon
¼ tsp.	ground cloves
1 tsp.	ground ginger
⅛ tsp.	ground allspice
⅛ tsp.	ground nutmeg
¼ tsp.	salt
4 Tbsp.	butter, at room temperature

Icing:

3 oz.	cream cheese, at room temperature
1 cup	powdered sugar, sifted
¼ cup	pure grade B maple syrup
¼ tsp.	salt

Preheat oven to 350 degrees. Oil a large, non-reactive bowl and set aside. Line a 13x9x2-inch metal baking pan with parchment paper.

In a mixing bowl, whisk together the first 5 ingredients for the dough until well combined. Set aside.

In a separate bowl or measuring cup, whisk together warm water, yeast, and sugar. Set aside for 5 minutes until the yeast is frothy and active. If after 5 minutes yeast does not appear active, discard mixture and start over with new ingredients.

Add flour to a large mixing bowl or bowl of a stand mixer. Add activated yeast mixture and pumpkin mixture to flour. Stir until ingredients form a dough. If using a stand mixer, attach dough hook and knead on medium speed for 5 minutes. If kneading by hand, turn dough out onto a clean, lightly floured surface and knead for 8 to 10 minutes. The desired consistency of the dough should be soft and just slightly sticky. Add more flour as necessary throughout the kneading process to achieve this consistency.

Form dough into a ball and transfer to oiled bowl. Toss dough around in the bowl to coat all sides lightly with oil. Cover with oiled plastic wrap and a kitchen towel. Place in a warm, draft-free spot. (*Note: I prefer somewhere near the preheating oven for a nice, warm spot.*) Let dough rise until nearly doubled, usually 1 to 1½ hours.

While dough is rising, whisk together first 7 filling ingredients and set aside.

Roll out dough into a 16-inch by 10-inch rectangle on a large, lightly floured piece of parchment or wax paper. (*Note: While rolling out the dough, make sure it doesn't stick to the surface. Occasionally lifting dough and, if necessary, add more flour underneath.*)

Schmear a thin layer of room-temperature butter over dough, leaving a ½-inch border on all sides. Sprinkle brown sugar mixture evenly over butter. Roll dough into a tight spiral—jelly-roll style—by rolling the 16-inch long edge closest to you over the filling. Continue rolling dough into a log until the opposite edge is on bottom. Slice dough into 12 even pieces and arrange on the parchment-lined baking dish, cut-side up. (*Note: Cinnamon rolls will touch in the pan and that's okay. The middle pieces are the best anyway!*) Cover pan with oiled plastic wrap and a kitchen towel. Let rolls rise for 30 minutes in a warm, draft-free area.

Remove towel and plastic wrap. Bake risen rolls at 350 degrees until tops and edges are golden and rolls are cooked through—30 to 35 minutes. Remove from oven and place on a wire rack to cool for at least 20 minutes before icing.

While rolls cool, prepare icing. Whisk together icing ingredients in a bowl until smooth. Set aside until ready for use.

Place a baking sheet over the dish of cinnamon rolls. Invert rolls onto the baking sheet and peel away parchment paper. Re-invert the rolls onto your choice of serving dish or another baking sheet. Spoon icing evenly over all of the cinnamon rolls, allowing it to dribble down the sides. Rolls are best when served fresh but are still good rewarmed the next day. Cinnamon rolls store better kept together because the edges will dry out if separated.

Pumpkin Cinnamon Rolls

with Maple Icing

These cinnamon rolls are perfect for Thanksgiving breakfast or any fall weekend. If you use fresh roasted pumpkin, make sure it's well pureed before adding it to the recipe.

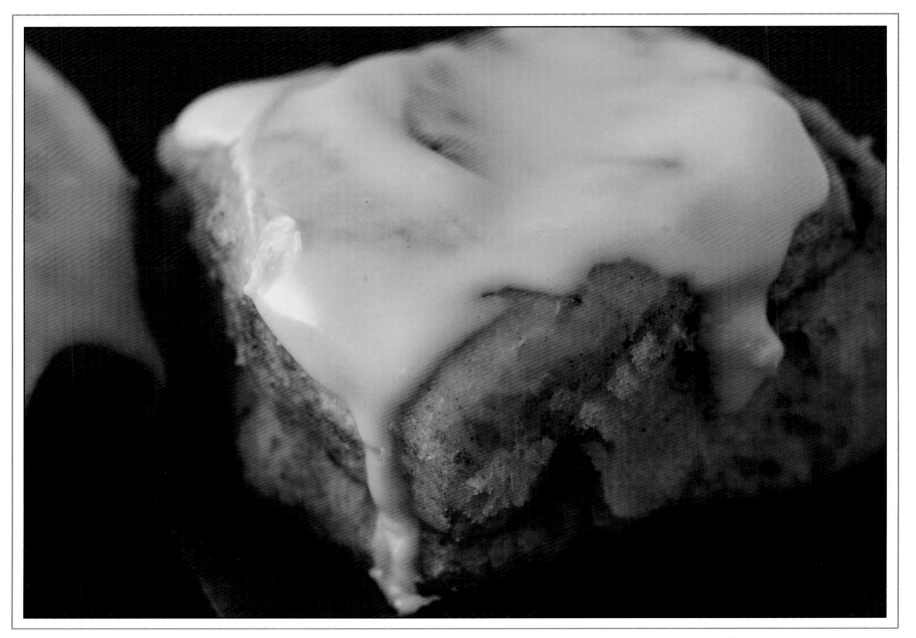

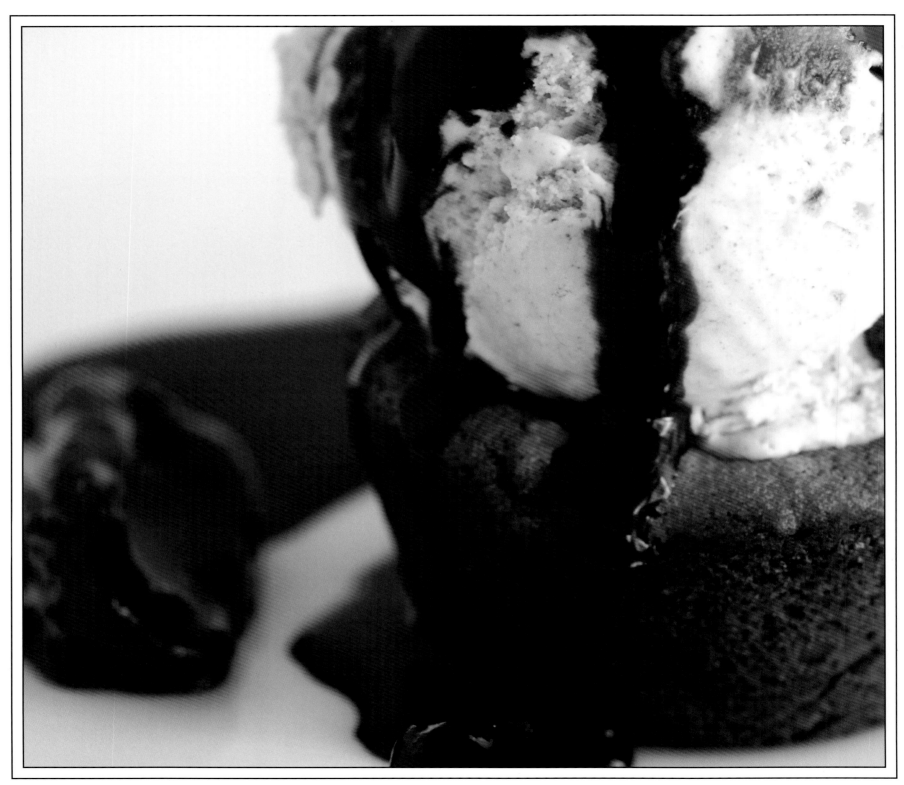

Brown Butter, Pine Nut, & Date Blondies

with Date Cream Cheese Ice Cream

The balsamic sauce has a strong flavor, so just drizzle a small amount over the ice cream until you've had a chance to taste it with the dessert. It's easy to add more if you love it but hard to remove it if you don't!

Blondies:

½ cup	(1 stick) butter
1 cup	(packed) brown sugar
½ tsp.	salt
1	egg
1 tsp.	high quality vanilla extract
⅓ cup	pine nuts, toasted (see page 243)
½ cup	Medjool dates, pits removed and chopped
1 cup	flour
½ tsp.	baking powder

Date & Balsamic Reduction:

1 cup	balsamic vinegar
2 Tbsp.	(packed) brown sugar
	pinch of salt
10	Medjool dates, pitted and halved
3 Tbsp.	heavy cream

Date Cream Cheese Ice Cream:

See Page 230

BLONDIES

Preheat oven to 350 degrees. Spray either an 8x8-inch baking dish or a regular 12-muffin tin with cooking spray.

Cook butter in a saucepan over medium heat until amber brown, stirring occasionally. (*Note: Be sure to not overcook—burnt butter will cause the dessert to taste bitter.*) Remove brown butter from heat and let cool for 10 minutes.

While brown butter cools, whisk together brown sugar, salt, egg, and vanilla in a mixing bowl until sugar dissolves into egg.

While whisking constantly, add brown butter to egg mixture in a slow stream. Add pine nuts and dates to batter. Stir with a rubber spatula to incorporate. Finally, add flour, stirring until just incorporated. The mixture will have the consistency of cookie dough.

Transfer, blondie dough to the prepared pan in an even layer or, if using a muffin tin, evenly distributed among the cups. Bake at 350 degrees for 20 minutes if using a baking pan or 15 minutes if using a muffin tin. (*Note: It's best to err on the side of being underdone.*)

Cool for at least 20 minutes on a wire rack before slicing or removing from the muffin tins.

To assemble desserts, place one blondie bar onto a plate and top with a scoop of date ice cream. Arrange 3 or 4 date halves around the blondie. Finish with a small drizzle of date and balsamic reduction over the ice cream.

DATES & BALSAMIC REDUCTION

Bring balsamic vinegar, brown sugar, and salt to a simmer in a saucepan over medium heat. Add date halves and simmer for 5 minutes.

Remove date halves from balsamic mixture and set aside.

Reduce remaining balsamic mixture to about ½ cup.

Remove from heat and stir in heavy cream and return dates to balsamic reduction. Use warm or cool to room temperature and store chilled for up to 3 days.

Crust:

1½ cups	flour
2 tsp.	granulated sugar
8 tbsp	(1 stick) butter, very cold, cut in ½-inch cubes
4 oz.	cream cheese, very cold, cut in ½-inch cubes
4 oz.	grated sharp cheddar cheese, very cold

Filling:

5–6 lbs.	Granny Smith apples, peeled, cored and cut in about ¼-inch thick slices
	juice from 1 lemon
1 cup	(packed) brown sugar
1 cup	granulated sugar
⅔ cup	flour
1½ tsp.	ground cinnamon
¼ tsp.	ground cloves
⅛ tsp.	ground allspice
¼ tsp.	freshly grated nutmeg
¼ tsp.	ground cayenne
½ tsp.	salt
2 Tbsp.	cold butter, cut into small pieces, to top the filling

Egg Wash

1	egg
1 Tbsp.	heavy cream

Cinnamon Ice Cream:

See Page 229

Prepare crust: process flour and sugar in a food processor to mix. Add butter, cream cheese, and cheddar cheese and process until ingredients come together in a ball and form a dough. Transfer dough to a lightly floured surface. Divide dough into equal halves and shape into compressed disks. Work quickly and do not overwork the dough. Wrap each disk tightly in plastic wrap and chill in the refrigerator for at least 1 hour before proceeding. Dough may be made up to 2 days in advance and stored in the refrigerator.

Preheat oven to 375 degrees with a rack positioned in the middle of the oven. Line a sheet pan with aluminum foil and place it on the middle rack.

While dough is chilling, prepare filling. Using your hands, toss all filling ingredients except butter in a very large mixing bowl until all apple slices are completely coated. Let sit for 30 to 60 minutes, stirring occasionally.

Remove first dough disk from fridge. Very lightly flour a large, clean work surface. Roll dough out with a rolling pin to form a 12-inch circle large enough to fit a 9-inch deep-dish glass or ceramic pie pan. If dough gets warm or starts sticking to the work surface, carefully place dough back into the refrigerator and chill for 5 to 10 minutes before proceeding. (*Note: It is important that the dough remains cool at all times and that not much flour gets worked into the dough during the rolling process.*) Carefully fit dough into the 9-inch pie pan. Chill bottom crust in refrigerator while working on top crust.

Remove second disk of dough from refrigerator.

Similar to the process described above, roll dough out into an approximate 12-inch circle. Chill in refrigerator until ready to use.

Add apple filling to crust-lined pie pan, making sure that all of the apples lie flat and are as compact as possible. Pour any juices left in the bowl over the apples. Scatter small pieces of cold butter evenly around the top of the filling.

Remove top crust from the fridge and gently place over the pie. Trim crust so only about 1-inch hangs off. Fold overhanging pieces under bottom crust and pinch to make edge stand up. To form a scalloped crust, use the thumb and forefinger of one hand to loosely press the outside edge of the crust inward while pressing outward from the opposite side using a finger of your other hand and work your away around the edge of the pie. Using a paring knife, cut four small slits in the middle of the pie so steam can vent during the baking process. Refrigerate prepared pie while preparing egg wash.

Whisk together 1 egg and 1 tablespoon heavy cream. Using a pastry brush, brush the crust of the pie with the egg wash. Bake pie at 375 degrees on the sheet pan positioned in the middle rack for about 1 hour and 10 minutes or until the apples feel tender when pierced with a knife. Check crust after about 50 minutes. If crust is getting too brown, loosely drape with aluminum foil. If crust is not browning evenly, rotate the sheet pan. Once apples are tender, cool on a wire rack for at least 1 hour before serving. Serve warm with a scoop of cinnamon ice cream.

Classic Apple Pie

with Cheddar Cheese Crust and Cinnamon Ice Cream

Because there is no water in the crust for this pie, there is little chance that you can mess it up. Making sure that the crust remains chilled at all times ensures that it will be super flaky as well.

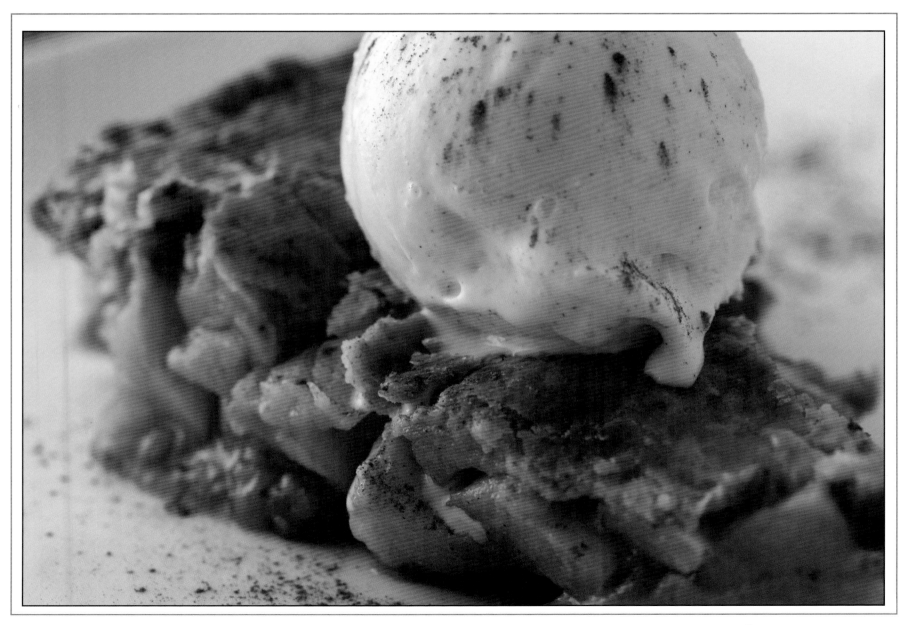

Triple Chocolate Macadamia Nut Cookie Sandwiches

with Java Buttercream Filling

Chocolate and coffee are naturally best friends with their similarly roasty flavor profiles. The java buttercream filling combined with the chocolate cookies is what really makes these cookie sandwiches special.

Cookie:

1¼ cups	flour
1 cup	unsweetened cocoa powder
1½ tsp.	baking soda
½ tsp.	kosher salt
1 cup	(2 sticks) butter, at room temperature
1	cup (packed) brown sugar
1	egg
1 tsp.	good vanilla extract
½ cup	macadamia nuts, roughly chopped
¾ cup	white chocolate chips or chunks
¾ cup	milk chocolate chips or chunks

Filling:

2 Tbsp.	instant coffee or instant espresso
2 Tbsp.	whole milk, plus extra
2 oz.	cream cheese, at room temperature
4 Tbsp.	(½ stick) butter, at room temperature
8 oz.	powdered sugar, sifted
1 Tbsp.	unsweetened cocoa powder
	small pinch salt

Ganache:

3 oz.	heavy cream
3 oz.	semi-sweet chocolate chips

DIRECTIONS

Preheat oven to 350 degrees. Line a baking sheet with parchment paper or Silpat.

Sift together first 4 ingredients. Set aside.

In a large mixing bowl, beat together softened butter and brown sugar until fluffy and mixed thoroughly. Add egg and vanilla and beat until completely incorporated. Stir sifted dry ingredients into butter mixture until completely incorporated. Add macadamia nuts and chocolate chips. Stir to evenly distribute throughout the dough.

Drop rounded tablespoons of cookie dough onto the prepared baking sheet with about 2 inches between each cookie. Once you've fill the sheet pan with cookies, gently flatten each cookie. Bake at 350 degrees for about 10 minutes until just cooked through. (*Note: With cookies, I always think it's better to err on the side of being underdone than overdone.*) Place sheet pan on a wire rack to cool.

Repeat baking process with remaining cookie dough—recipe yields about 3 sheets of cookies. Cool all cookies completely before filling.

While cookies cool, prepare filling. In a small microwave safe bowl, whisk together instant coffee and whole milk. Microwave for 15 seconds until milk is hot. Whisk again to dissolve all coffee granules into milk. Beat milk mixture with remaining ingredients in a large mixing bowl until fluffy. If filling is too thick or a little chalky from the powdered sugar, add more whole milk, 1 teaspoon at a time, beating until incorporated, until desired consistency is reached. Let filling rest for 30 minutes at room temperature before proceeding.

Make ganache:

Heat heavy cream in a small saucepan over medium heat to a near-boil. Pour cream over chocolate chips in a heat-safe bowl. Stir until chocolate melts completely and ganache achieves a satiny texture. (*Note: If you continue to stir too long after chocolate has melted, the ganache will take on an undesirable grainy texture.*)

Spread about 1½ tablespoons filling per cookie on the flat sides of half of the cookies. Complete cookie sandwiches by topping the filled cookies with an unfilled cookie, flat-side down. Drizzle cookie sandwiches with ganache. Let ganache set before serving, about 2 to 3 hours. Cookie sandwiches may be stored in an airtight container at room temperature for 3 to 4 days.

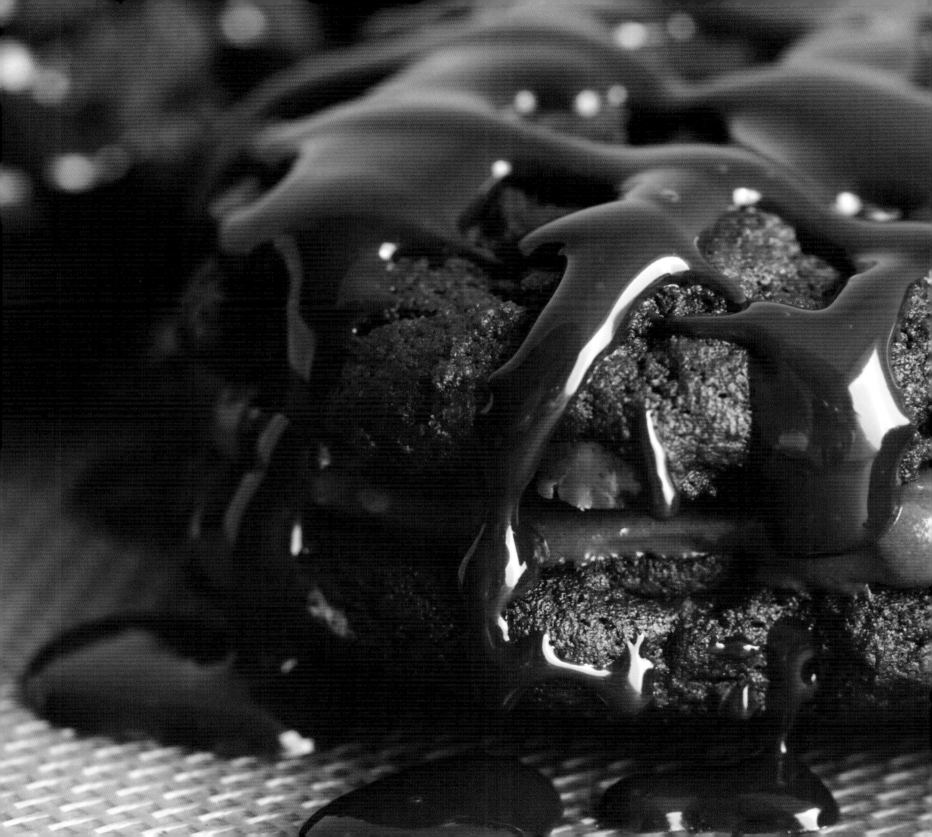

Moist Ginger Cake

with Wasabi Frosting and Sesame Brittle

To make quick work of peeling the ginger for the cake, simply use the tip of a spoon to scrape the peel off. Not only does it come off effortlessly, you will save more of the "meat" of the ginger using this technique than you would using a knife or vegetable peeler. Also, you can thinly slice the peeled ginger and mince it in a food processor, if you have one. Skipping this step will result in undesirable long, fibrous ginger "hairs" throughout the cake.

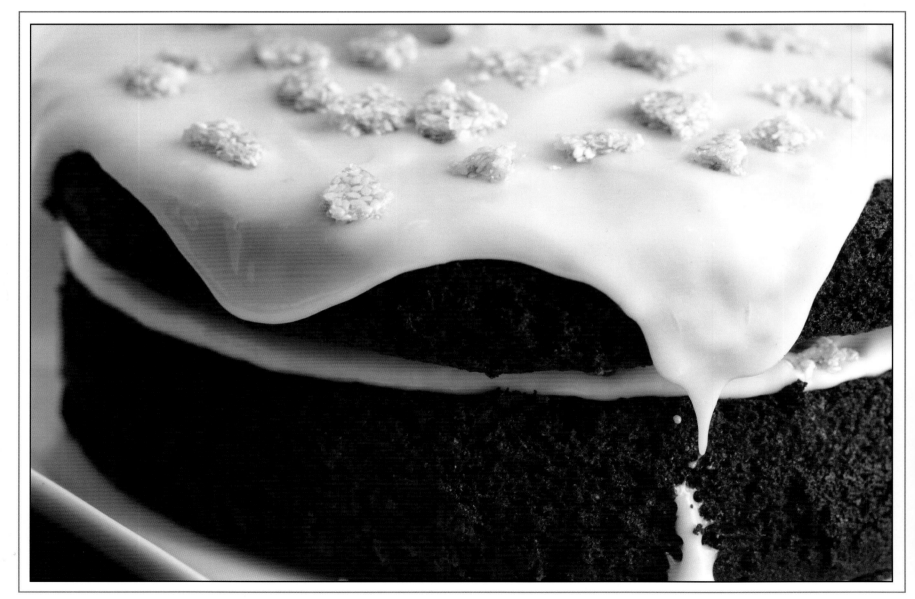

Cake:

2½ cups	cake flour
1 tsp.	ground cinnamon
½ tsp.	ground cloves
½ tsp.	salt
2 tsp.	baking soda
½ cup	fresh ginger, peeled and finely minced or grated with a Microplane
1 cup	molasses
1 tsp.	pure vanilla extract
1 cup	buttermilk
½ cup	(1 stick) butter, at room temperature
1 cup	brown sugar
¼ cup	toasted sesame oil
2	eggs

Wasabi Buttercream:

5 Tbsp.	butter, at room temperature
2 cup	powdered sugar, sifted
3 Tbsp.	milk, plus extra
½ tsp.	pure vanilla extract
¼ tsp.	salt
2½ tsp.	wasabi powder

Wasabi Glaze:

4 oz.	cream cheese, at room temperature
2 tsp.	wasabi powder
¼ tsp.	kosher salt
2 Tbsp.	milk
½ tsp.	pure vanilla extract
1 cup	powdered sugar, sifted

Sesame Ginger Brittle:

See Page 241

Preheat oven to 350 degrees. Line two 9-inch cake pans with parchment paper and grease with butter. Dust lightly with flour. Knock out any excess flour.

Sift together first five ingredients and set aside.

In a separate bowl, whisk to combine grated ginger, molasses, vanilla, and buttermilk and set aside.

In a large mixing bowl, beat butter until fluffy. Add brown sugar and beat again until fluffy. Add sesame oil and beat until incorporated. Next add eggs, one at a time, beating until fully incorporated after each addition. Add a third of the dry ingredients and stir until just incorporated. Add half of the wet ingredients and stir until just incorporated. Repeat this process, ending with the final third of dry ingredients. (*Note: Do not overwork the batter. Once the flour has been added, it is important to only stir until just incorporated or the cake will become tough and dense.*)

Divide cake batter between prepared cake pans and bake at 350 degrees until a toothpick inserted into the center of the cake comes out clean with only a few crumbs—but *NO* batter—about 30 minutes.

Cool cake pans on a wire rack for at least 30 minutes before removing cakes from pan. To remove cake, gently run a knife around the edge of the pan to loosen. Place a plate over the cake and invert to flip the cake onto the plate. Carefully peel away the parchment paper.

Place one cake onto a serving dish. Spread wasabi buttercream in an even layer on only the top of the cake. Place the second cake on top of the buttercream to form a layer cake. Pour wasabi glaze over the cake, allowing some to drip over the edges and run down the sides of the cake. Directly before serving, sprinkle with chopped pieces of sesame brittle for decoration. (*Note: Do not add the sesame brittle early, or it will get softened from the moisture in the glaze.*) Serve at room temperature.

WASABI BUTTERCREAM

Beat together all ingredients until completely smooth. If the consistency is too stiff after beating, thin it out by adding single teaspoons of milk at a time until a thick yet silky, spreadable consistency is reached.

WASABI GLAZE

Using a rubber spatula, beat cream cheese until fluffy. Add wasabi, salt, milk, and vanilla and beat until smooth. Add sifted powdered sugar and beat until smooth and fully incorporated. If consistency is too thick for drizzling, add single teaspoons of milk at a time until glaze reaches desired consistency but without letting it get too runny.

Peanut Butter Crust:

1	package peanut butter sandwich cookies
½ cup	(1 stick) butter, melted

Peanut Butter Cheesecake Filling:

2	(8-oz.) packages cream cheese, at room temperature
1¼ cups	creamy peanut butter, NOT natural
1 cup	sugar
¼ tsp.	salt
8 oz.	sour cream
1 Tbsp.	pure vanilla extract
3	eggs

Chocolate Ganache Topping:

8 oz.	semi-sweet chocolate chips
8 oz.	heavy cream
½ Tbsp.	instant coffee granules
2 Tbsp.	sugar
½ cup	salted dry roasted peanuts, roughly chopped

Preheat oven to 325 degrees with a rack positioned in the middle of the oven. Wrap the outside of a deep 9-inch springform pan with several layers of aluminum foil to prevent the water bath from seeping in when baking.

Make crust: Process peanut butter cookies in a food processor until cookies are in fine crumbs. (*Note: If you don't have a food processor, you can crumble cookies by putting them in a plastic resealable bag and mashing with a rolling pin or meat mallet.*)

Pour cookie crumbs into a large bowl and stir in melted butter until well combined.

Pour cookie crumb mixture into springform pan. Using a straight-sided cup, work crumbs into an even layer on the bottom of the pan and up onto the sides to form cookie crust. Set aside.

Bring a large kettle of water to a boil for water bath.

Add cream cheese, peanut butter, sugar, and salt to the bowl of a stand mixer or a large mixing bowl with electric beaters and beat until fluffy and well combined, scraping down the sides as necessary.

Add sour cream and vanilla to cream cheese mixture. Beat until fully incorporated. Add one egg at a time, beating until fully incorporated after each addition, scraping down the sides as necessary.

Once eggs are incorporated, pour cheesecake batter onto cookie crust. Place cheesecake into a roasting pan or other large baking dish with high sides. Pour enough boiling water into roasting pan to surround springform pan with about 1 inch of water.

Carefully place cheesecake into preheated oven on the middle rack. Bake at 325 degrees until cheesecake is completely set, about 1 hour.

Remove from oven. Carefully remove cheesecake from water bath and cool on a wire rack for at least 1 hour.

While the cheesecake is cooling, prepare topping.

Bring heavy cream, sugar, and instant coffee granules to a boil in a small saucepan over medium-high heat, stirring frequently and scraping bottom to prevent scalding. Once cream has reached a simmer, pour over chocolate chips in a heat-safe bowl. Whisk slowly until chocolate melts into cream and forms a glossy ganache. Let cool for 15 minutes.

Pour ganache over cheesecake in an even layer. Sprinkle chopped peanuts over ganache layer to decorate. Chill cheesecake in the refrigerator for at least 12 hours before serving. Cheesecake can be made up to 2 days in advance and stored chilled.

Creamy Peanut Butter Cheesecake

with Rich Chocolate Ganache

I am normally a proponent of using ingredients in as natural a form as you can find them, but to achieve a silky texture, this recipe requires that you use a creamy peanut butter such as Jif or Skippy rather than natural peanut butter. The recipe has been tested using both varieties, and the consistency of the cheesecake is far superior using one of the ultra-processed peanut butters. Besides, there is *no way* that the peanut butter sandwich cookies in the crust are made with all-natural peanut butter.

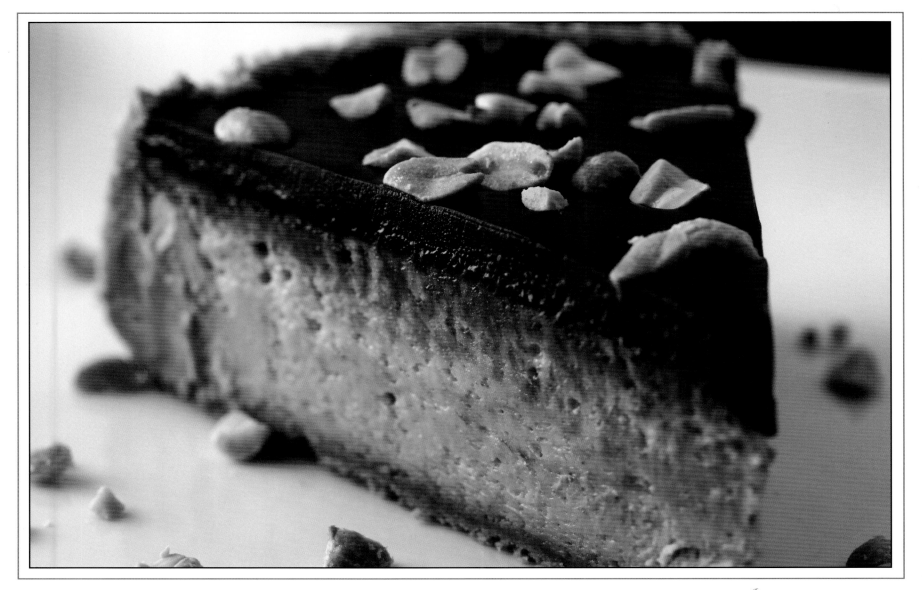

Sparkling Kiwi Limeade

Kiwifruit season begins in November. As soon as the first ripe kiwis of the season are available, we make a batch of this concentrate to freeze in ice cube trays and have kiwi limeade whenever the urge hits us over the next month.

KIWI LIMEADE

6   ripe kiwifruit, peeled

1 cup fresh squeezed lime juice

1 cup granulated sugar (if you like tart limeade, only use ¾ cup)

½ tsp. kosher salt

sparkling water

2   ripe kiwis, sliced about ¼-inch thick, for garnish

Puree kiwis in a blender. Whisk together lime juice, sugar, and salt until all sugar has dissolved. Whisk together kiwi puree and sweetened lime juice, Kiwi-lime concentrate can be made one day in advance and refrigerated. Alternately, kiwi concentrate can be frozen for up to 1 month. (Try freezing in ice cube trays if you want to defrost single servings at a time.)

Fill a glass with ice. Pour kiwi concentrate about a third of the way up the glass. Fill the remainder of the glass with sparkling water. Use more or less concentrate, depending on your tastes. Stir lightly to mix water and concentrate. Garnish glass with kiwi slices.

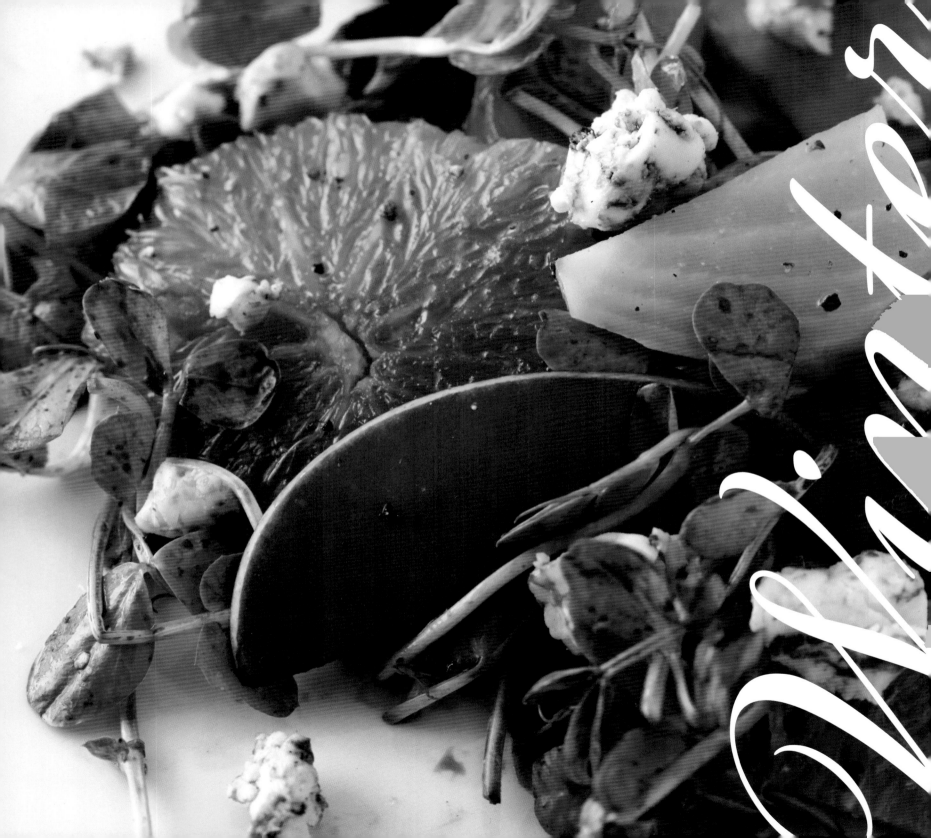

Openers

Main

Breakfast

Dessert

Drinks

Buttermilk Beer Battered Onion Rings

with Horseradish-Blue Cheese Dipping Sauce

Onion rings are good year round, but I tend to crave heavier foods during the colder winter months. Having eaten at a shamefully high number of chain restaurants in my childhood, I particularly enjoy the slightly sweet, zesty horseradish dipping sauce that often accompanies onion rings. This horseradish-blue cheese dip is my take on that sauce.

Buttermilk-Beer Batter:

	peanut oil, for frying
¾ cup	buttermilk
¾ cup	beer
1 cup	flour
1 tsp.	kosher salt
¼ tsp.	freshly cracked black pepper
½ tsp.	granulated garlic
2	sweet onions, peeled, cut in 1-inch thick rounds

Horseradish-Blue Cheese Sauce:

⅓ cup	mayonnaise
2 Tbsp.	ketchup
2 Tbsp.	prepared horseradish
1 Tbsp.	Worcestershire sauce
1 tsp.	Sriracha hot chile sauce
¼ tsp.	granulated garlic
¼ tsp.	onion powder
¼ tsp.	ground cayenne
2 oz.	blue cheese, crumbled
1 Tbsp.	white vinegar
¼ tsp.	freshly cracked black pepper, plus extra
¼ tsp.	kosher salt, plus extra

BUTTERMILK BEER ONION RINGS

Preheat oil for deep frying to 360 degrees.

Combine all batter ingredients a large mixing bowl. Whisk until smooth.

Separate onion slices into individual rings. Coat onion rings thoroughly in batter.

Carefully add several battered onion rings to preheated oil so that they sit in a single layer at the top of the oil. Do not overcrowd the pan. Fry onion rings until golden—about 3 minutes per batch—carefully flipping onion rings after about 2 minutes. Drain fried onion rings on a paper towel to drain. Repeat frying process with remaining onions, working in batches. Serve immediately once all rings have been fried.

HORSERADISH-BLUE CHEESE SAUCE

Whisk together sauce ingredients in a mixing bowl, breaking up blue cheese as much as possible. Adjust seasoning to taste with more kosher salt and freshly cracked black pepper. Refrigerate until ready for use. Can be stored in the refrigerator for up to 1 week.

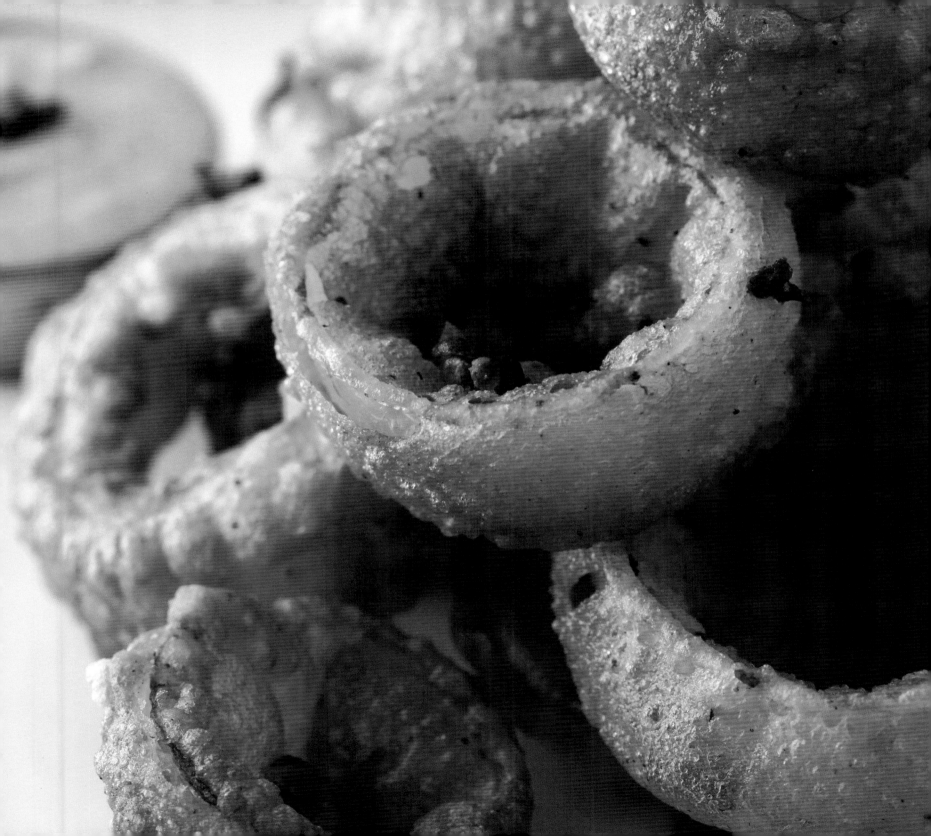

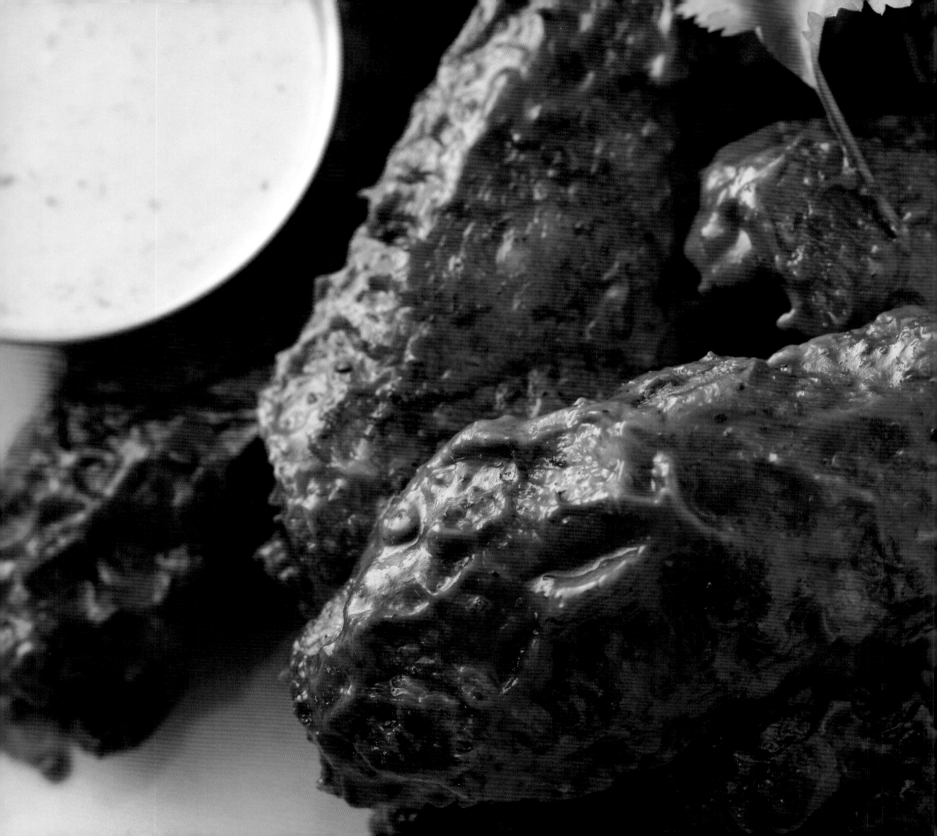

Spicy Chipotle Buffalo Wings

with Cilantro Ranch Dressing

I find that wings taste best immediately after being tossed in the sauce, so I serve each batch as soon as they are finished rather than waiting for all of the batches to fry before plating. Just make sure that the people you are feeding know that at least half of the last batch has your name on it!

BUFFALO WINGS

Spicy Chipotle Sauce:

½ can	pureed chipotle in adobo
2 Tbsp.	white distilled vinegar
1	small clove garlic, minced
2 Tbsp.	vinegary hot sauce like Texas Pete, Krystal or Louisiana Brand
2 tsp.	packed brown sugar
½ tsp.	kosher salt
¼ tsp.	freshly cracked black pepper
4 oz.	melted butter

	peanut oil for deep frying
3 lbs.	chicken wings
	kosher salt
	freshly cracked black pepper
	celery sticks, for serving

Cilantro Ranch Dressing:

½ cup	buttermilk
½ cup	mayonnaise
½ cup	(packed) cilantro leaves
½	jalapeño, seeds removed for less heat
2	cloves garlic, peeled
1 tsp.	onion powder
2 Tbsp.	chives, chopped
1 Tbsp.	flat leaf parsley
½ tsp.	freshly cracked black pepper
1 tsp.	kosher salt

Heat oil for deep frying to 350 degrees. If frying on the stove top, make sure oil only comes halfway up the side of the pot but is at least 3 inches deep.

Blend all sauce ingredients *except* butter in a blender until smooth. While blender is running, drizzle in melted butter until fully incorporated to form an emulsified sauce. Set aside.

Pat chicken wings dry with paper towels. Toss wings with kosher salt and freshly cracked pepper. Working in batches to prevent oil temperature from falling too low, fry wings until crispy, golden, and cooked through, about 8 to 10 minutes per batch.

Drain wings briefly on paper towels and then toss with some spicy chipotle sauce in a bowl to coat evenly. Serve with a side of cilantro ranch (see below) and celery sticks. Repeat process with remaining wings. Serve immediately after each batch.

CILANTRO RANCH DRESSING

Blend all dressing ingredients in a blender until smooth. Store in an airtight container, refrigerated, for up to 1 week.

Golden and Red Beet Salad

with Cara Cara Orange, Granny Smith Apple, and Crumbled Blue Cheese

Beets are one of the most polarizing foods I've come across. For the most part, people either really love or really dislike beets. I grew up eating them from my dad's garden and happen to fall in the "beet lover" category. If you are a "beet hater" and the only beets you've ever eaten came from a can or a jar, give this salad a try and reassess your opinion.

BEET, ORANGE, AND BLUE CHEESE SALAD

Salad:

3	golden beets
3	red beets
	oil, for drizzling
	kosher salt
	freshly cracked black pepper
2	Cara Cara navel oranges (or any large, ripe orange)
½	Granny Smith apple, core removed and cut in half lengthwise
3 cups	pea tendrils, micro greens, or watercress
2–3 oz.	crumbled blue cheese

Dressing:

¼ cup	Cara Cara orange juice
	juice from 1 small lemon
1 Tbsp.	Dijon mustard
¼ tsp.	kosher salt
¼ tsp.	freshly cracked black pepper
2 Tbsp.	canola oil

Preheat oven to 350 degrees.

Drizzle beets with oil and sprinkle with kosher salt and freshly cracked black pepper. Toss to coat. Bake beets on a sheet pan at 350 degrees for 45 to 60 minutes or until tender when pierced with a knife. Let beets cool until able to handle.

Trim ends off beets and then, using a paring knife, peel/scrape off outer layer of skin. Cut beets in half and slice them ¼-inch thick lengthwise. Separate red beets and golden beets into two different bowls to prevent dying the golden beets red.

Whisk together first 5 dressing ingredients. While whisking continuously, drizzle in canola oil. Pour half of dressing over red beets and half over golden beets, tossing each bowl to coat. Let beets marinate, chilled, for at least 30 minutes.

While beets are marinating, peel oranges, leaving inside "meat" intact. Slice peeled orange into ¼-inch thick rounds. Set aside

After beets are done marinating, remove from refrigerator. Slice apple into ⅛-inch thick slices, using a mandoline, if you have one. Divide apple slices evenly between red and golden beets. Toss each bowl separately. Adjust seasonings in both bowls to taste with kosher salt and freshly cracked black pepper.

Directly before plating, toss your choice of greens with some dressing from either (or both) bowls of beets.

To plate, divide greens, beets, apple slices, and orange slices among four plates. Sprinkle each salad with equal amounts of blue cheese crumbles. Drizzle leftover vinaigrette around the plates as a garnish.

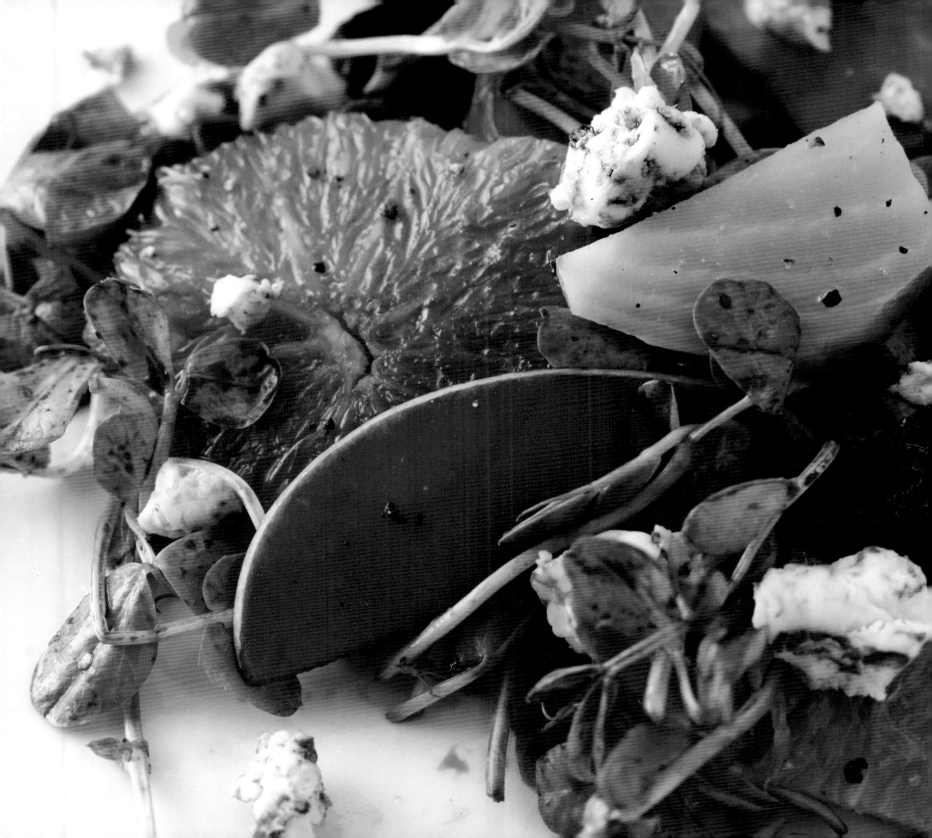

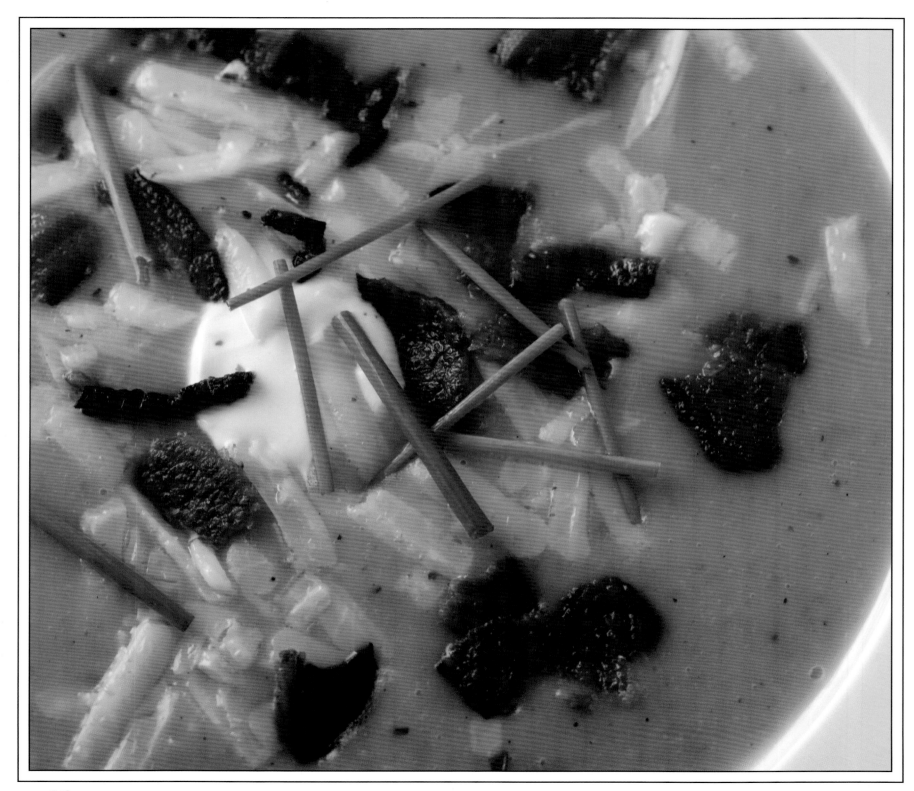

Loaded Potato Soup

with Bacon, Sharp Cheddar, Sour Cream, and Chives

The first time I had my good friend Nicole's potato-leek soup, I realized that it was possible for a soup to taste just like a baked potato□.□.□.□but in comforting liquid form. This loaded baked potato soup is directly inspired by that delicious bowl of potato-leek soup. The soup itself is relatively healthy, but the add-ins are less so. You can make the soup as decadent as you like by "loading" it up with your preference of garnishes.

POTATO SOUP

1½ Tbsp.	butter
1	yellow onion, peeled and diced
2	leeks, white part only, cleaned and diced
5	cloves garlic, peeled and minced
1½ tsp.	fresh rosemary, minced
3 lbs.	Yukon gold potatoes, cut in half and sliced ¼-inch thick
6 cups	homemade or low-sodium chicken, plus extra
1 tsp.	kosher salt, plus extra
½ tsp.	freshly cracked black pepper, plus extra
¼ cup	heavy cream

To garnish:

shredded sharp cheddar cheese

sour cream

crumbled cooked bacon

chopped chives or thinly sliced green onions

Melt butter in a large pot over medium heat. Once the pan is hot and butter has melted, add onion and leeks. Stir. Sauté veggies over medium heat, stirring occasionally, until onions are translucent and leeks are soft, about 10 minutes.

Add garlic and rosemary to veggies and sauté for another minute. Add potatoes, chicken stock, salt, and pepper and raise the heat to medium-high. Stir. Bring soup just to a boil and then reduce heat to low. Simmer soup over low heat until potatoes are very tender and starting to disintegrate—1½ to 2 hours. Transfer half of soup to a blender and blend until smooth. Stir blended soup back into the pot. Using a potato masher, mash up remaining potatoes so that there are bite-sized chunks of potato disbursed throughout the soup. Stir in heavy cream. If soup is thicker than desired, thin it out with a small amount of extra chicken stock. Adjust seasoning to taste with more kosher salt and freshly cracked black pepper.

To serve, ladle soup into a bowl and top with a dollop of sour cream, shredded cheese, crumbled bacon, and chives.

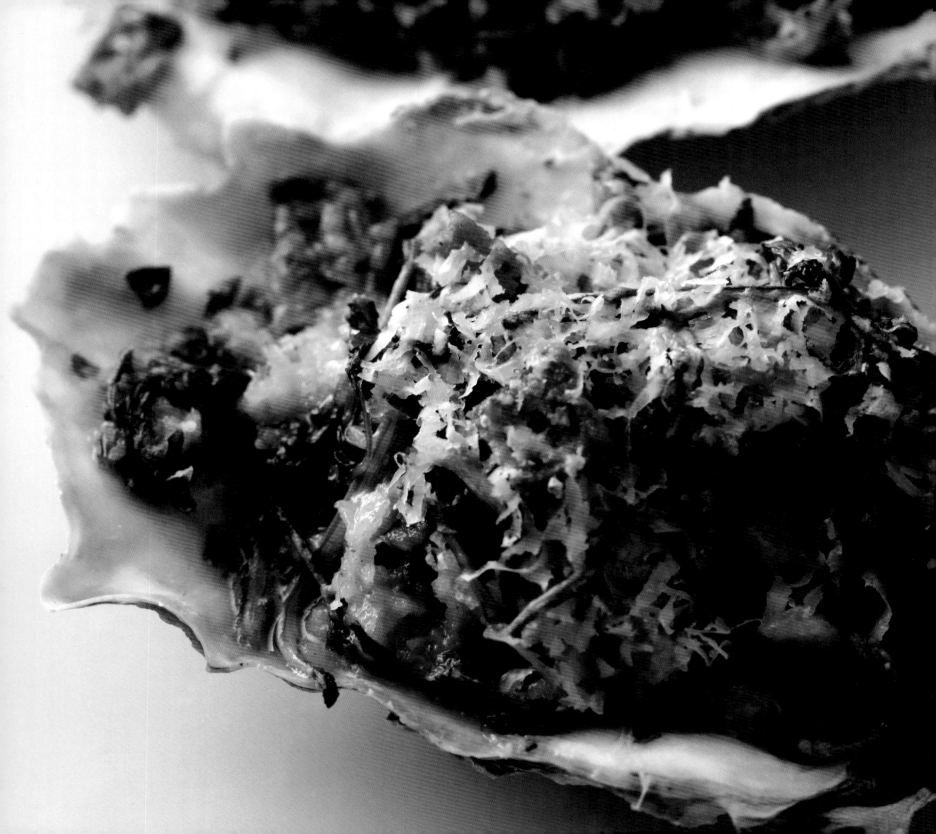

Arugula Oysters Rockefeller

My version of Oysters Rockefeller uses arugula rather than spinach—providing a little extra flavor. To change things up further, replace the bacon with your choice of browned sausage or the Parmesan with any variety of grated cheese, like aged Manchego or Gruyère.

OYSTERS

Arugula Filling

3	thick slices bacon
1	large clove garlic, minced
2 cups	(packed) cups arugula leaves, roughly chopped
1 Tbsp.	fresh parsley, minced
¼ cup	panko
¼ cup	Parmigiano Reggiano, freshly grated
	juice from ½ lemon
¼ tsp.	freshly cracked black pepper

3 Tbsp.	freshly grated Parmigiano Reggiano,
12	very fresh oysters on the half shell
8–10	cups kosher salt, for serving

Preheat oven to 475 degrees.

Cook bacon in a sauté pan over medium heat, flipping occasionally, until fat renders out and bacon is crispy. Drain on paper towels.

Drain off all but 1 tablespoon bacon drippings. Sauté garlic in bacon drippings over medium heat, stirring often, for 1 minute. Add arugula and parsley to garlic and sauté until wilted. Remove from heat and add remaining filling ingredients. Stir to combine. Let filling cool for 10 minutes.

Line a shallow baking pan with 5 cups of kosher salt. Nestle oysters on the half shell into salt bed Distribute filling evenly among oysters. Sprinkle with freshly grated Parmigiano Reggiano cheese.

Bake oysters at 475 degrees for about 10 minutes or until topping is golden and the oysters are just cooked through. To serve, pour another 4 or so cups of kosher salt onto a serving plate. Nestle the cooked oysters into salt bed. Serve immediately.

Braised Short Ribs:

8	bone-in short ribs (3 to 4 lbs.)
	kosher salt
	freshly cracked black pepper
1 Tbsp.	flour, for dusting
⅓ cup	oil, for browning (will drain off most oil)

To Sauté:

5	cloves garlic, peeled and minced
1-inch	piece ginger, peeled and minced
1	jalapeño pepper, minced (use less, depending on desired heat)

Braising Liquid:

½ cup	soy sauce
¾ cup	freshly squeezed orange juice
2 Tbsp.	rice wine vinegar
	juice from 1 lime
1½ tsp.	sesame oil
1 Tbsp.	brown sugar
¾ cup	low-sodium chicken stock
1	star anise
1	bay leaf
2 tsp.	lemongrass, tough outer layer removed and minced

2 Tbsp.	cornstarch
1½ Tbsp.	cold water

Crispy Sushi Rice Cakes (see page 232)

sliced scallions, for garnish

Toasted Sesame Seeds, for garnish (see page 243)

Preheat oven to 275 degrees.

Preheat a large oven-safe pot over high heat for 4 minutes.

While pan is preheating, season short ribs on all sides with kosher salt and freshly cracked black pepper. Dust with flour and toss to coat.

Once the pan is hot, add the oil to the pan. (*Note: The oil should heat quickly to the point of rippling. Do not let the oil smoke or burn.*) Once oil ripples with heat, brown half of seasoned short ribs on all sides, about 2 minutes per side—12 minutes total—until well browned. Remove from pan and set aside. Repeat browning process with remaining short ribs.

While short ribs are browning, whisk together all ingredients for the braising liquid and set aside.

Reduce heat to medium. After short ribs have all been browned, drain off all but 1 teaspoon oil. Add garlic, ginger, and jalapeño to the pan. Sauté for about 30 to 60 seconds, stirring continuously, until the fragrance of the aromatics is released.

Add braising liquid to the pan with aromatics. Using a wooden spoon, scrap the bottom of the pan, making sure to release anything that may have stuck to the bottom while browning ribs. Bring liquid to a boil

and add short ribs back to the pan, making sure they are all nestled down into liquid. Cover and braise in the oven at 275 degrees for 3 to 4 hours or until "fall off the bone" tender.

Cool to room temperature, cover, and chill overnight in the refrigerator. (*Note: During the chilling process, all of the fat will rise to the surface and solidify in a hard layer. Using a spoon or your fingers, remove this layer of hardened fat, leaving all the congealed pan juices and short ribs beneath.*)

Heat ribs, covered, over medium-low heat until warmed through, stirring occasionally.

While ribs are rewarming, whisk together cornstarch and cold water until cornstarch has completely dissolved.

Stir cornstarch solution into simmering short ribs, taking care to evenly distribute cornstarch in the pan sauce. Simmer for 1 to 2 minutes until liquid has thickened and become viscous.

To assemble: Place one rice cake in the middle of a plate. Top rice cake with 1 or 2 short ribs. Spoon sauce over ribs and rice cake. Garnish with sliced scallions and toasted sesame seeds

Savory Asian Braised Short Ribs

Over Crunchy Sushi Rice Cakes

The crisp texture of the sushi rice cakes are the perfect complement to the falling-apart savory short ribs. When frying the cakes, place them carefully into the hot oil—they will splatter due to the high water content of the rice. Also, if you cannot find lemongrass for the short ribs, substitute 1 teaspoon lemon zest. The flavor won't be exactly the same, but it will still add a brightness to the dish that would otherwise be missing.

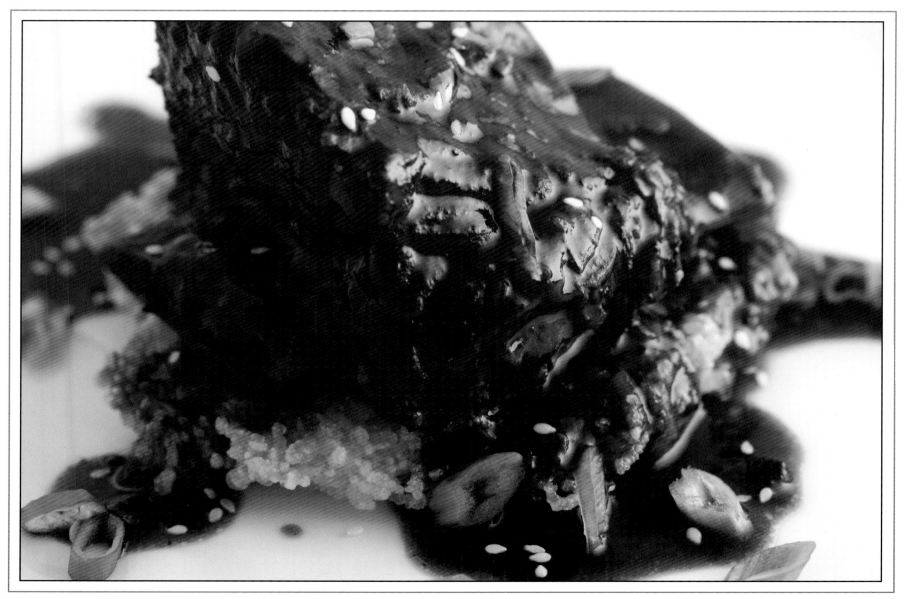

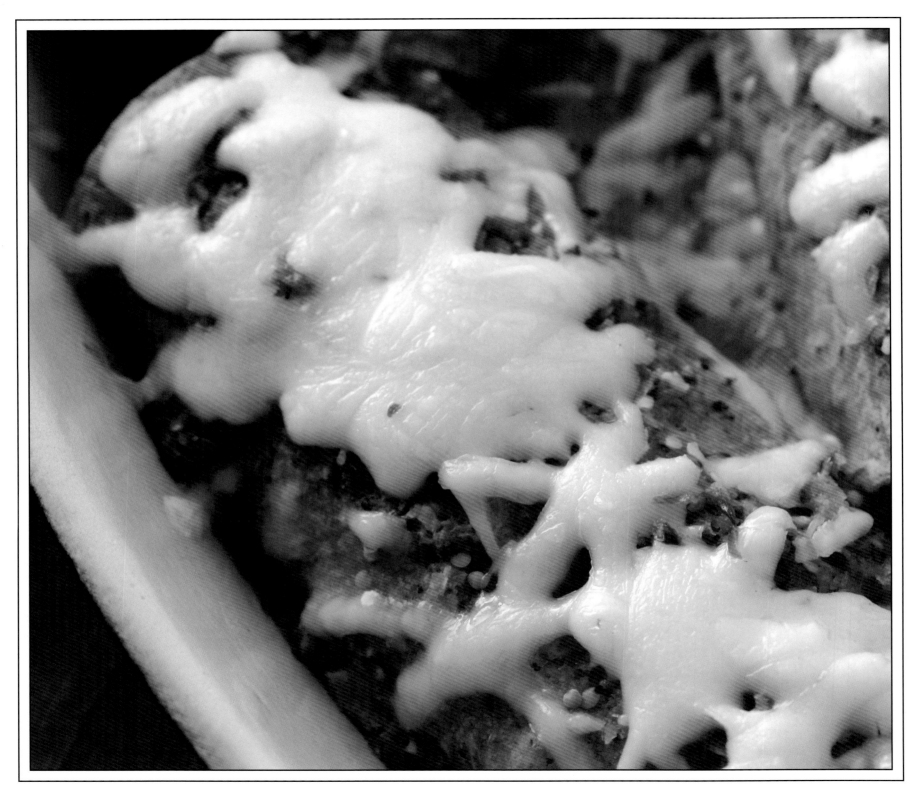

Chicken Enchiladas Verde

with Roasted Poblano-Tomatillo Sauce

Even though it adds extra work, using homemade corn tortillas for this recipes makes these enchiladas melt in your mouth. If you like your enchiladas particularly saucy, try doubling the Poblano-Tomatillo Sauce recipe. This recipe is a great way to use leftover turkey from Thanksgiving or rotisserie chicken.

Enchiladas:

6 oz.	Monterey jack cheese, grated
1 recipe	corn tortillas (see page 90).
1 recipe	Poblano-Tomatillo Sauce

Filling:

6 oz.	cream cheese, at room temperature
2 cups	shredded leftover cooked chicken or turkey
1	roasted poblano (see page 239) peeled, seeds and stems removed, and diced
¼ tsp.	ground cumin
¼ tsp.	freshly cracked black pepper, plus extra
¼ tsp.	kosher salt, plus extra

Poblano-Tomatillo Sauce:

1	roasted poblano (peel, seeds, and stems removed), diced (see page 239)
1 lb.	fresh tomatillos, husks removed and rinsed
1	serrano chile (use less depending on desired heat)
	juice from 1 large lime (or two small)
⅓ cup	fresh cilantro leaves
½	small yellow onion, peeled and chopped roughly
2	cloves garlic, chopped roughly
¼ cup	water
½ tsp.	kosher salt, plus extra
¼ tsp.	freshly cracked black pepper, plus extra

CHICKEN ENCHILADAS

Preheat oven to 400 degrees. Lightly grease a rectangular glass or ceramic baking dish. Set aside.

Using a rubber spatula, cream filling ingredients together in a mixing bowl until thoroughly mixed. Adjust seasoning to taste with more kosher salt and freshly cracked black pepper.

Place about 2 tablespoons filling mixture in a line down the middle of one corn tortilla. Roll tortilla around filling as tightly as possible without breaking tortilla. Place enchilada seam-side down into the greased baking dish. Repeat process with more corn tortillas until all of the filling has been used.

Pour Poblano-Tomatillo Sauce evenly over enchiladas. Sprinkle with grated Monterey jack cheese. (*Note: At this point, the tray of enchiladas can be tightly wrapped with plastic wrap and aluminum foil and frozen for up to 3 months.*)

Bake enchiladas at 400 degrees until cheese is melted and beginning to turn golden and filling is bubbly and heated through—25 to 45 minutes. Remove from oven and serve immediately.

If baking frozen, bake at 350 degrees for 1 to 1½ hours until cooked through. Cover the pan with foil if cheese turns too brown before the filling has cooked through.

POBLANO-TOMATILLO SAUCE

Blend all ingredients together until smooth. Adjust seasonings to taste with more kosher salt and freshly cracked black pepper.

Grits:

1½ cups	whole milk
1½ cups	water
1½ tsp.	kosher salt, plus extra
1 tsp.	freshly cracked black pepper, plus extra
4	sprigs thyme, tied into a bundle with butcher's twine
¾ cup	yellow corn grits
2½ oz.	cream cheese, cubed
1 cup	raw hazelnuts, toasted (see page 243)
1 cup	flour
2	eggs
2 Tbsp.	water

kosher salt

freshly cracked black pepper

peanut oil, for deep frying

Prepare grits the day before serving:

Line a 9x9-inch baking dish with parchment paper.

Heat milk, water, salt, pepper, and thyme in a medium saucepan over medium-high heat, stirring occasionally and scraping the bottom of the pot to prevent burning, until the liquid just begins to boil and foam up. (*Note: Keep a watchful eye on the liquid because once it reaches a boil the milk will curdle if the heat isn't reduced immediately.*)

As soon as liquid begins to boil, pour in grits while whisking constantly to prevent any lumps. Reduce heat to low and simmer until liquid absorbs completely and grits are tender and thick. (*Note: For this dish, you do not want the grits to be at all runny.*) Discard thyme sprigs. Remove from heat and stir in cream cheese until melted and completely incorporated. Adjust seasonings to taste with more kosher salt and freshly cracked black pepper.

Pour grits into the lined baking dish and spread into an even layer. Cool to room temperature and cover with foil or plastic wrap and refrigerate. Chill grits at least 12 hours or up to 2 days before proceeding.

Fill a deep fryer with peanut oil to the manufacturer's fill line and preheat for 20 minutes until hot.

While oil is preheating, process toasted hazelnuts in a food processor and pulse until nuts have been ground into crumbs. (*Note: Do not over process, or the nuts will turn into a paste/nut butter.*)

Pour hazelnut crumbs into a bowl. Season nuts with ½ teaspoon kosher salt and ¼ teaspoon freshly cracked black pepper. Stir.

In a separate bowl, mix together flour, ½ teaspoon kosher salt and ¼ teaspoon freshly cracked black pepper. Stir.

In a third bowl beat eggs, 2 tablespoons water, ½ teaspoon kosher salt and ¼ teaspoon freshly cracked black pepper. Arrange bowls in a row in the following order: flour mixture, egg mixture, and hazelnut crumbs.

Remove grits from the refrigerator. Run a butter knife around the edges of the pan to loosen the sides. Place a large plate or cutting board over the pan and invert grits. Remove pan and peel away parchment paper. Cut grits into 4 even rows and cut each row into 4 equal 2¼-inch squares.

Dredge grit cakes one at a time. Dip one square into flour mixture, coating all sides with flour and shaking off any excess flour. Dip floured square into egg mixture and coat completely. Finally, dip grit cake into hazelnut mixture and coat all sides evenly with hazelnut crumbs. Set aside on a large plate or sheet pan while repeating process with remaining cakes.

Fry cakes, 2 or 3 at a time, for 3 to 4 minutes per batch until golden brown, carefully stirring occasionally to prevent cakes from sticking together or burning on the bottom. Using a spider or slotted spoon, remove cakes from oil and drain on paper towels. Continue frying in batches of 2 or 3, until all the cakes have been fried. Serve immediately.

To assemble: Lean two grits cakes up against each other in the middle of a plate. Spoon mushroom-beet ragu behind the grits cakes. Stack three lemon chips on top of cakes and ragu. Garnish plate with a drizzle of chive oil.

Continued on Next Page

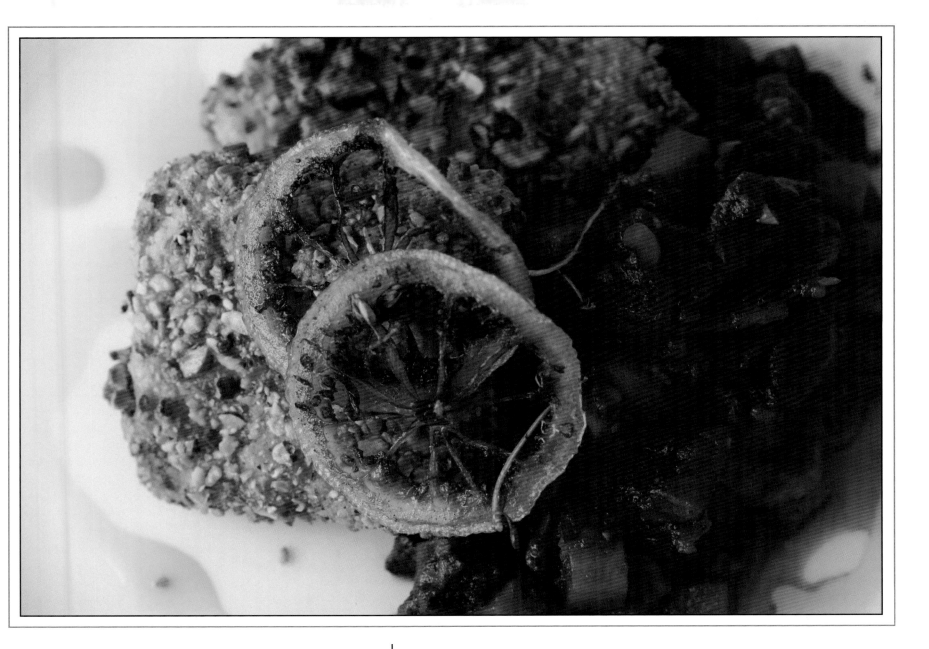

Hazelnut-Crusted Thyme and Cream Cheese Grit Cakes

with Wild Mushroom & Golden Beet Ragu

The flavors of this dish are so bold that I never miss the meat. A mouthful that consists of grit cake, wild mushroom-beet ragu, and a little piece of fried lemon chip is sheer heaven.

Wild Mushroom & Golden Beet Ragu:

2½ Tbsp.	safflower, canola or peanut oil, separated in ½-tablespoon portions
1 lb.	assorted wild mushrooms, roughly chopped
	(use a variety of whatever is in season—morels, chanterelles, oyster, or the always available cremini mushrooms)
1	golden beet, peeled and diced
2	cloves garlic, peeled and minced
6	sprigs fresh thyme, bundled with butcher's twine
1½ cups	canned crushed tomatoes, preferably San Marzano if you can find them
¾ cup	dry red wine
¼ tsp.	crushed red pepper flakes
	kosher salt and freshly cracked black pepper

Chive Oil:

1 cup	chives, roughly chopped
½ cup	canola or safflower oil
½ tsp.	kosher salt
	cheesecloth

Preheat a large sauté pan over medium to medium-high heat for 4 minutes. Add ½ tablepsoon oil to the pan. Once oil ripples with heat, add a fourth of the chopped mushrooms. Sprinkle with kosher salt and freshly cracked black pepper. Stir. Sauté mushrooms, stirring occasionally, until caramelized and cooked through, usually 7 to 9 minutes. Do not stir constantly, or mushrooms will never caramelize. Transfer from the pan to a bowl or plate while continuing to sauté remaining mushrooms.

Return pan to heat. Repeat sautéing process above 3 more times, each time using ½ tablespoon oil and ¼ of mushrooms, making sure to season each batch and sauté until well caramelized for best flavor.

Once all mushrooms have been sautéed and set aside, return pan to heat. Add final ½ tablespoon oil. Heat until oil ripples. Add diced beet to hot oil and season with kosher salt and pepper. Sauté, stirring occasionally, until beets begin to caramelize, 6 to 8 minutes. Add minced garlic to pan and sauté for another minute, stirring constantly.

Return sautéed mushrooms to the pan with beets. Add thyme bundle, crushed tomatoes, red wine, and pepper flakes. Stir. Raise heat to medium-high and bring to a boil. As soon as the ragu reaches a boil, reduce heat to low. Simmer over low heat until liquid has nearly all cooked away, stirring occasionally, about 40 to 50 minutes. Adjust seasoning with kosher salt and freshly cracked black pepper as desired.

CHIVE OIL

Fill a bowl with ice water. Set aside.

Bring a medium-sized pot of water to a boil.

Once water is boiling, blanch chives for 30 seconds to 1 minute. Strain and transfer immediately to ice water to shock. Remove from ice water and wring out as much liquid as possible. Pat dry.

Place chives, kosher salt, and oil in a high-powered blender such as a Blendtec or Vita-Mix—cheap blenders will not puree as finely. Blend until completely pureed.

Line a fine mesh sieve with cheesecloth and place over a bowl or cup. Pour chive oil into the lined sieve. Place sieve and bowl or cup in the refrigerator and allow oil to strain slowly through cheesecloth for 12 hours. Do not press oil through the cloth or try to speed up the straining process. Once strained, store in an airtight container in the refrigerator for 2 weeks.

Manchego, Bacon, and Cremini-Stuffed Brined Pork Loin Roast

with Roasted Garlic Smashed Red Potatoes and Grilled Asparagus

This stuffed pork roast makes a great main course for a holiday meal and pairs well with other holiday favorites. As a side note, in both California and Louisiana, the two places we've spent the last nearly fifteen years of our lives, winter is rather mild, and grilling season is year-round. If you live in a climate that does not allow for winter grilling, feel free to roast the asparagus rather than braving the elements to throw them on the grill.

BRINED PORK LOIN ROAST

Brine:

½ cup	kosher salt
½ cup	(packed) brown sugar
1	star anise
2	sprigs rosemary, crushed with the back of a knife
3	cloves garlic, peeled and smashed
1 tsp.	crushed red pepper flakes
1 cup	water
6 cups	cold water
2 cups	ice

Stuffing:

4	slices thick-cut bacon
2 cups	cremini mushrooms, chopped
¼ tsp.	kosher salt, plus extra
¼ tsp.	freshly cracked black pepper, plus extra
3	cloves garlic, peeled and minced
1 tsp.	fresh rosemary leaves, minced
2 Tbsp.	sherry vinegar
½ cup	panko bread crumbs
3 oz.	Manchego cheese, shredded

Bring first 7 brine ingredients to a boil in a saucepan over high heat. Remove from heat and add cold water and ice. Once ice has melted and brine has cooled to at least room temperature, pour into a large container with a lid.

Add butterflied pork roast to brine. Brine, in the refrigerator, for 12 to 18 hours.

Remove from brine and let sit at room temperature on a wire rack for 1 hour to drain before cooking. Pat dry before stuffing.

MANCHEGO, BACON & CREMINI STUFFING

Prepare stuffing: Cook bacon in a sauté pan over medium heat until brown and crispy—8 to 10 minutes—flipping halfway through cooking. Remove from pan and drain on paper towels.

Drain off all but 1 tablespoon bacon fat from the pan. Return pan to heat. Add chopped cremini mushrooms and sprinkle with kosher salt and freshly cracked black pepper. Stir. Sauté mushrooms over medium heat until caramelized—about 10 minutes— stirring occasionally. Add garlic and rosemary to mushrooms. Sauté another

60 seconds, stirring continuously to prevent garlic from burning. Deglaze the pan with sherry vinegar, scraping the bottom of the pan with a wooden spoon to get up any bits that may be stuck.

Remove from heat and let cool for 10 minutes. Place cooled mushrooms into a mixing bowl with the panko bread crumbs and Manchego cheese. Stir to combine thoroughly. Adjust seasoning to taste with more kosher salt and freshly cracked black pepper.

Continued on Next Page

Pork Loin

1 (3-lb.)	pork loin roast, butterflied
2 Tbsp.	canola oil
¼ tsp.	freshly cracked black pepper
1 tsp.	fresh rosemary, minced
	butcher's twine

Gravy:

1 Tbsp.	sherry vinegar
1 Tbsp.	flour
1 cup	chicken stock

Roasted Garlic Smashed Red Potatoes

See Page 240

Grilled Asparagus

See Page 233

Preheat oven to 350 degrees.

Stuff pork roast: Lay brined butterflied pork roast out flat onto a cutting board with butterflied center facing up. Place stuffing mixture in an even layer over half of butterflied roast. Fold butterflied pork back over stuffing to form a whole stuffed pork roast. Using butcher's twine, tightly tie roast about every 1½ inches to ensure that the roast stays together and cooks evenly.

In a small bowl, mix together minced rosemary and freshly cracked black pepper. Set aside.

Preheat canola oil in an oven-safe large sauté pan over medium-high heat. Once oil ripples with heat, but before it begins to smoke, add pork roast to the pan to brown, fat-side down. Sear over medium-high heat for about 3 minutes until well browned. While top is browning, sprinkle bottom of roast with half of the rosemary-black pepper mixture.

Flip roast and sprinkle remaining rosemary-black pepper mixture over top of roast. Insert a digital meat thermometer into the middle of the roast at the thickest part of the meat. If the thermometer has an alarm, set it for 140 degrees. Place sauté pan with pork loin roast into the oven. Bake roast at 350 degrees for about 20 minutes per pound until the roast's internal temperature reaches 140 degrees. Remove roast from the oven and place on a board to rest, loosely covered in foil, for at least 10 minutes.

While pork is resting make gravy. Drain off all but 1 tablespoon pork fat from sauté pan. Place pan over medium heat. Deglaze the pan with sherry vinegar and cook off liquid. Add flour to form a roux. Cook roux, stirring constantly, for 3 minutes. While whisking continuously, slowly drizzle in chicken stock to form a gravy. Simmer gravy until thickened, about 3 to 4 minutes, scraping up any bits of deliciousness from the bottom of the pan to be incorporated into the sauce.

Remove twine and slice pork roast. To serve, spoon mashed potatoes into the middle of a plate. Lean a slice of pork roast up against the pile of mashed potatoes. Spoon gravy over roast and potatoes. Lay asparagus next to potatoes. Serve immediately.

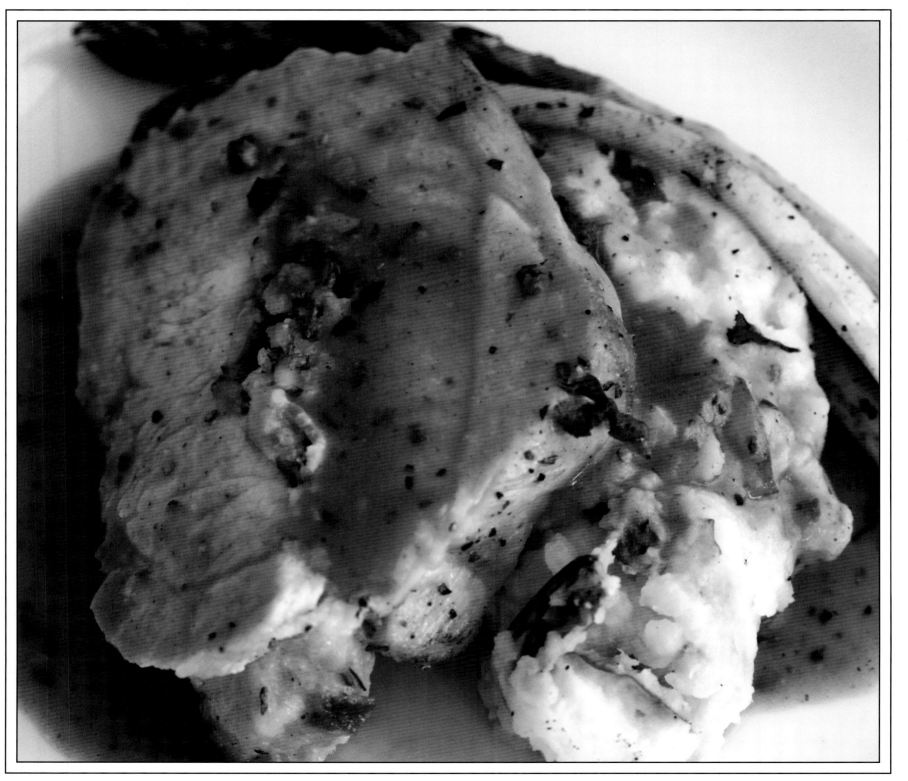

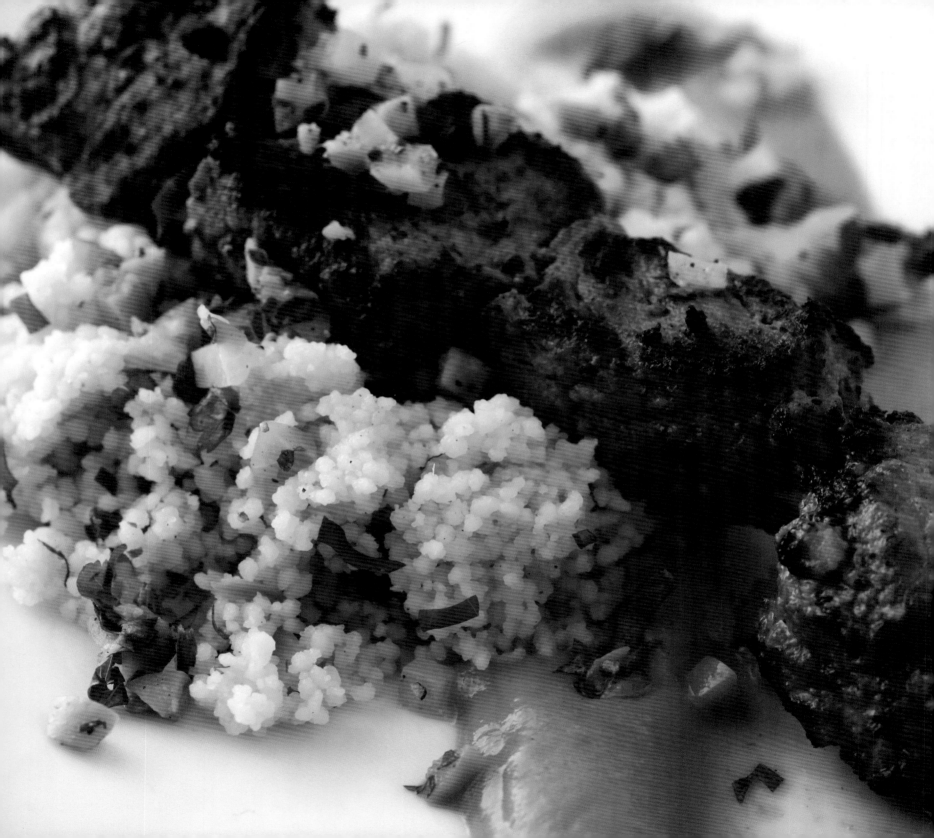

Moroccan New York Strip Kebabs

with Cilantro-Pine Nut Couscous and Roasted Carrot Sauce

Preserved lemon is an ingredient common to Moroccan cuisine. They are made by simply packing lemons in a jar with kosher salt and lemon juice. The rind of the preserved lemon is the only part consumed; the pulp is discarded. While they are easy to make, they take weeks to preserve. So, if you're in a rush, look for them in specialty gourmet and middle eastern/Moroccan markets or online.

1½ lbs.	boneless New York Strips, trimmed of fat and cut in 1½-inch cubes
4	wooden skewers, soaked in water for at least 1 hour

Marinade:

2 Tbsp.	tahini
	juice from 1 lemon
½	preserved lemon, pulp removed, rinsed and diced
2	cloves garlic, peeled and roughly chopped
½	jalapeño, seeded if you don't like too much spice, minced
¼ cup	cilantro
¾ tsp.	kosher salt
½ tsp.	freshly cracked black pepper
½ tsp.	ground cumin
⅛ tsp.	ground ginger
⅛ tsp.	ground cinnamon
⅓ cup	olive oil

Couscous:

1 tsp.	olive oil
¼ cup	pine nuts
1¼ cups	low sodium chicken stock
½ tsp.	ground cumin
1 tsp.	kosher salt, plus extra
¼ tsp.	freshly cracked black pepper, plus extra
1 cup	couscous
¼ cup	fresh cilantro, chopped

Roasted Carrot Sauce

See Page 239

Preserved Lemon-Olive Garnish

See Page 238

NEW YORK STRIP KEBABS

Whisk to combine all marinade ingredients *except* olive oil to a mixing bowl. While whisking continuously, slowly drizzle in the olive oil.

Pour marinade over steak cubes in a resealable plastic bag. Toss to evenly coat meat. Seal the bag, removing as much air as possible to emulate a vacuum seal. Marinate beef in the refrigerator for 2 to 3 hours.

Prepare grill for high heat.

While grill is heating, remove beef from marinade. Thread beef onto the soaked skewers to make kebabs.

Grill kebabs directly over high heat for 2 to 3 minutes per side, rotating skewers a quarter turn each time, for a total cook time of 8 to 12 minutes (8 for medium-rare; 11 to 12 for medium). Remove from heat and let rest 5 minutes before serving.

COUSCOUS

Preheat olive oil in a 1-quart pot over medium heat for 3 minutes. Add pine nuts to the pot. Toast pine nuts until golden, stirring frequently, for 4 to 5 minutes. Add chicken stock, cumin, salt, and pepper to the pot. Raise heat to high and bring to a boil. Stir in couscous. Return to a boil and cover the pot with a lid or aluminum foil and remove from heat. Let couscous steam in the pot for 15 to 20 minutes until all liquid is absorbed. Fluff with a fork and toss in chopped cilantro. Adjust seasonings to taste with kosher salt and freshly cracked black pepper.

Chile puree:

3	dried ancho chiles, stems and seeds removed
3	dried new Mexican chiles, stems and seeds removed
1 Tbsp.	chile pequin
⅓ cup	steeping liquid

Soup:

2	slices bacon
2½ lbs.	boneless short ribs
1 tsp.	flour, for dusting
1	large yellow onion, diced
1	red bell pepper, stem and seeds removed, diced
2	Anaheim chiles, stem and seeds removed, diced
5	cloves garlic, minced
¼ tsp.	dried thyme
½ tsp.	dried oregano
1 tsp.	kosher salt, plus extra for seasoning
½ tsp.	freshly cracked black pepper, plus extra for seasoning
1 Tbsp.	chili powder
1½ Tbsp.	ground cumin
¾ cup	dried black beans
¾ cup	dried navy beans
2 tsp.	brown sugar
4 cups	chicken or beef stock
1 (12-oz.)	can beer
1 (28-oz.)	can whole tomatoes, preferably San Marzano tomatoes
⅓ cup	fresh cilantro, chopped

Garnish:

diced red onion

fresh cilantro leaves

shredded sharp cheddar

sour cream

Mexican Cornbread:

See Page 235

Preheat oven to 275 degrees with a rack positioned in the bottom of the oven.

Bring a pot full of water to a boil. Remove water from heat and add dried chiles. Cover submerged chiles and let steep for 30 minutes. Reserve ⅓ cup steeping liquid and drain off remaining water from chiles. Blend rehydrated chiles and reserved steeping liquid at high speed until smooth. Set aside until ready to use.

While chiles are steeping, Cook bacon in a large stock pot over medium heat until most fat has rendered out and slices are crisp—about 10 minutes—flipping halfway through cooking. Remove bacon from pan, leaving only rendered fat.

While bacon is cooking, season short ribs liberally with kosher salt and freshly cracked black pepper. Sprinkle meat with 1 teaspoon flour. Toss to coat.

Raise heat to medium-high. When bacon fat is nearly to the smoking point, brown one batch of short ribs on all sides, making sure not to overcrowd the pan. Remove from pan and set aside. Repeat browning process with remaining ribs. Once all ribs have been browned, remove from pan and reduce heat to medium.

Sauté diced onion, red bell pepper, and Anaheim chiles over medium heat, stirring occasionally, until the onions are translucent and the peppers are soft—about 10 minutes. Add minced garlic, dried thyme, oregano, kosher salt, black pepper, chili powder, and cumin to the pan. Sauté for another 60 seconds, stirring continuously.

Add black and navy beans to seasoned vegetables. Stir and sauté another 2 minutes. Add brown sugar, stock, beer, and canned tomatoes, crushing each tomato with your hands as you add it to the pot. Raise the heat to high and bring to a boil, stirring occasionally.

Once liquid has reached a boil, add chile puree and the browned short ribs to the pot. (*Note: If you prefer a chili with less heat, add only half of the chile puree.*) Stir. Cover pot with an oven-safe lid and place chili in the oven.

Braise chili at 275 degrees for 2 hours. After 2 hours, remove the lid and stir in fresh cilantro. Return pot to oven and continue braising for another 1 to 2 hours until beans are soft and ribs are "fall-apart" tender.

Remove short ribs from pot and shred with two forks, leaving some meat in chunks. Discard any connective tissue that didn't melt away in the braising process. Add shredded meat back to chili. Stir to combine. Adjust seasoning to taste with kosher salt and freshly cracked black pepper. (*Note: Chili is best when made the day before it's served.*) Rewarm over medium heat and garnish with a combination of diced red onion, cilantro leaves, shredded cheddar, and sour cream. Serve with freshly baked cornbread muffins.

Hearty Short Rib Chili

with Mexican Cornbread

When testing this recipe, the main complaint I received was that there wasn't more of it. This recipe may not satisfy those chili purists who believe that beans or tomatoes should never make an appearance in chili, but fortunately I haven't run into too many of those folks. As I suggest with most soups, stews, or braised dishes, wait a day to eat it—the chili will taste best the day after it's made.

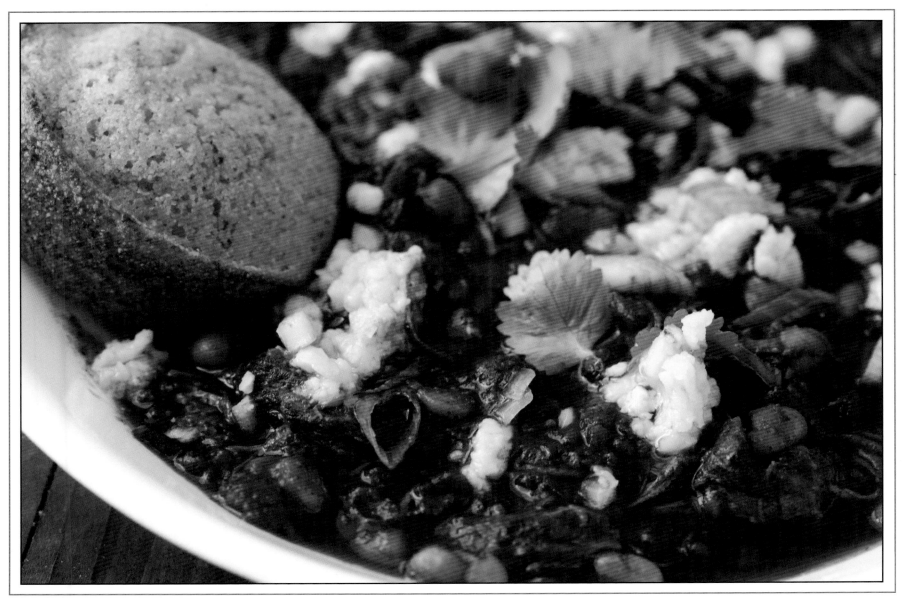

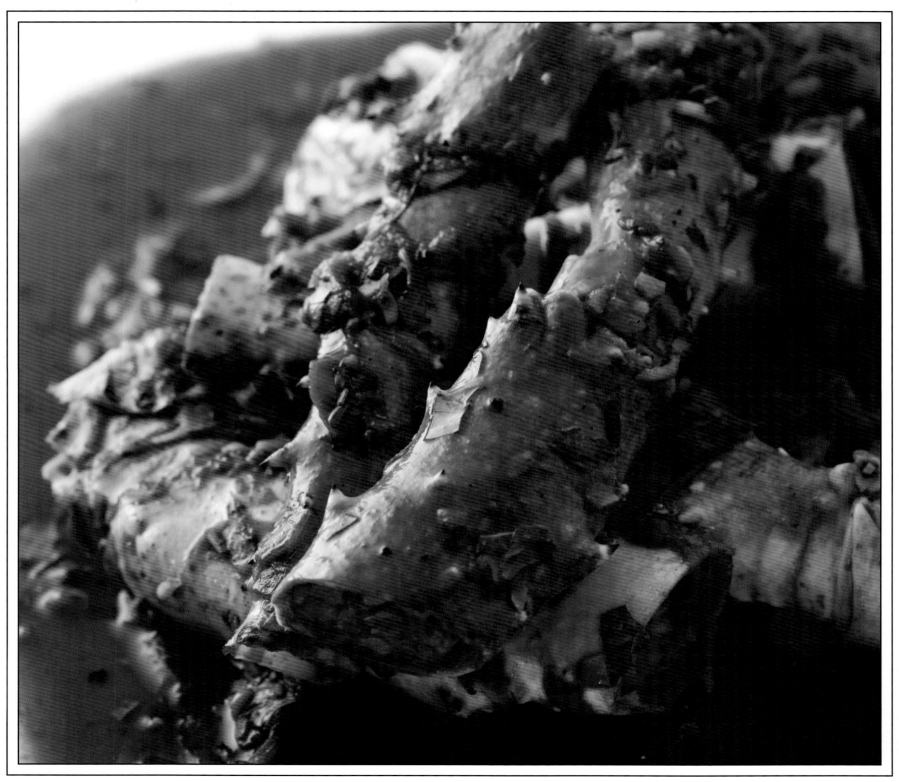

New Orleans' Style Barbecue King Crab Legs

This is a play on the traditional "New Orleans-Style Barbecue Shrimp." Instead of using shrimp, I like to use king crab legs. If you've ever had New Orleans-Style Barbecue Shrimp, you know very well that what people commonly associate with barbecue sauce has nothing to do with this dish. Make sure you have a nice loaf of French bread for sopping up all of the extra sauce. There is no way I would let that go to waste.

BARBECUE KING CRAB LEGS

4 Tbsp.	cold butter, divided in half and cut into ½-inch cubes
3	cloves garlic, minced
¼ tsp.	dried thyme
¼ tsp.	dried oregano
½ tsp.	freshly cracked black pepper
⅛ tsp.	cayenne
¼ cup	IPA beer
¼ cup	Worcestershire sauce
	juice from ½ a lime
1 tsp.	vinegary hot sauce, like Crystal or Texas Pete
½ tsp.	anchovy paste
2 lbs.	defrosted cooked king crab legs, cut into segments
¼ cup	fresh parsley, chopped
1	loaf french bread, warmed

Melt 2 tablespoons butter in a sauté pan over medium heat. Once butter has melted and foam has subsided, add minced garlic. Sauté for two minutes, stirring constantly. If garlic begins to brown, reduce the heat.

Add dried thyme, oregano, black pepper, cayenne, and beer to garlic. Stir. Raise heat to medium-high and reduce beer by half. Add Worcestershire sauce, lime juice, hot sauce, and anchovy paste. Whisk to combine thoroughly. Reduce heat to medium and simmer crab legs in liquid for 10 to 15 minutes until heated through, tossing or stirring occasionally. Add parsley and stir.

While whisking continuously, add remaining cold butter to crab legs, one cube at a time, allowing each cube to completely incorporate before adding the next cube in order to keep butter emulsified with cooking liquid. Serve with warm French bread.

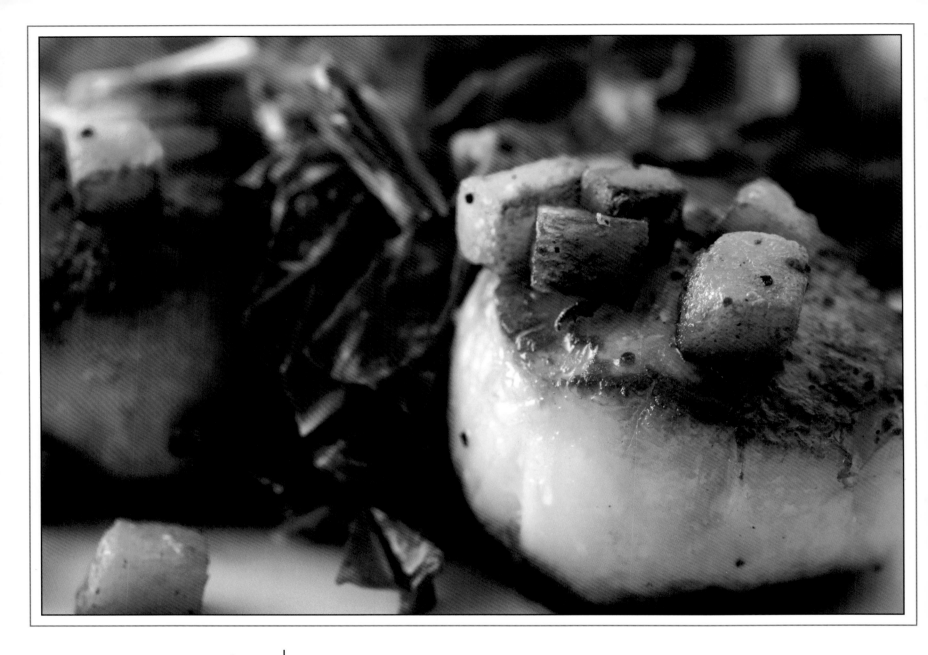

Seared Scallops

with Creamed Collards and Brown Butter-Sage Butternut Squash

The perfect bite of this dish will include a little bit of each element. The sweetness of the sea scallops plays beautifully off of the caramelized butternut squash. When cooking the squash, try to remember not to stir too frequently so that the caramelizing has a chance to occur without raising the heat above medium, which would cause the butter to go from browned to burnt.

Seared Scallops:

12	sea scallops, side muscles removed if still present
3 Tbsp.	canola or peanut oil
	kosher salt
	freshly cracked black pepper

Brown Butter-Sage Butternut Squash:

3 Tbsp.	butter
3 cups	butternut squash, peeled, seeded, and cut in ¼-inch cubes
4	fresh sage leaves, minced
	kosher salt
	freshly cracked black pepper

Creamed Collard Greens:

2	bunches collard greens, thick middle stems removed, ⅓-inch thick shred
¾ cup	heavy cream
¼ tsp.	freshly ground nutmeg
	kosher salt
	freshly cracked black pepper

Heat a large sauté pan over high heat for 2 minutes and add canola oil. While pan is heating, liberally season sea scallops with kosher salt and freshly cracked black pepper.

Once oil ripples from heat, but before it starts smoking, sear 6 sea scallops over high heat, undisturbed, for 3 minutes until a golden brown crust has formed. Flip scallops and cook for another 3 minutes, undisturbed, until scallops are just opaque in the middle. Remove from pan and loosely cover with foil. Repeat searing process with remaining 6 scallops. (*Note: Searing in* two batches keeps from overcrowding the pan and allows for a hotter pan and a better crust.)

To plate:

Place a pile of creamed collards in the middle of a plate and arrange three scallops around the outside of the pile. Scattered butternut squash over the scallops and around the plate. Repeat plating process three more times for a total of 4 servings.

BROWN BUTTER-SAGE BUTTERNUT SQUASH

Melt butter in a large sauté pan over medium heat and let it brown slightly. After the butter has turned light amber, add butternut squash to the pan, stir, and spread in an even layer over the bottom of the pan. Sprinkle with kosher salt, freshly cracked black pepper, and sage but do not stir. Let squash cook without stirring for 4 or 5 minutes until bottom of squash has had a chance to caramelize. Toss squash so that a different side has a chance to caramelize. Sauté for another 4 or 5 minutes and toss again. Sauté until squash is cooked through and caramelized on all sides, about 5 more minutes. Adjust seasonings to taste with more kosher salt and freshly cracked black pepper.

CREAMED COLLARD GREENS

Bring a large pot of salted water to a boil over high heat. Add shredded collards to boiling water. Stir. Boil for 4 minutes. Reduce heat to low. Drain off all water and place collards back over low heat. Add cream, nutmeg, and a liberal pinch of kosher salt and freshly cracked black pepper. Stir. Let collards simmer in cream, stirring occasionally, until nearly all liquid in the cream has cooked away, about 30 minutes. Adjust seasoning to taste with more kosher salt and freshly cracked black pepper.

Lamb Bolognese:

3 Tbsp.	canola or peanut oil
4 lbs.	lamb shanks
	flour, for dusting
2	carrots, roughly chopped
1	yellow onion, roughly chopped
3	stalks celery, roughly chopped
5	cloves garlic, smashed
	stems from 1 bunch of parsley
1	(3-inch) sprig of rosemary
1 cup	basil leaves and stems
1	(14.5-oz.) can fire-roasted tomatoes
2 cups	low sodium beef or lamb broth
½	bottle dry red wine
½ tsp.	freshly cracked black pepper, plus extra
1 tsp.	kosher salt, plus extra
¾ cup	tomato sauce (recipe below)

Tomato Sauce:

1 Tbsp.	olive oil
1	yellow onion, peeled and finely diced
4	cloves garlic, peeled and minced
1 cup	dry red wine
1	(28-oz.) can crushed tomatoes, preferably San Marzano
1	(28-oz.) can diced tomatoes, preferably San Marzano
¼ cup	fresh basil, torn
¼ cup	fresh flat leaf parsley, chopped
¼ tsp.	crushed red pepper
	kosher salt
	freshly cracked black pepper

Preheat oven to 350 degrees.

Preheat a large, oven-safe pot over medium-high heat for 3 minutes. Add canola oil to the pan.

While pan is heating, liberally season lamb shanks on all sides with kosher salt and freshly cracked black pepper and dust lightly with flour.

Once oil ripples with heat, brown half of the lamb shanks for 2 to 3 minutes per side until well caramelized. Remove from pan and brown remaining lamb shanks. Remove from pan and set aside.

Pour off all but 1 tablespoon oil. Return pan to heat. Reduce heat to medium. Add carrots, onions, and celery. Stir. Sprinkle with a pinch of kosher salt and freshly cracked black pepper. Sauté vegetables over medium heat for about 10 minutes, stirring occasionally, until veggies are soft and onions translucent. Add garlic to vegetables and sauté another 2 minutes, stirring occasionally.

Add remaining bolognese ingredients *except* tomato sauce to the pan. Raise heat to high and bring ingredients to a boil. Add browned lamb shanks to boiling liquid and submerge completely. Cover pot and cook in preheated 350 degree oven for about 2 hours or until fork-tender and falling apart.

Let shanks sit in cooking liquid for 15 minutes. Remove from liquid and let cool enough to handle. Shred meat from shanks, discarding the bones and any fat or connective tissue. Set aside in a mixing bowl.

While shanks are cooling, strain cooking liquid through a fine mesh sieve. Add strained liquid to a pan and place over medium-high heat. Reduce by half.

Add ½ cup reduced liquid and half of the tomato sauce to bowl with shredded lamb. Stir to moisten evenly. Adjust seasoning to taste with more kosher salt and freshly cracked black pepper. (*Note: You likely won't need to add much—if any—salt. You can prepare bolognese up to 1 day in advance, if desired. Just rewarm before assembling the lasagna.*)

TOMATO SAUCE

Preheat olive oil in a large pan over medium heat for 3 minutes. Sauté onion in oil over medium heat for about 10 minutes, stirring occasionally, until onion turns translucent. Add minced garlic to pan and sauté for another 60 seconds, stirring frequently, making sure to not to let garlic brown. Deglaze pan with red wine, scraping up any bits on the bottom of the pan. Cook off almost all of the wine, stirring occasionally.

Once only a small amount of liquid is left, add remaining ingredients for tomato sauce. Stir. Simmer tomato sauce until thickened, about 30 minutes. Adjust seasoning to taste with kosher salt and freshly cracked black pepper. (*Note: You can make the sauce up to 2 days in advance. Just rewarm before assembling the lasagna.*)

Continued on Next Page

Lamb Bolognese Lasagna

There's just something so warm and comforting about lasagna that makes it a perfect dish for winter. If lamb isn't your favorite, try replacing the meat in the bolognese with veal or pork shanks or a combination of the two. Any of these meats will create a delicious lasagna.

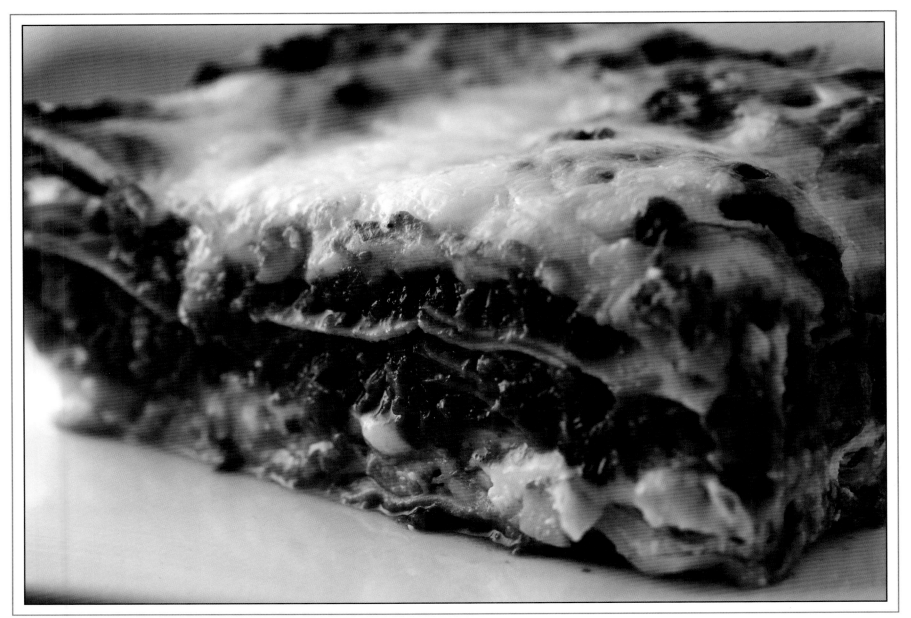

Ricotta Mixture:

1	(15-oz.) container of Ricotta
1	egg, beaten
⅓ cup	freshly grated Parmesan cheese
¼ tsp.	kosher salt
¼ tsp.	freshly cracked black pepper
¼ cup	basil leaves, cut in a chiffonade

Mornay Sauce:

1 Tbsp.	butter
1 Tbsp.	flour
1 cup	milk, lukewarm
1	pinch of nutmeg
1 cup	Gruyère, grated
¼ cup	freshly grated Parmesan
	kosher salt
	freshly cracked black pepper

Assembly:

1	box no-boil lasagna noodles (you won't use all the noodles)
4 oz.	part-skim mozzarella, shredded
¼ cup	freshly grated Parmesan
	Tomato Sauce
	Ricotta Mixture
	Mornay Sauce
	Lamb Bolognese

RICOTTA MIXTURE

Whisk together all ingredients in a mixing bowl until well incorporated. Chill for at least 30 minutes before assembly so Ricotta has time to absorb the other flavors.

MORNAY SAUCE

Melt 1 tablespoon butter in saucepan over medium heat. Once butter has completely melted, add flour to make a roux. Whisk continuously for about 1 minute. While continuing to whisk vigorously, slowly drizzle in milk. (*Note: Adding milk too quickly or all at once will result in lumps in the sauce.*) Stir in nutmeg. Cook sauce until thickened slightly, whisking frequently, about 7 minutes. Once thickened, remove from heat and add cheese. Whisk until cheese has completely melted and sauce is smooth. Adjust seasoning to taste with kosher salt and freshly cracked black pepper. (*Note: Wait until just before you're ready to assemble the lasagna before making this sauce.*)

ASSEMBLY

Preheat oven to 350 degrees.

Butter a deep 9x9-inch baking dish. Add 1 cup tomato sauce to the bottom of the dish in an even layer. Next, add a layer lasagna noodles to completely cover bottom, overlapping noodles as necessary. Spread all of ricotta mixture over noodles in an even layer. Pour Mornay sauce ricotta mixture. Add another layer of lasagna noodles to completely cover the Mornay sauce, gently pressing down to ensure a compact lasagna. Pour lamb bolognese over lasagna noodles in an even layer. Top with another layer of lasagna noodles. To finish the lasagna, spoon 2 to 2½ cups tomato sauce over the top layer of noodles. Sprinkle tomato sauce with mozzarella and Parmesan cheese.

Place assembled lasagna onto a baking sheet. *Loosely* cover lasagna with foil. Bake on the center rack at 350 degrees for 20 minutes. Remove foil and bake for another 25 to 35 minutes until cheese is bubbly and golden around the edges and noodles are tender. Remove from oven and let cool for *at least 25 minutes before cutting and serving.* (*Note: If you cut into the lasagna too soon, the liquid won't have a chance to reabsorb into the dish and will run out of the lasagna.*)

Low-and-Slow Oven-Roasted Pulled Pork Sandwiches

with Virginia-Style Barbecue Sauce

Call me crazy, but my hankerings for barbecue don't stop when winter rolls in. When it's too cold to smoke a pork shoulder outside all day (or when I'm just feeling lazy), making pulled pork using the low-and-slow oven-roasting method gets the job done tastily. Growing up in the mountains of Virginia, it's only natural that the sauce I prefer for pulled pork is the typical vinegar-based Virginia/Carolina style, but feel free to drizzle some of your favorite barbecue sauce over the coleslaw before closing the sandwiches.

PULLED PORK

Rub:

2 Tbsp.   kosher salt

1 Tbsp.   freshly cracked black pepper

2 Tbsp.   brown sugar

1 Tbsp.   smoked paprika

1 Tbsp.   granulated garlic

1   (4–6 lb.) bone-in pork shoulder roast

Virginia-Style Barbecue Sauce

Coleslaw

vinegary hot sauce, like Texas Pete, Crystal, or Louisiana Brand

High-quality buns or hoagie rolls, sliced in half for sandwiches

Stir together rub ingredients. Coat pork roast liberally and evenly on all sides with rub. Wrap rubbed roast tightly in plastic wrap and let sit in the refrigerator for 12 to 24 hours. Remove from fridge and let sit at room temperature for 1 hour before roasting.

Preheat oven to 240 degrees. Remove plastic wrap from roast and place on a foil-lined baking sheet. Insert a meat thermometer into the middle of the thickest part of the roast, not touching any bones. If you have a digital thermometer with an alarm, set the alarm to go off when the pork reaches 200 degrees.

Roast pork, undisturbed, at 240 degrees until internal temperature reaches 200 degrees, about 1 hour 15 minutes to 2 hours per pound. (*Note: Cooking times will vary due to size of roast. At an internal temperature of 200 degrees, the meat will be nearly falling apart and come off bone easily.*) Cool until able to handle. Using your hands, shred pork into bite-sized hunks, discarding any bones, large pieces of fat, or connective tissue. (*Note: Pork will shred into smaller pieces when it's heated with the sauce, so don't worry about the pork being finely shredded initially.*)

At this point, pork can be stored refrigerated in an airtight container until ready to serve, for up to 2 days.

Simmer pulled pork in a pot over medium heat with 1 to 1½ cups Virginia-style barbecue sauce until almost all liquid has been simmered off and absorbed into pork, stirring occasionally, usually 15 to 20 minutes.

To assemble sandwiches, place a heaping scoop of pulled pork onto the bottom half of a bun. Pile coleslaw on top of pulled pork. Douse top bun with hot sauce and place over coleslaw to close sandwich. Make as many sandwiches as you can eat and serve immediately.

Continued on Next Page

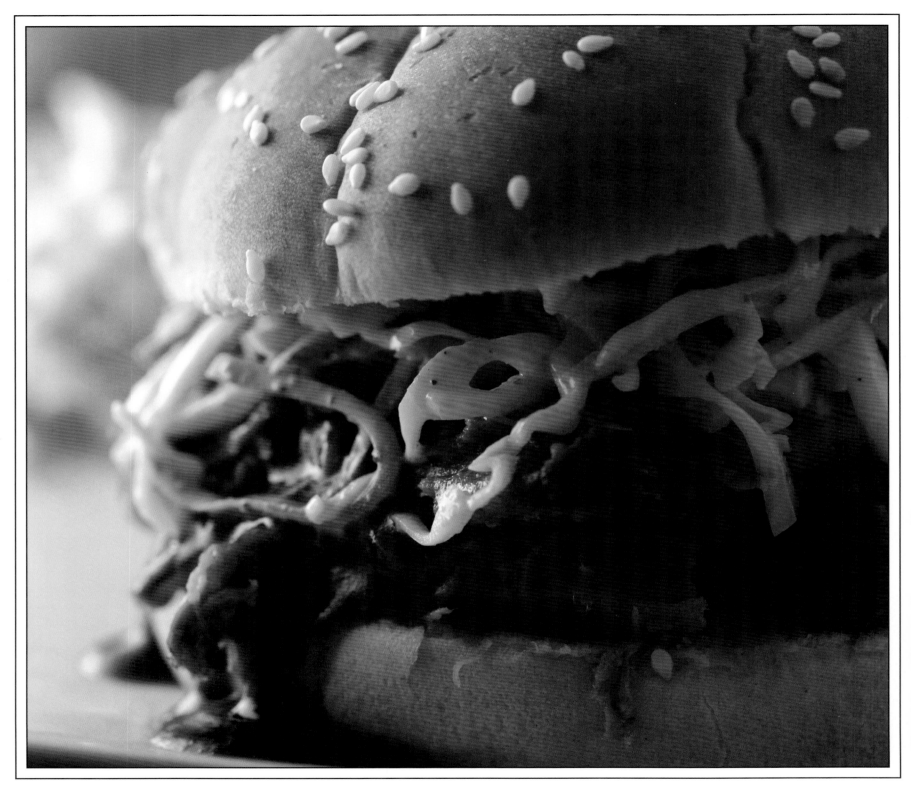

VIRGINIA-STYLE BARBECUE SAUCE

Virginia-Style Barbecue Sauce:

1 cup	apple cider vinegar
½ cup	water
¼ cup	(packed) brown sugar
1 Tbsp.	kosher salt
1 tsp.	red pepper flakes
1½ tsp.	freshly cracked black pepper
⅓ cup	ketchup
1 Tbsp.	Dijon mustard
1 Tbsp.	Worcestershire sauce
½ Tbsp.	vinegary hot sauce, like Texas Pete, Crystal, or Louisiana Brand

Coleslaw:

¼ cup	Virginia-Style Barbecue Sauce
¼ cup	mayonnaise
½ tsp.	sugar
½ tsp.	kosher salt, plus extra
½ tsp.	freshly cracked black pepper, plus extra
½	head green cabbage, finely shredded
½	head red cabbage, finely shredded
1	large carrot, peeled and finely julienned
1	Granny Smith apple, cored and finely julienned
2	green onions, thinly sliced

Whisk together all ingredients in a medium-sized saucepan over medium heat until brown sugar has dissolved into vinegar. Heat just until vinegar comes to a simmer and remove from heat. Cool to room temperature. Barbecue sauce stored in an airtight container in the refrigerator will last indefinitely. Let sit for at least 6 hours before using for flavors to marry.

COLESLAW

Whisk together first 5 coleslaw ingredients in a small mixing bowl until thoroughly combined.

Combine remaining ingredients in a large mixing bowl. Pour mayonnaise mixture over shredded veggies. Toss to evenly coat all veggies with dressing. Adjust seasoning to taste with more kosher salt and freshly cracked black pepper. Let rest, chilled, for 30 minutes to 2 hours before serving for flavors to marry.

Chermoula:

⅓ cup	(packed) fresh cilantro leaves
½ cup	(packed) flat parsley leaves
2	cloves garlic
½	preserved lemon, rind only, rinsed and roughly chopped
¾ tsp.	ground cumin
¾ tsp.	sweet paprika
¼ tsp.	ground cayenne
½ tsp.	kosher salt, plus extra
	juice from 1 small lemon
⅓ cup	high quality olive oil

Fish:

4	(4- to 5-oz.) U.S.–caught swordfish steaks, skin removed
2 Tbsp.	canola oil
	kosher salt
	freshly cracked white (or black) pepper

Salad:

1 Tbsp.	extra virgin olive oil
2	cloves garlic, minced
4	anchovy filets, minced
2 cans	chickpeas, drained and rinsed (or 3 cups cooked dried chickpeas)
⅓ cup	(packed) sun-dried tomatoes, julienned
10	kalamata olives, pitted and roughly chopped
¼ cup	(packed) flat leaf parsley, roughly chopped
3 oz.	feta, crumbled
	kosher salt
	freshly cracked black pepper

crumbled feta, for garnishing

Process chermoula sauce ingredients in a food processor until smooth. Adjust seasoning to taste with more kosher salt. Set aside.

Preheat a large sauté pan over medium-high to high heat to cook fish and another large sauté pan over medium-low heat for salad.

While pans are preheating, season swordfish steaks on all sides with kosher salt and freshly cracked white pepper. Add 2 tablespoons canola oil to pan over high heat. Once oil ripples with heat, but before it starts to smoke, sear swordfish—in batches, if necessary—over high heat for 3 minutes until golden. Flip and sear for another 3 minutes or until just cooked through.

As soon as you start searing fish, add olive oil to the sauté pan over medium heat. Heat oil for 60 seconds and add garlic and anchovies. Sauté for about 60 seconds, stirring constantly. Add chickpeas to garlic and anchovies and stir. Cook for 3 minutes. Remove from heat and add remaining ingredients, stirring to combine. Adjust seasoning to taste with kosher salt and freshly cracked black pepper.

To plate, divide chickpea salad among 4 plates, piling salad in the middle of each plate. Lean a swordfish steak on top or up against the salad. Drizzle chermoula around the plate and over the fish. Garnish with crumbled feta.

Seared Swordfish

with Chermoula Sauce and Chickpea, Sun-Dried Tomato and Kalamata Olive Salad

I realize that to some chefs and gourmands there is no greater offense than to serve fish and cheese in the same dish. Fortunately, I'm not from that same school of thought. To me, as long as it tastes good and the flavors are well-balanced I have no qualms about throwing some crumbled feta or shaved Parmesan into a seafood dish. As a side note, in other parts of the world, over-fishing has caused swordfish populations to decline to dangerously low levels. If you cannot find swordfish caught in the United States, opt for different fish in this recipe altogether. Try to choose a firm, meaty fish caught as local as possible if you can.

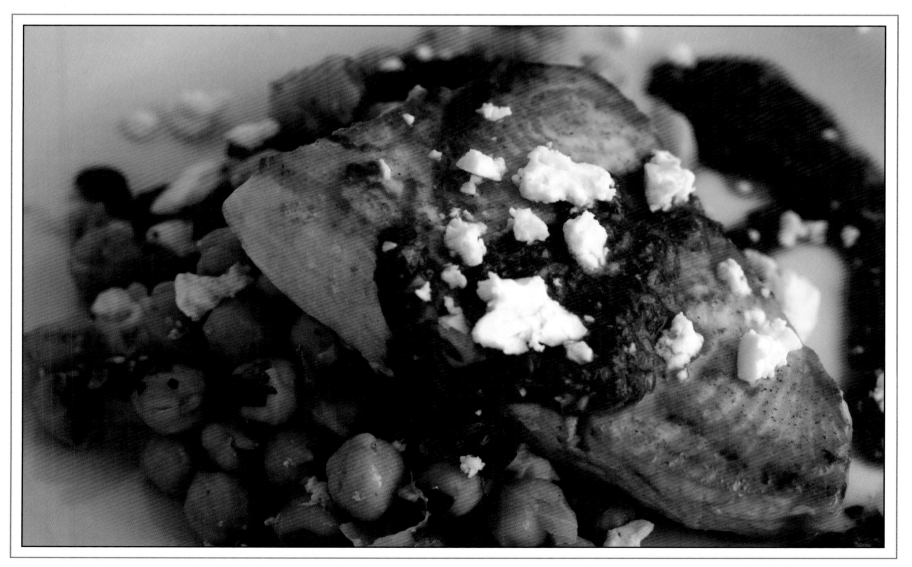

Uber-Creamy Salami and Chevre Macaroni and Cheese

Instead of throwing in bacon or pancetta, salami adds the meaty element to this macaroni and cheese. I suggest cooking the pasta just a wee little bit past al dente for the best macaroni and cheese. If the pasta is cooked to al dente and then added to the sauce, it will absorb too much of the liquid from the dish resulting in a drier, less velvety casserole after baking.

MACARONI & CHEESE

Cheese Sauce

1 tsp.	extra virgin olive oil
4 oz.	salami, diced into ¼-inch (not deli sliced)
2 Tbsp.	butter
3 Tbsp.	flour
2 cups	whole milk, at room temperature
½ cup	heavy cream, at room temperature
⅛ tsp.	freshly ground nutmeg
1 tsp.	Coleman's mustard powder
¼ tsp.	crushed red pepper flakes
1	sprig fresh thyme
¼ tsp.	freshly cracked black pepper
¼ tsp.	kosher salt, plus extra
4 oz.	herbed chevre, crumbled
5 oz.	sharp cheddar, shredded

10 oz.	medium shells pasta, cooked to tender according to package directions

Topping:

½ cup	panko bread crumbs
1 Tbsp.	olive oil

Preheat oven to 450 degrees. Spray a deep glass or ceramic loaf pan with cooking spray. Set aside.

In a small bowl, toss together panko bread crumbs and olive oil. Work oil into bread crumbs with your fingers until evenly disbursed with no lumps. Set aside.

Bring a large pot of salted water to a boil over high heat. Boil pasta until tender according to package directions. Drain thoroughly.

While pasta is cooking, make cheese sauce: Preheat a medium-sized saucepan over medium heat. Once the pan is hot, add olive oil and heat until oil ripples. Add diced salami to oil. Cook salami for 5 to 7 minutes, stirring occasionally, until caramelized and some of fat renders out. (*Note: Do not render out all of the fat or the salami will become tough and hard to chew.*)

Remove salami from pan and drain off all but 1 tablespoon rendered fat. Add butter and melt over medium heat. Once butter has melts, add flour to form roux. Whisk. Cook roux, whisking constantly for 2 to 3 minutes. If roux takes on any color, briefly remove from heat.

Slowly drizzle in milk while whisking constantly to dissolve roux into liquid. (*Note: When the liquid is first introduced, the roux will seize up, but as more liquid is added, it will return to a smooth paste. Adding the liquid too quickly will result in a very lumpy sauce.*) Once milk as been incorporated, add heavy cream, nutmeg, mustard powder, crushed red pepper, thyme, and freshly cracked black pepper. Whisk to combine. Bring mixture to a simmer over medium heat, stirring frequently and scraping the bottom of the pan to prevent liquid from scalding. Once liquid reaches a simmer—*not* a boil—simmer for 2 to 3 more minutes until thickened slightly. Add salt, herbed chevre, and sharp cheddar. Whisk until cheese melts into sauce. Adjust seasonings to taste with more kosher salt and freshly cracked black pepper.

Pour cheese sauce over drained pasta. Toss to evenly coat all shells with sauce. Pour pasta and sauce into prepared loaf pan, scraping every last drop of sauce out with a rubber spatula. Sprinkle oiled panko over macaroni and cheese. Bake at 450 degrees until crumb topping is golden brown and cheese sauce is bubbly, about 15 minutes. Remove from oven and let set for 10 minutes before serving.

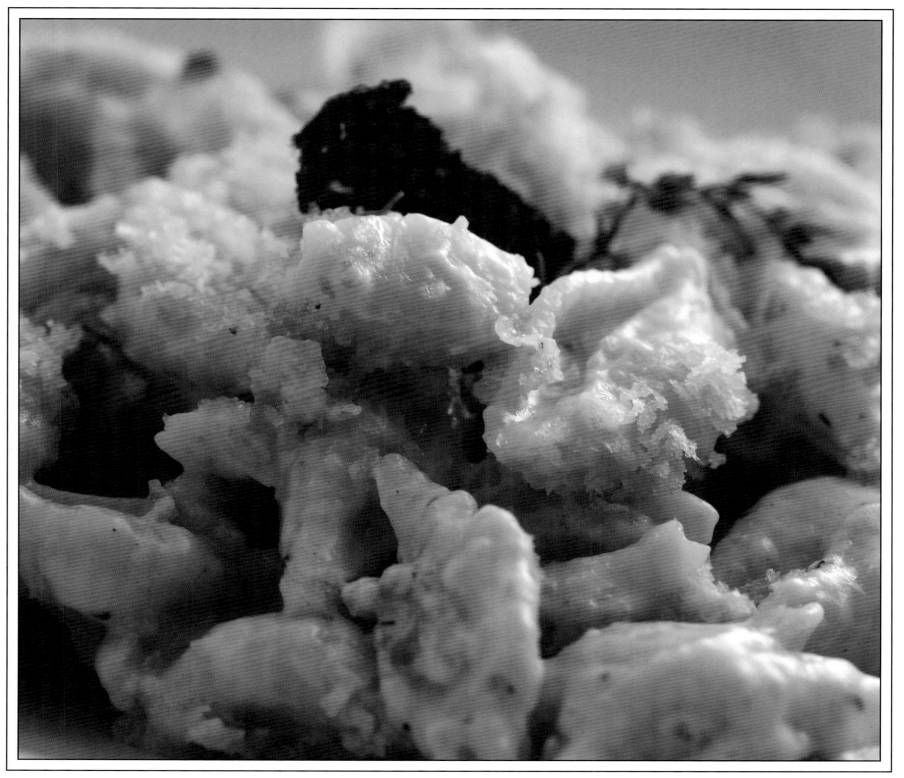

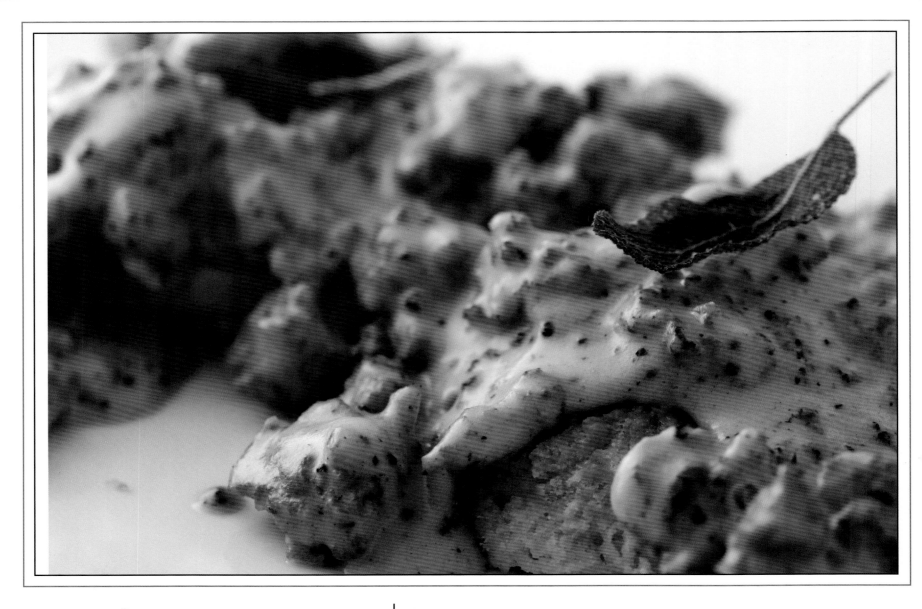

Southern-Style Biscuits and Sausage Gravy

If you're lucky enough to live in an area that carries White Lily flour, by all means, use 2 cups of it instead of the flour listed in the recipe. White Lily has a lower protein content than all-purpose flour and a higher protein content than cake flour, which makes it the ideal flour for biscuits. More protein in flour equals more gluten bonds and thus chewier, more elastic bread. If you've ever eaten a Southern-style biscuit, you know that it should be fluffy, moist, crumbly, and not in the least bit chewy. Since White Lily isn't available too far out of the South, this recipe calls for 1 part flour and 1 part cake flour to achieve a similar protein content.

Biscuits:

1 cup	all-purpose flour
1 cup	cake flour
½ tsp.	baking soda
1½ tsp.	baking powder
1½ tsp.	kosher salt
4 Tbsp.	butter, very cold and cut in small cubes
¾ cup + 2 Tbsp. buttermilk	

For Brushing

2–4 Tbsp. melted butter

White Sausage Gravy:

1	thick-cut slice bacon
12 oz.	breakfast sausage
1 tsp.	fresh sage, minced
1 Tbsp.	butter
2½ Tbsp.	flour
2½ cups	whole milk, at room temperature
½ tsp.	freshly cracked black pepper, plus extra kosher salt

Preheat oven to 500 degrees—or as high as your oven will go—for 1 hour before baking biscuits to ensure a super hot oven.

Sift first 5 ingredients together in a mixing bowl.

Incorporate cold butter into flour mixture by blending ingredients together using your hands, a fork, or a pastry blender until it resembles a course meal with pea-sized lumps. (*Note: If using your hands, work extra quickly so that the butter doesn't melt during the blending process. You can also process the flour mixture and butter in a food processor and pulse until the butter is cut into the flour and pea-sized crumbs appear. Return the butter-flour mixture to the mixing bowl before proceeding with the recipe.*)

Add buttermilk to flour and butter. Stir just until all the ingredients have come together in a ball of dough. (*Note: Try not to overwork the dough or you'll have tough biscuits!*)

Turn dough out onto a lightly floured surface. Press or roll dough into a 1-inch thick circle, working the dough as little as possible. Using a round cutter or ring mold dipped in flour, carefully cut out biscuits and arrange them on a sheet pan in a circle, with the edges of each biscuit nearly touching one another and 1 biscuit situated in the middle of the circle. Loosely form the remaining dough scraps into 1 biscuit.

Brush biscuits with melted butter. Bake in super hot oven for 10 to 12 minutes or until tops are golden brown.

Remove from oven and brush with more melted butter. Serve immediately. Biscuits are best eaten the day they are made.

WHITE SAUSAGE GRAVY

Cook bacon slice in a large sauté pan over medium heat until all fat has rendered out and the bacon is crispy, flipping after the first side has browned. Remove bacon from the pan and eat or save for another use.

Leaving bacon drippings in the pan, raise heat to medium-high. Once pan has heated and bacon fat is almost to the smoking point, add breakfast sausage to the pan, breaking it up into hunks as you drop it in. Brown sausage, stirring occasionally, and further breaking it up into smaller pieces, until well browned and just cooked through—6 or 7 minutes. Remove sausage from the pan.

Reduce heat to medium. Drain off all but 1 tablespoon rendered fat. Add butter and fresh sage to drippings. Once butter has melted, whisk in flour. Cook flour, whisking continuously, for about 2 minutes. If roux takes on any color, briefly remove from heat.

While whisking constantly, slowly drizzle in milk. Continue whisking until smooth. Stir in black pepper. Cook gravy until it just begins to boil. Reduce heat to low and simmer, stirring frequently, until thickened— 2 or 3 minutes. Add browned sausage back to gravy. Simmer for another minute. Adjust seasoning to taste with kosher salt and more freshly cracked black pepper. Serve immediately over split buttermilk biscuits.

Maple and Dry-Roasted Peanut Bars

with Chevre Shortbread Crust

There is a small amount of chevre in the shortbread crust, and while you can't necessarily detect its specific flavor, it adds a really nice element that would otherwise be missing. If you want a more pronounced chevre flavor, simply substitute more of the butter in the shortbread with more chevre.

MAPLE & DRY-ROASTED PEANUT BARS

For the shortbread base:

2 cups	flour
½ cup	(packed) brown sugar
½ tsp.	kosher salt
2 oz.	chevre, cubed
8 Tbsp.	(1 stick) butter, cut in cubes

For the filling:

8 Tbsp.	(1 stick) butter
1 cup	(packed) brown sugar
½ cup	pure maple syrup
3 Tbsp.	light corn syrup
2 Tbsp.	heavy cream
2¼ cups	salted dry roasted peanuts

For the glaze:

3 oz.	cream cheese, at room temperature
⅓ cup	pure maple syrup
⅔ cup	powdered sugar, sifted

Preheat oven to 350 degrees with the rack positioned in the middle of the oven.

Process first 3 shortbread ingredients in a food processor. Add butter and chevre and process until mixture forms pea-sized lumps. Pour mixture into a 9x13-inch metal baking pan. Using a flat-bottomed metal or plastic spatula, press shortbread crumbs into an even, compact layer. Bake shortbread at 350 degrees on the middle rack for 20 minutes until edges are golden.

While shortbread is baking, prepare filling. Whisk together first 5 filling ingredients in a saucepan over medium heat. Bring mixture to a simmer, stirring occasionally. As soon as mixture reaches a simmer, turn off heat and stir in peanuts.

Pour peanut filling over hot shortbread base as soon as base comes out of the oven. Return pan to the oven and bake for another 20 minutes until filling bubbles and edges start browning. Cool on a wire rack until room temperature.

While bars are cooling, whisk together glaze ingredients until smooth.

Once bars have cooled, run a knife around edges to loosen. Cut into 24 evenly sized bars. Once cut, drizzle with glaze in a zig-zag pattern. Let glaze set for 4 hours before serving. (*Note: Bars can be eaten as soon as they are glazed, but the topping won't set and may smudge if you are storing them for later.*)

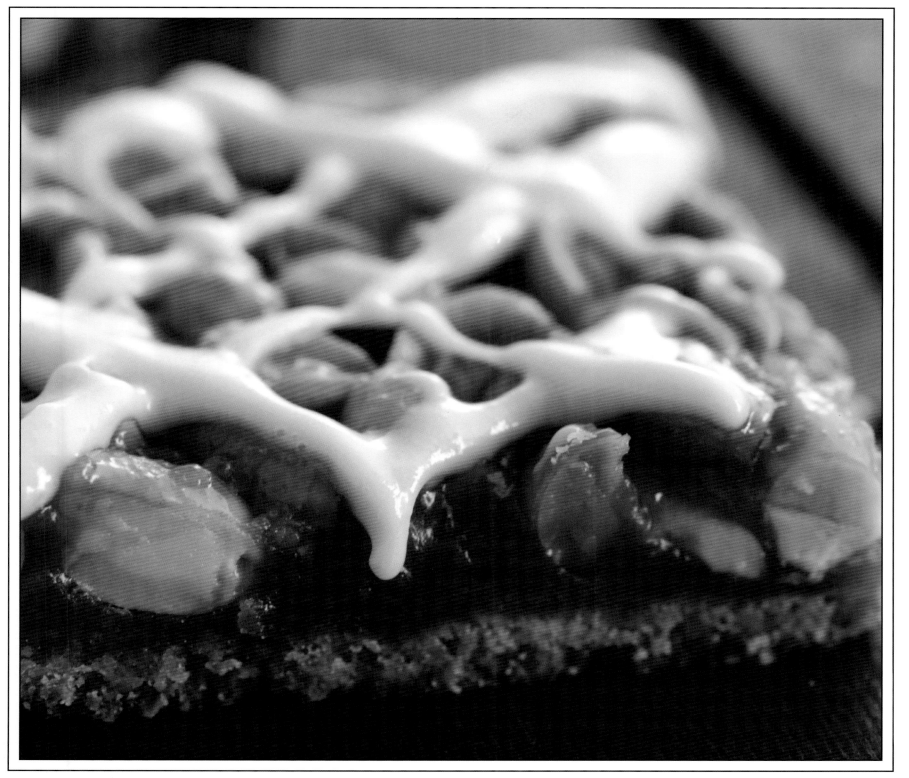

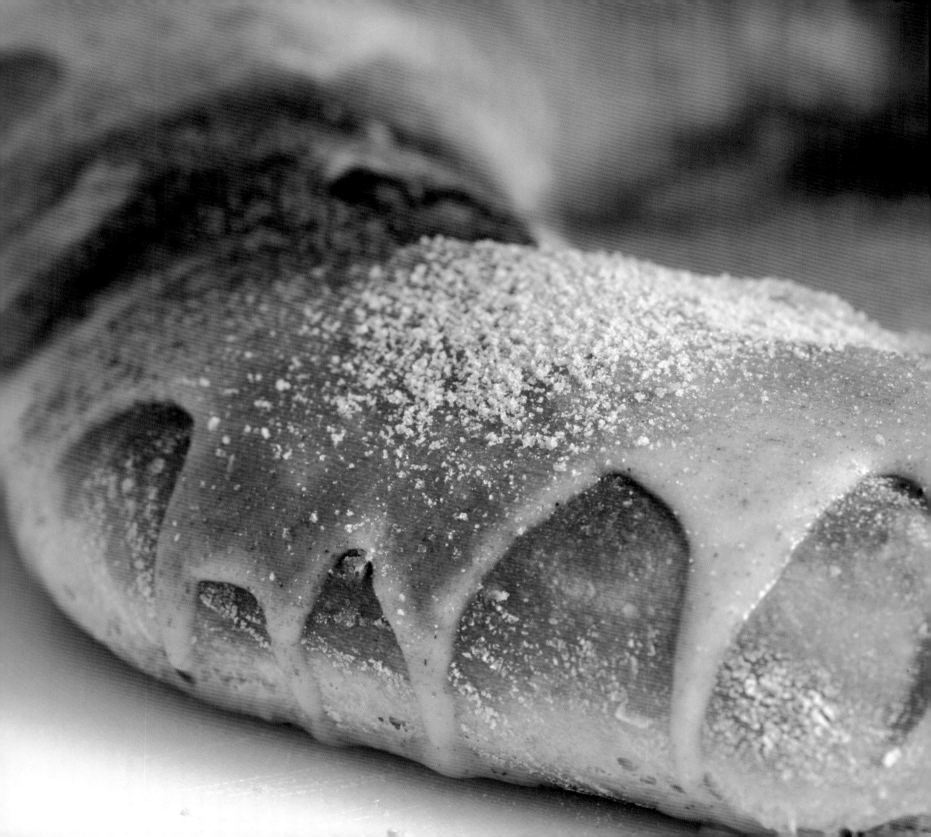

New Orleans' Style King Cake

with Apple-Cream Cheese Filling

It is traditional to hide a little plastic baby in the king cake after it has been baked. Whoever receives the slice with the baby is supposed to buy or bake the next cake for everyone to eat. With homemade king cakes, people will often insert a dried bean in lieu of the plastic baby. I've never actually done this because I'm always afraid that someone will accidentally chip a tooth or choke on it! As a side note, king cake should only be consumed during Mardi Gras season (after Twelfth Night and before Ash Wednesday). Eating or making a king cake out of season is unheard of!

COLORED SUGARS

Colored Sugars:

1 cup	Superfine/Caster Sugar, NOT powdered sugar
	red, yellow, and blue food coloring

For the dough:

2 Tbsp.	butter
¼ cup + 1 Tbsp.	sugar
½ tsp.	salt
8 oz.	sour cream
1	packet active dry yeast
¼ cup	lukewarm water, about 105 degrees
2¾–3¼	cups flour
	oil, for greasing the bowl

Divide caster sugar among 3 separate bowls. Dye one bowl purple with red and blue food coloring, one bowl yellow, and one bowl green using blue and yellow food coloring. Simply add food coloring to sugar and work dyes in with the back of a spoon until completely incorporated. You can make your colors as vivid as you like. Let the dyed sugar dry out for at least 2 hours before using, stirring occasionally to break up any clumps.

DOUGH

Grease a large, non-reactive mixing bowl liberally with oil for dough to rise in. Set aside.

Melt butter in a small saucepan over medium heat, and add ¼ cup sugar and salt. Stir to dissolve. Add sour cream and whisk until smooth. Heat sour cream mixture until lukewarm—about 105 degrees—stirring occasionally. Remove from heat. If sour cream heats over 110 degrees, allow it to cool to about 105 before proceeding.

While sour cream mixture is heating, add yeast to a large mixing bowl. Add warm water and 1 tablespoon sugar to yeast and stir. Let yeast mixture set for 5 minutes to activate (it should begin foaming and bubbling). If after 5 or so minutes, the yeast does not activate, discard mixture and start with new ingredients.

Add lukewarm sour cream mixture and 1 cup flour to activated yeast. Stir thoroughly. Add another 1¾ cups flour. Mix until fully incorporated. (*Note: The desired texture of the dough is soft, but not sticky or wet. During the kneading process, you will be able to incorporate more flour, so if the dough is just slightly sticky at this point, that's okay. It is much harder to add liquid once the dough has been formed, so I suggest adding less flour in the beginning and working it in as you knead. I find that just about three cups of flour gives me the soft dough texture desired.*)

Continued on Next Page

For the filling:

1	egg, beaten
8 oz.	cream cheese, at room temperature
¼ cup	sugar
2	Granny Smith apples, peeled, cored, and diced
½ tsp.	cinnamon
¼ tsp.	salt
⅓ cup	brown sugar
1 tsp.	corn starch
	juice from half a lemon

For the icing:

1 oz.	cream cheese, at room temperature
1½ cups	powdered sugar, sifted
2 Tbsp.	milk, plus extra as needed
	pinch of salt

Turn dough out onto a clean surface, lightly dusted with flour. Knead for 7 minutes, adding more flour as necessary. Shape dough into a ball and transfer to the oiled bowl. Flip the dough ball around so that all sides get evenly coated. Spray a sheet of plastic wrap with cooking spray, or grease with oil. Cover bowl with plastic wrap, greased-side down. Place a kitchen towel over plastic wrap to block out light. Let dough rise in a warm, draft-free location—I find that a spot near the preheating oven works well—until doubled in size, about 1 hour. While dough is rising, make fillings.

FILLING

Beat together first three filling ingredients until egg and sugar have been completely incorporated into cream cheese. Set aside. In a separate bowl, combine remaining filling ingredients, tossing until apple cubes are evenly coated.

Once dough has doubled, line a 2-foot long work surface with parchment paper. Dust parchment with flour to prevent dough from sticking. After lightly oiling your hands, carefully stretch dough out into an approximately 20-inch by 6-inch wide rectangle. (*Note: Ideally, the middle section of dough will be thicker than the edges, although that is easier said than done. If you find the dough sticking to the parchment paper, simply dust surface with a little more flour.*)

Leaving a 1-inch border on all edges, spread cream cheese mixture onto dough in a thin, even layer. Next, add apple mixture over cream cheese layer, maintaining a border. Starting with the edge closest to you, roll the dough—jelly-roll fashion—into a log. About 3 inches from the far side, wrap the unrolled edge to the top of the roll to complete the log. Press down on the seam firmly enough to adhere the two pieces together, but not hard enough to pierce the dough.

Very carefully, connect the ends of the log together to form an oval. Press the edges together firmly to completely seal off the oval. At this point, you should have a completely assembled king cake, seam-side up.

Slide king cake (on parchment paper) onto a large, flat, moveable surface, such as a cutting board. Line a sheet pan with parchment paper. Place lined sheet pan over cake. Being careful not to smash the cake, quickly invert the two surfaces, transferring king cake, now seam-side down, onto the parchment-lined baking sheet. Peel off top piece of parchment. Cover with a kitchen towel and let cake rise for another 30 minutes.

Bake at 375 degrees for 25 to 30 minutes or until golden. Remove from oven and on a wire rack for at least 30 minutes.

ICING

Whisk together icing ingredients until a smooth consistency suitable for drizzling. If icing is too thick, simply whisk in a *small* amount of milk until you've reached your desired consistency.

Once cake has cooled, drizzle icing evenly over cake, allowing it to run down the sides. Using a wire sieve, dust stripes of colored sugar in rotating colors, yellow, green, and purple. Best eaten the day it's made.

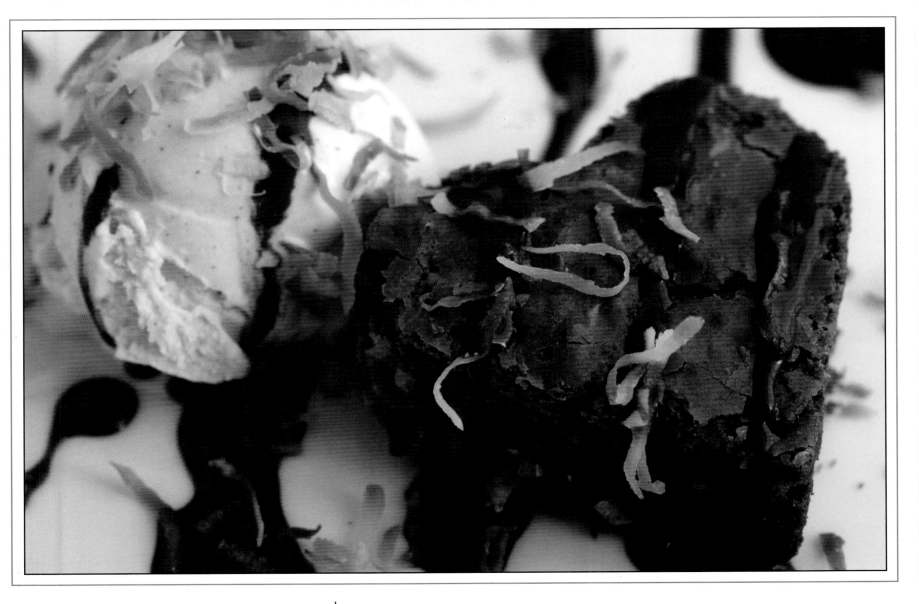

Coconut-Pecan Swirl Brownie Sundaes

with Vanilla Bean Ice Cream, Chocolate Sauce, and Toasted Coconut

My inspiration for this dessert originally came from taking the delicious coconut-pecan frosting element of a classic German Chocolate cake and swirling it into brownies. The outcome wasn't exactly what I had originally planned because the coconut mixture kind of melts into the batter, but every time I make these brownies they are eaten in a flash.

Continued on Next Page

Coconut-Pecan Swirl:

3 oz.	chopped pecans
1 can	sweetened condensed milk
7 oz.	sweetened flaked coconut
¼ tsp.	salt

Brownies:

8 oz.	semi-sweet chocolate chips
1 cup	(2 sticks) butter, cut in cubes
½ Tbsp.	instant espresso or coffee (optional)
4	eggs
1 Tbsp.	vanilla
¼ tsp.	salt
1 cup	(packed) brown sugar
¾ cup	granulated sugar
1 cup	flour

Special Equipment: heart-shaped cookie cutters

Toasted Coconut:

1 cup	sweetened coconut flakes

Preheat oven to 350 degrees. Spray a 9x13-inch metal baking pan with cooking spray. Set aside.

Stir all Coconut-Pecan Swirl ingredients in a mixing bowl until thoroughly combined. Set aside.

Bring 1 inch water in a large saucepan to a boil over medium-high heat.

While water is coming to a boil, combine chocolate chips, butter, and instant espresso to a heat proof bowl. (*Note: I always use a metal bowl.*)

Place bowl with chocolate and butter over the top of boiling water to create a double boiler. Stir constantly until chocolate and butter have melted completely. Scrape the sides of the bowl to prevent chocolate from burning. Remove from heat.

Beat eggs in a separate bowl. Add vanilla, salt, brown sugar, and granulated sugar. Whisk until thoroughly combined. Add melted chocolate mixture to egg mixture. Whisk to combine thoroughly.

Gently fold in half of flour until most of it has been incorporated. Fold in remaining flour until just incorporated. Do *not* overmix batter—overmixing leads to tough brownies.

Pour half of the brownie batter into the prepared baking dish. Add half of the coconut pecan swirl mixture in dollops into the brownie mix. Using a butter knife, swirl brownie batter and coconut mixture together. Pour remaining brownie batter into the pan and add remaining coconut in dollops. Again, swirl coconut and brownie batter together.

Bake brownies at 350 degrees for 30 to 40 minutes until a toothpick inserted into the middle of the brownies comes out mostly clean. (*Note: A few crumbs are okay but no batter should be visible on the toothpick.*) Do not overcook.

Cool on a wire rack for at least 30 minutes before slicing.

To plate, use a heart-shaped cookie cutter (optional) to cut out brownies. Place on a plate with a scoop of ice cream. Drizzle with chocolate sauce and garnish with a sprinkle of toasted coconut flakes.

TOASTED COCONUT FLAKES

Preheat oven to 350 degrees.

Spread coconut flakes out in a single layer on a baking sheet. Place into preheated oven. Toast for 8 to 9 minutes until golden, stirring occasionally.

Vanilla Bean Ice Cream:

3 cups	heavy cream
1 cup	whole milk
⅔ cup	granulated sugar
1/2 tsp.	salt
1	vanilla bean, sliced in half lengthwise
4	egg yolks
1 Tbsp.	pure vanilla extract

Special Equipment: ice cream machine

Chocolate Sauce:

4 oz.	semisweet chocolate chips
4 oz.	milk
4 oz.	heavy cream
1 Tbsp.	sugar

Heat first 5 ingredients in a large saucepan over medium-high heat, stirring frequently and scraping the bottom of the pan to prevent burning, until cream mixture is just about to come to a boil. While mixture is heating, beat egg yolks in a mixing bowl. As soon as cream is almost boiling, reduce heat to medium and remove pan from heat. Pull out vanilla bean and scrape beans from the inside of the pod. Discard or rinse and save to make vanilla sugar.

While whisking egg yolks constantly, slowly drizzle in 1 cup cream mixture to temper eggs. Stir tempered egg mixture back into pan with remaining heavy cream. Cook over medium heat for about 5 minutes, stirring constantly, until custard is thick enough to coat the back of a spoon—about 170 degrees, if you want to use a thermometer. Do not let mixture simmer, or eggs will curdle and you'll need to start over.

Strain ice cream base through a wire-mesh sieve. Cool for 30 minutes at room temperature. Chill base in the refrigerator, ideally overnight. (*Note: If you are in a time crunch, you can use an ice bath to cool the mixture quicker.*)

Pour chilled mixture into an ice cream machine and freeze according to the manufacturer's directions. Transfer frozen ice cream to an airtight container and place in freezer. Freeze for at least 2 hours or until firm, before serving.

BASIC CHOCOLATE SAUCE

Place chocolate chips in a heat-safe metal bowl.

Heat milk in a small saucepan over low heat. Heat to a bare simmer, stirring frequently.

Heat heavy cream and sugar in a separate small saucepan over medium heat, stirring frequently, until nearly at a boil.

Pour cream over chocolate chips. Slowly whisk chocolate and hot cream until chocolate has completely melted into cream. Add warmed milk to sauce and stir until completely incorporated. Cool to room temperature if using with ice cream. Store chilled for up to 7 days. Reheat using a double boiler.

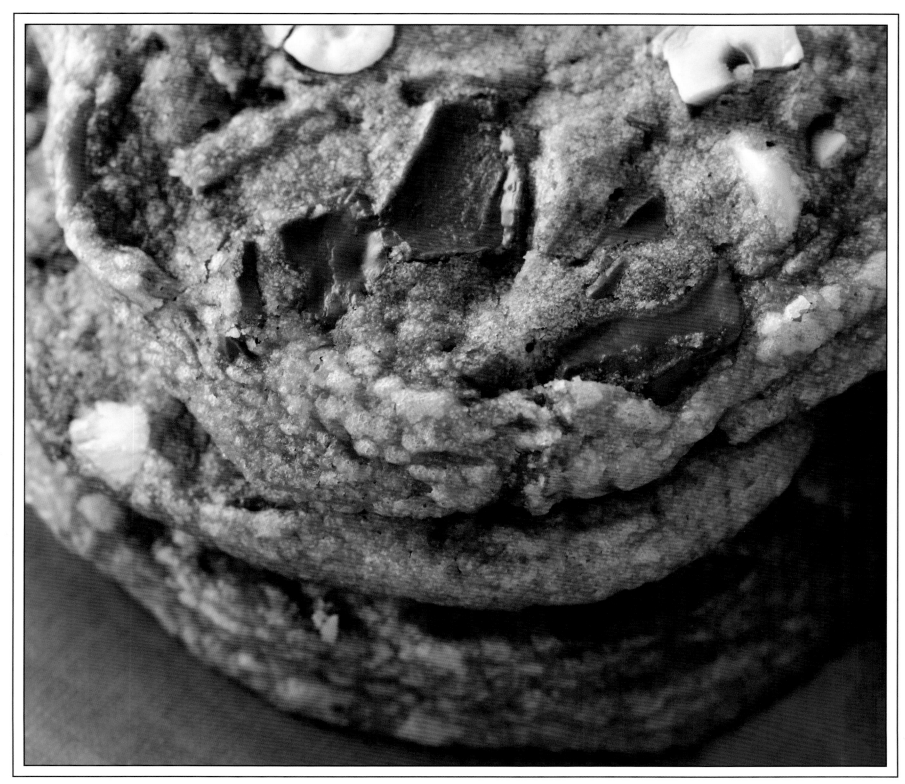

Chewy Brown Butter Cookies

with Milk Chocolate Chunks, Toffee, and Hazelnut

Shaping these cookies into a log serves two purposes in this recipe. If the dough is cooked as a drop cookie the ingredients won't be able to spread as much, causing the cookies to be thicker. By shaping the dough into a thick log you can slice off thinner portions of round dough solving this problem. Secondly you get the added bonus of having self-made "slice-n-bake" cookies in the fridge so you can bake as many or as few cookies as you're craving at the moment. These cookies should not be over-baked. For best results, remove them from the oven after 11 minutes. The middle of the cookie will look almost completely uncooked but as they cool to room temperature they will have the perfect consistency of a soft, chewy chocolate chip cookie.

CHEWY BROWN BUTTER COOKIES

1 cup	(2 sticks) butter
1½ cups	golden brown sugar
1 tsp.	salt
2	eggs
1½ tsp.	good vanilla extract
2¼ cups	flour
½ tsp.	baking soda
6 oz.	milk chocolate, either chips or chunks
3	Skor or Heath candy bars, roughly chopped
1 cup	hazelnuts, toasted, papery outer casing removed, and roughly chopped (see page 243)

Melt butter in a small saucepan over medium heat. Simmer melted butter, stirring occasionally, until it turns brown, about 5 minutes after the butter has melted. Be sure to stir and scrape the bottom of the pan while simmering to gauge the color of the butter. Do not allow the butter to burn. If the butter burns, discard and start over.

Let brown butter cool for 30 minutes at room temperature. Pour cooled brown butter into a large mixing bowl. Stir in brown sugar and salt until well blended. Add eggs one at a time, stirring after each addition until fully incorporated. Stir in vanilla. Next add flour and baking soda, stirring until flour is completely incorporated into cookie dough. Stir in chocolate chunks, chopped toffee, and hazelnuts until evenly disbursed throughout the dough.

Cover a flat work surface with a long piece of plastic wrap. Form cookie dough into a log with a diameter of about 3½-inches down the middle of the plastic wrap. Wrap plastic tightly around cookie log and twist ends, sealing like a Tootsie Roll. Chill cookie dough in the refrigerator for at least 4 hours and up to 3 days before proceeding. Cookie dough can be frozen in the log form for up to 1 month. Defrost before slicing and baking.

Preheat oven to 350 degrees.

Line a baking sheet with either parchment paper or Silpat.

Slice log into ½-inch wide slices. Arrange up to 6 portions of cookie dough onto the lined sheet pan, evenly spaced. The cookies will spread out while cooking, so don't overcrowd the pan. Bake cookies at 350 degrees for 11 to 13 minutes or until edges are golden. At 11 minutes, the cookies will look undercooked, but this is when the cookies should be removed from the oven if you want perfect cookies that will maintain softness for days. At 13 minutes, the cookies will look closer to cooked through and will still be soft in the middle but will have a little crispness around the edges. Remove from oven and cool on the pan on a wire rack for at least 20 minutes before transferring to another plate or eating. Toffee with be liquefied when first removed from the oven and will burn your mouth if eaten immediately.

Bake as many or as few cookies as desired. Store remaining cookie dough log, tightly wrapped in plastic in the fridge for up to 4 days.

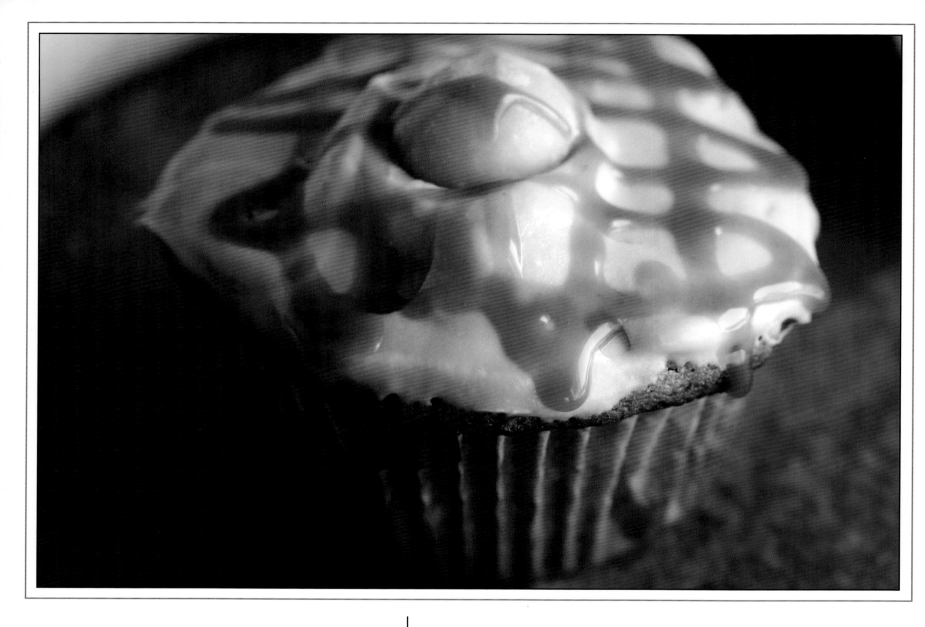

Banana, White Chocolate, & Macadamia Nut Cupcakes

Although not a cookie, white chocolate macadamia banana cupcakes make a great addition to the Christmas "cookie" plates I hand out to friends and family every year. Frankly, I make these any time of year when I find myself with bananas that are verging on "too ripe" to eat on their own. If you want to make the recipe a little healthier, substitute half of the butter with buttermilk.

BANANA, WHITE CHOCOLATE, AND MACADAMIA NUT CUPCAKES

Cupcakes:

2¼ cups	cake flour
¾ tsp.	baking soda
¼ tsp.	baking powder
½ tsp.	salt
3	very ripe bananas, peeled and mashed
⅓ cup	buttermilk
1 tsp.	pure vanilla extract
1½ cups	(3 sticks) butter
½ cup	granulated sugar
½ cup	(packed) brown sugar
2	eggs
1 cup	white chocolate chips
¾ cup	salted macadamia nuts, roughly chopped

Garnish:

24	whole salted macadamia nuts

Salted Caramel Sauce:

1¼ cup	granulated sugar
¼ cup	water
2 tsp.	kosher salt
⅔ cup	heavy cream

Salted Caramel Cream Cheese Frosting

See Page 241

Preheat oven to 350 degrees with rack positioned in the center of the oven. Line two 12-cup muffin tins with cupcake liners. Set aside.

Sift together first 4 ingredients. Set aside.

In a separate bowl, whisk together mashed bananas, buttermilk, and vanilla extract until well combined and set aside.

In a large mixing bowl, beat butter at medium speed until light yellow and fluffy. Add granulated sugar and brown sugar. Beat until fully incorporated and fluffy.

Add eggs one at a time, beating after each addition until egg is fully incorporated into the butter-sugar mixture before adding the next egg.

Once all eggs have been incorporated, add a third of the sifted flour mixture. Beat until flour is just barely incorporated. Add half of the banana mixture, beating again until just barely incorporated. Continue additions of a third of flour, remaining half of banana mixture, and final third of flour, beating each addition until just barely incorporated. Do not overwork the batter, or the cupcakes will be tough and dense rather than moist and crumbly.

After last addition of flour has been incorporated, fold in white chocolate chips and macadamia nuts.

Fill lined muffin tins about two-thirds full with batter. Bake at 350 degrees for 20 to 25 minutes until a toothpick inserted into the center of one of the cupcakes comes out clean—a few crumbs are okay but *no* batter should be on the toothpick. Remove pan from oven and cool on a wire rack for at least 30 minutes before removing cupcakes from tin. (*Note: If your oven isn't large enough to bake both pans of cupcakes on the middle rack at the same time, bake in batches.*)

Once cupcakes have cooled to room temperature, frost with Salted Caramel Cream Cheese Frosting, place a macadamia nut on top of each frosted cupcake, and drizzle with Salted Caramel Sauce.

SALTED CARAMEL SAUCE

Stir sugar, salt, and water in a medium (at least 2-quart) saucepan over medium-high heat. Stir, cooking over medium-high heat, until sugar has dissolved. Allow syrup to boil, untouched, until it reaches a deep amber color, about 350 degrees. Swirl pan occasionally to help distribute heat around the pan without stirring. Brush down sides of the pan as necessary with a pastry brush dipped in water to prevent sugar from crystallizing on the sides of the pan.

As soon as the syrup turns a deep amber color, remove pan from heat and add heavy cream. Caramel will bubble up furiously, which is why having a large pan is necessary. Reduce burner to low and return the pan to the heat. Stir until caramel has dissolved into cream. Boiled sugar/caramel is extremely hot and will cause bad burns if not handled carefully. Remove from heat and let cool to room temperature, at least 1 hour. Store in an airtight container in the refrigerator for up to 2 weeks. Allow caramel sauce to return to room temperature before using.

Blood Orange, Ginger Beer, and Tequila Cocktail

One of the strongest and, in my opinion, best ginger beers on the market is Stewart's brand. Stewart's ginger beer is one of the few that will actually make your mouth tingle and turn warm from the strength of the ginger. While any brand of ginger beer will work, this recipe was formulated with Stewart's and if you can find it, I would suggest using it.

BLOOD ORANGE, GINGER BEER, AND TEQUILA COCKTAIL

For garnishing all drinks:

¼ cup	blood orange juice
	zest from one blood orange
¼ cup	granulated sugar
	slices of blood orange for garnish

For each individual drink:

1 cup	ice
2 oz.	blood orange juice
1.5 oz.	tequila
	juice from 1 wedge of lime
3 oz.	strong ginger beer

Place ¼ cup blood orange juice into a bowl. In a separate bowl, combine blood orange zest and sugar.

Dip the rim of a high ball glass into orange juice first and then into orange zest-sugar mixture to coat the rim evenly.

In a cocktail shaker, combine a cup of ice, 2 ounces blood orange juice, 1.5 ounces tequila, and a squeeze of lime juice. Close the shaker and shake vigorously. If you don't have a cocktail shaker, combine ingredients in a liquid measuring cup and stir well. Pour beverage from shaker into the prepared high ball glass. Top drink off with ginger beer and stir lightly with a mixing stick or small spoon. Garnish the rim with a blood orange slice and serve immediately. (Repeat recipe over . . . and over . . . and over . . . as desired—and responsibly.)

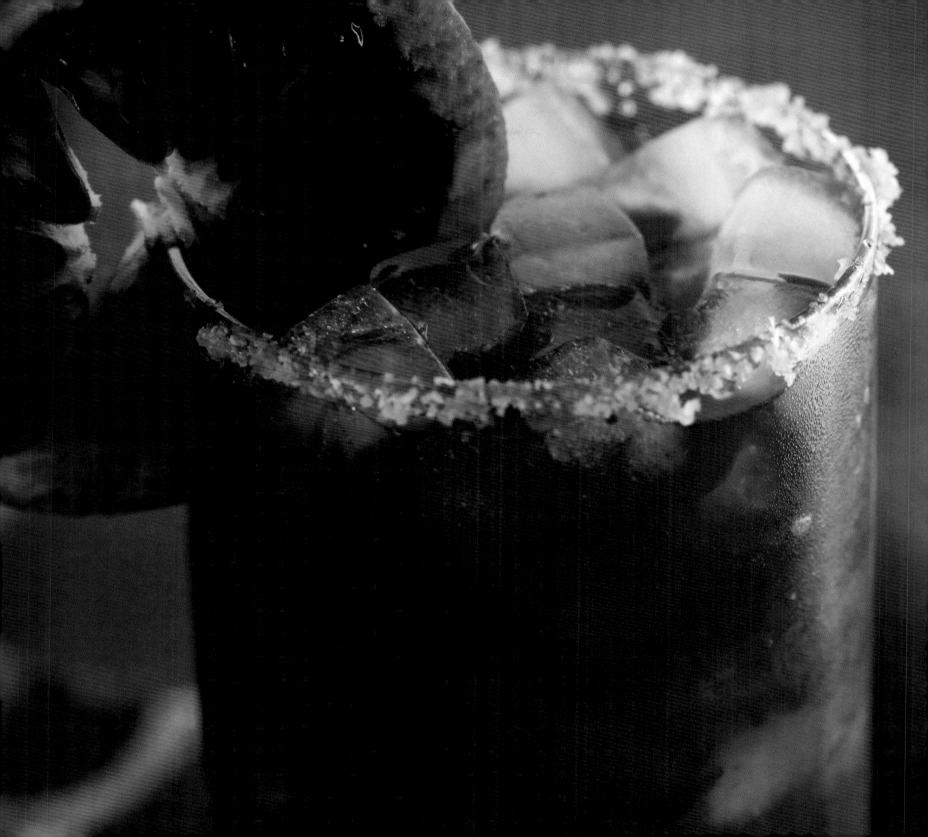

Basic Recipes & Techniques

ANCHO CHILE PIZZA SAUCE:

3 dried ancho chiles, stems and seeds removed

¼–½ cup steeping liquid

1 (14.5-oz.) can diced fire-roasted tomatoes, drained

1 clove garlic, peeled

¼ tsp. ground cumin

¼ tsp. kosher salt, plus extra

¼ tsp. freshly cracked black pepper

juice from ½ lime

Bring a large pot of water to a boil. Add chiles to boiling water and remove from heat. Place a plate or other heavy item on top of chiles to keep them submerged beneath the surface of the water. Steep chiles for 20 to 30 minutes until rehydrated. Reserve ½ cup steeping liquid then drain rehydrated chiles

Blend chiles with remaining ingredients and ¼ cup reserved steeping liquid until smooth. If sauce is too thick, thin out with a little more steeping liquid. Because this is a pizza sauce, it shouldn't be too thin so try not to over-dilute. Adjust seasonings to taste with kosher salt and freshly cracked black pepper.

ANCHO TOMATO SAUCE:

2 shallots

1 tsp. extra virgin olive oil

½ tsp. kosher salt, plus extra

¼ tsp. freshly cracked black pepper, plus extra

3 dried ancho chiles, stems and seeds removed

1 (14.5-oz.) can diced tomatoes

1 clove garlic

⅛ tsp. ground cinnamon

½ cup steeping liquid

Preheat oven to 350 degrees.

Cut shallots in half, leaving the peel on. Drizzle with 1 teaspoon olive oil and season with kosher salt and freshly cracked black pepper. Wrap shallots in aluminum foil. Roast at 350 degrees for 60 to 75 minutes until caramelized and tender. Remove from oven and let cool enough to handle. Squeeze shallots out of their peel and into a blender.

While the shallots are roasting, bring a large pot of water to a boil. Add chiles to boiling water and remove from heat. Place a plate or other heavy item on top of chiles to keep them submerged beneath the surface of the water. Steep chiles for 20 to 30 minutes until rehydrated. Reserve ½ cup steeping liquid and then drain rehydrated chiles

Add chiles, reserved steeping liquid and remaining ingredients for the sauce to the blender with roasted shallots. Pulse until smooth. Adjust seasonings to taste with more freshly cracked black pepper and kosher salt.

APPLE & TART CHERRY CHUTNEY:

1 cup cider vinegar

1 cup brown sugar

½ oz. (an inch-long piece) fresh ginger, peeled and roughly chopped

6 cloves garlic

½–1 serrano chile, stem removed, depending on desired heat

1 lb. Granny Smith apples, peeled, cored, and diced into ½-inch cubes

½ small yellow onion, peeled and diced

¾ cup dried tart cherries or cranberries

2 tsp. brown mustard seeds

1 star anise

⅛ tsp. ground cloves

⅛ tsp. ground allspice

½ tsp. kosher salt, plus extra

Bring cider vinegar and brown sugar to a boil in a large sauté pan over medium-high heat. Reduce heat to medium-low and simmer for 5 minutes until sugar has dissolved and vinegar has reduced slightly.

While vinegar is simmering, process ginger, garlic, and serrano chile in a food processor until finely minced. (*Note: If you don't have a food processor, chop by hand.*) Stir in remaining ingredients, including minced garlic mixture, to vinegar. Simmer, stirring occasionally, over medium-low heat until chutney thickens and water has almost all cooked away—40 to 50 minutes. Remove from heat and cool to room temperature. Serve at room temperature or chilled. Chutney will store for up to 2 weeks refrigerated.

ARUGULA PESTO:

1 clove garlic

2 Tbsp. toasted almonds, roughly chopped

1 ½ cups arugula leaves

juice from ½ lemon

¼ tsp. kosher salt

¼ tsp. freshly cracked black pepper

3 Tbsp. olive oil

1 oz. freshly grated Parmigiano Reggiano

Process garlic and almonds in a food processor until minced. Add remaining ingredients, except cheese. Process until completely pureed. Add cheese and process again. Store in an airtight container, chilled, until ready for use, up to 1 day in advance.

AVOCADO-YOGURT SAUCE:

1 ripe avocado, peel and pit removed

½ cup whole milk plain yogurt

juice from 1 lemon

½ serrano chile (or less if you don't like spice)

1 small clove of garlic

½ tsp. kosher salt, plus extra

Blend all ingredients in a blender until silky smooth. Adjust seasoning to taste with more kosher salt.

BAILEY'S BUTTERCREAM:

4 oz. cream cheese, at room temperature

½ cup (1 stick) butter, at room temperature

16 oz. powdered sugar, sifted

¼ tsp. salt

¼ cup plus 2 Tbsp. Bailey's Irish Cream liqueur

Beat all ingredients in a mixing bowl until smooth.

BUTTERY ROASTED POTATOES:

2 extra large or 3 large Yukon gold potatoes (about 1½ lbs.)

4 Tbsp. butter

kosher salt and freshly cracked black pepper

Preheat oven to 400 degrees.

Bring a large pot of heavily salted water to a boil over high heat.

Slice potatoes in ¾-inch thick slices. Add potato slices to water and boil for 5 minutes. Drain.

Arrange boiled potatoes on a baking sheet. Toss with butter to coat. Once butter has melted from the heat of the potatoes, it should pool around potatoes on the baking sheet. Season both sides of potato slices liberally with kosher salt and freshly cracked black pepper. Bake seasoned potatoes 400 degrees for 20 minutes until caramelized on the bottom. Flip potatoes and bake for another twenty minutes until both sides are golden and buttery. Remove from oven and serve immediately.

CINNAMON ICE CREAM:

3 cups heavy cream

1 cup whole milk

⅛ cup granulated sugar

½ tsp. salt

1 vanilla bean, sliced in half lengthwise

1 cinnamon stick

1 ½ tsp. ground cinnamon

4 egg yolks

1 tsp. pure vanilla extract

Special Equipment: ice cream machine

Heat first 7 ingredients in a large saucepan over medium-high heat, using the tip of a knife to scrap seeds from vanilla bean into cream. Stir frequently and scrape bottom of the pan to prevent burning until cream mixture is about to come to a boil. While mixture is heating, beat egg yolks in a separate mixing bowl. As soon as cream is near boiling, reduce heat to medium and remove pan from heat. Discard cinnamon stick and vanilla bean pod.

While whisking egg yolks constantly, slowly drizzle in 1 cup hot cream mixture to temper eggs. Stir tempered egg mixture back into pan with remaining heavy cream. Place the pan over medium heat and cook for about 5 minutes, stirring constantly, until custard is thick enough to coat the back of a spoon (about 170 degrees if you want to use a thermometer). Do not let the mixture reach a simmer or eggs will curdle and you will need to start over.

Strain ice cream base through a wire-mesh sieve. Cool for 30 minutes at room temperature. Chill thoroughly in the refrigerator, ideally overnight. If you're in a time crunch, you can use an ice bath to cool the mixture more quickly.

Pour chilled mixture into an ice cream machine and freeze according to the manufacturer's directions. Transfer frozen ice cream to an airtight container and freeze for at least 2 hours, or until firm, before serving.

CORNMEAL PIZZA CRUST

1½ cups bread flour, plus extra for dusting

½ cup cornmeal, plus extra for dusting

1 tsp. kosher salt

¾ cup + 2 Tbsp. warm water, about 105 degrees

1 tsp. sugar

1 packet active dry yeast

2 Tbsp. olive oil

Preheat oven to 500 degrees or as high as it will go.

Liberally oil a large mixing bowl and set aside.

Whisk together flour, cornmeal, and salt in a mixing bowl or the bowl of a stand mixer.

In a separate bowl, dissolve sugar and yeast in water. Stir to combine. Let yeast mixture sit for about 5 minutes until foaming and bubbling. If the yeast is not clearly active at this point, discard mixture and start again with fresh ingredients.

Once yeast is active, add it and the olive oil to the flour mixture. Stir until flour pulls away from the bowl and forms a ball of dough. If using a stand mixer, attach dough hook and mix at medium speed for 6 minutes. If kneading by hand, turn dough out onto a lightly floured surface and knead for 10 minutes. Form kneaded dough into a ball and place in oiled bowl. Turn dough around to coat with oil. Cover the bowl with greased plastic wrap, greased side down, and a kitchen towel. Place in a warm, draft free area to rise. (*Note: I often place it by the preheating oven.*) Let dough rise until doubled in size, about 1 hour. Punch down dough and let rise for another 30 minutes until it's doubled again. Alternately, you can punch down dough and refrigerate overnight to allow yeast to ferment longer and have a better flavor. If refrigerated, let sit at room temperature until it doubles in size, about 1½ hours.

Divide dough in half; recipe will make 2 pizzas.

Line a large sheet pan with parchment paper on a large sheet pan and dust with cornmeal.

Dust your hands with flour and dough ball with cornmeal. Take one dough ball in your hands. Working from the outer ½-inch edge of dough, begin pinching and lightly pulling dough, working in a circle, until you have formed the outer crust. This dough is relatively loose, so be careful not to rip it. Carefully stretch dough into a circle and place on the parchment-lined sheet pan.

Top as desired. Bake in a super hot oven for 10 to 12 minutes or until crust is crisp and golden on the bottom and cheese is golden and bubbly.

CUTTING CITRUS SUPREMES:

First, slice off the top and bottom ends of the citrus fruit, removing all of the pith down to the actual flesh. Set the trimmed, flat edge of the fruit onto a cutting board. Working from the top, carefully slice off remaining pith and skin by cutting off strips, following the curve of the citrus. Once all of the skin and pith has been removed, holding the citrus over a bowl to collect the juice and carefully run your knife between each segment of membrane, working your way around the entire fruit, to extract the citrus supremes, leaving the membrane behind. Try not to squeeze the fruit during this process. Place the supremes into a separate bowl from the juice. Once all of the supremes have been cut, squeeze any excess juice from the remaining membranes. Discard membranes.

DATE CREAM CHEESE ICE CREAM:

For the Base:

1 cup half-and-half

1 cup heavy cream

½ vanilla bean

¼ tsp. ground cinnamon

⅔ cup Medjool dates,
    pitted and roughly chopped

¾ cup sugar

¼ tsp. salt

2 eggs

For Step Two:

8 oz. cream cheese, at room temperature

½ cup Medjool dates,
    pitted and roughly chopped

Special Equipment: ice cream machine

Bring first 5 base ingredients to a simmer in a small saucepan over medium heat, using the tip of a knife to scrape seeds from vanilla bean into cream. Stir occasionally, being sure to not allow base mixture to reach a boil. Remove vanilla bean pod from cream. Rinse and let air dry. Save for making vanilla sugar if so desired.

While cream is coming to a simmer, whisk sugar, salt, and eggs in a mixing bowl until fluffy and light yellow.

While whisking eggs constantly, *slowly* drizzle in hot cream in small amounts to temper eggs. If you add hot cream all at once, eggs will scramble and you will need to start over. Once half of cream has been incorporated, pour in remaining ingredients. Stir to combine. Pour ice cream base into a blender. Blend until very smooth. Cover ice cream base and place in the refrigerator to cool for at least 4 hours or up to 1 day.

Beat room temperature cream cheese in a mixing bowl until fluffy with a rubber spatula.

Add ½ cup chilled ice cream base to cream cheese. Beat until fully incorporated and smooth. Add another ½ cup liquid and whisk until smooth. Add remaining ice cream base and whisk until fully incorporated. Stir in chopped dates, separating chunks as you go. Stir.

Pour ice cream base into the bowl of the ice cream maker. Freeze the ice cream according to the manufacturer's directions. Once frozen, transfer ice cream to an air tight container. Freeze ice cream for at least 3 hours before serving.

DEMI-GLACE:

Although this recipe is specifically for lamb demi-glace, you can replace the lamb bones with beef, veal, buffalo, duck, or chicken bones to make whatever variety of demi-glace you require. While demi-glace takes a long time to make, it is very easy and requires little active cooking time other than skimming.

For **Bouquet Garni:**

2 sprigs thyme

1 dried bay leaf

6 stems flat leaf parsley

½ tsp. black peppercorns

cheesecloth and butcher's twine

5 lbs. lamb bones

2 carrots, roughly chopped

1 large yellow onion, cut in quarters

1 leek, discard green part

¼ cup tomato paste

Place thyme, bay leaf, parsley stems, and peppercorns into the middle of a piece of cheesecloth. Tie into a sealed bundle using butcher's twine. Set aside.

Preheat oven to 450 degrees.

Place bones into a roasting pan large enough so that they can sit in a single layer without any overlapping. Roast bones until lightly browned, about 1½ to 2 hours. Scatter carrots, onion, and leek around bones. Return to oven and roast for another 40 to 50 minutes until well browned. Don't let anything burn or caramelize to the point of turning black. This will turn entire stock bitter and ruin your demi-glace.

Transfer bones and vegetables to a large stock pot. Place roasting pan on burners over medium heat. Add 2 cups water to roasting pan to deglaze, scraping the pan to dissolve any flavorful bits stuck to the bottom of the pan. Pour liquid from the roasting pan into the stock pot with bones and vegetables. Add tomato paste, bouquet garni, and enough cold water to cover bones by two inches. You can continue to add

more water to stock as it simmers, if necessary.

Simmer stock over medium-high heat. It's important not to try to heat the stock too quickly or to simmer the water too rapidly. This will cause the impurities to be swirled back into the stock. Simmer stock for 12 to 24 hours. Skim any fatty froth that arises about every 10 minutes for the first hour. For the remainder of the simmering process, skim every 30 to 45 minutes. Skimming will help prevent a cloudy stock. Add more cold water as necessary during simmering process to keep bones completely submerged.

Once stock has finished simmering, strain through a fine mesh sieve or chinois into a new, clean stock pot. Don't force any liquid through the sieve using a utensil; rather, tap the sides of the sieve to loosen the particles that are clogging the strainer. Using force or pressing the liquid through will lead to an impure stock. Discard bones and other solids.

Reduce strained stock over medium-high heat until only 1 cup of demi-glace remains, skimming occasionally. Keep a watchful eye to make sure you do not over-reduce the stock. Cool to room temperature and store in an airtight container, refrigerated for up to 1 week or frozen for up to 6 months.

DRIED BEANS:

Instead of buying canned beans, you can easily cook them yourself. To cook any kind of dried bean—other than lentils or split peas—soak beans overnight in a large pot of cold water. Soaking is an optional step but it will dramatically reduce cooking time. Drain beans. Bring a large pot of liberally salted water to a boil over high heat. Add beans and return liquid to a boil. Reduce heat to low and gently simmer until beans are soft and cooked through. Do not try to cook beans above a gentle simmer or exterior shells will crack, and beans will turn to mush. Any desired spices can be added to the braising liquid, or you can sauté aromatics like onions, celery, or carrots in the pot before adding water. Once cooked, drain beans and eat plain or use in recipes or salads.

DUCK STOCK:

2 ducks, skin removed

1 bottle dry red wine

1 large yellow onions, cut in quarters

2 carrots, roughly chopped

3 stalks celery, roughly chopped

stems from 1 bunch of parsley

1 tsp. dried oregano

1 tsp. dried basil

1 tsp. dried thyme

2 tsp. whole black pepper corns

2 Tbsp. kosher salt

lots of water

Cover all ingredients in a large stock pot with at least 3 or 4 inches water. Bring to a boil over medium-high heat. Once stock has reached a boil, reduce heat to medium-low and simmer for 1½ hours, occasionally skimming off any froth or scum that rises to the surface.

While stock is simmering, preheat oven to 400 degrees.

Remove duck carcasses from stock and let cool enough to handle, about 20 minutes. Remove all meat from ducks, reserving for gumbo or another use. Roast remaining duck bones on a baking sheet at 400 degrees for 45 minutes to 1 hour or until bones begin to brown.

Transfer browned bones back into stock pot. Continue to simmer for another 2 hours, adding more water if necessary. Strain. Allow stock to cool to almost room temperature and chill overnight in the refrigerator. Skim off any hardened fat from stock before using. Stock can be stored frozen for up to 1 year.

FRIED LEMON SLICES:

1 lemon

peanut oil for frying

kosher salt

Heat oil in a deep-fryer filled to the manufacturer's "fill line" until hot, about 20 minutes.

While oil is heating, slice lemon into whole ring slices as thin as possible—$\frac{1}{16}$- to $\frac{1}{8}$-inch thin—using a mandoline. Discard slices that are all pith or stem.

Once oil is hot, fry lemon slices in batches of 3 for about 1 minute per batch, stirring occasionally, until pulp of lemon has fried away and turned brown and the rind and pith begin to turn golden. Remove from oil using a spider or slotted spoon and drain on paper towels. Sprinkle with a small amount of kosher salt. Repeat frying and draining process two more times with remaining lemon slices.

FRIED SUSHI RICE CAKES:

1 cup Calrose rice (or other sticky sushi rice)

1 tsp. kosher salt

1 cup & 2 Tbsp. water

canola or peanut oil for frying

Place rice in a large bowl. Fill bowl with cold water. Using your hand, swish rice around until the water turns cloudy, gently rubbing the grains together with your fingers as if you were polishing them. Drain and repeat this process 3 more times until the water runs nearly clear.

Pour rice into a wire mesh sieve and let drain for at least 30 minutes or up to 6 hours.

Place rice and 1 cup + 2 Tbsp. water into a small saucepan or rice cooker. Let rice soak in water for 30 minutes. If using a rice cooker, add salt, stir, and simply cover and turn on the rice cooker. If using a pan, add salt, stir, and bring water to a boil over high heat. Cover and let cook for 1 minute at high heat. After 1 minute, reduce heat to medium and cook for 5 minutes. Reduce heat to low and cook for another 10 minutes. Do not peek at the rice during the cooking process. Remove rice from heat and let steam in the pan for another 10 minutes. Fluff with a fork. Rice should be sticky and tender.

Allow rice to cool enough to handle. Rice may be made up to 1 day in advance.

Grease a sheet pan and set aside. Form rice into four evenly sized patties. Set on the greased

pan until ready to use.

Fill a large pot or deep sauté pan with ½-inch oil and preheat over medium-high heat. To test oil temperature, stick the end of a wooden spoon into the oil. If oil is hot, lots of bubbles will form around the wood. Once oil is hot, fry 2 rice patties for 2 to 4 minutes until golden on the bottom. Carefully flip patties and fry for another 2 to 4 minutes until second side is golden as well. Remove from heat and place on paper towels to drain. Repeat frying and draining process with remaining 2 rice patties. Serve immediately once all patties are fried.

GREEN OLIVE TAPENADE:

1 cup pitted green olives

1 anchovy filet

1 Tbsp. capers

¼ cup flat leaf parsley

1 clove garlic

juice and zest from ½ lemon

1 Tbsp. olive oil

¼ tsp. freshly cracked black pepper

Process all ingredients in a food processor until well pureed—about 30 seconds. Store chilled for up to 4 days.

GRILLED OR ROASTED ASPARAGUS:

1½ lbs. asparagus spears, fibrous ends trimmed

2 tsp. canola oil

kosher salt and freshly cracked black pepper

Prepare grill for medium-high heat.

If asparagus spears are fat, use a peeler to peel stalks, leaving only the top 2½ inches unpeeled. Drizzle with oil and sprinkle with kosher salt and freshly cracked black pepper. Toss to coat.

Grill seasoned asparagus until beginning to char, 3 to 4 minutes, flip and continue grilling for another 3 minutes until grill marks appear on other side and asparagus is cooked through. Remove from heat and serve immediately.

Alternately, if it's too cold outside to grill the asparagus, you can roast it. Preheat oven to 425 degrees. Arrange seasoned asparagus spears on a sheet pan. Roast at 425 degrees for 12 to 15 minutes until spears begin to caramelize on the bottom and are just cooked through. Serve immediately.

HARISSA PASTE:

4 dried chile de árbol or cayenne chiles

4 dried ancho chiles

4 dried guajillo chiles

4 cloves garlic, peeled

½ tsp. ground coriander

1 tsp. ground caraway seeds

½ tsp. ground cumin

½ tsp. dried mint

1 tsp. kosher salt

juice from 1 lemon

3 Tbsp. extra virgin olive oil, plus extra

Bring a pot of water to a boil over high heat. Once boiling, remove pot from heat and add all dried chiles to hot water. Place a plate or other heavy object on top of chiles to keep them submerged. Rehydrate dried chiles in hot water for about 20 minutes.

Drain off all water from rehydrated chiles. Remove stems from chiles and most seeds from larger ones. Puree chiles in a blender with remaining Harissa ingredients until very smooth. Transfer Harissa to an airtight container. Cover top of paste with a thin layer of oil to help preserve color during storage. Seal container and store in refrigerator for 3 to 4 weeks.

HOMEMADE BARBECUE SAUCE:

1 Tbsp. canola oil

1 small yellow onion, diced

1 Tbsp. fresh ginger, peeled & minced

1 (14.5-oz) can diced tomatoes

1 bulb roasted garlic, separated into cloves

3 Tbsp. brown sugar

1 Tbsp. molasses

3 Tbsp. yellow mustard

3 Tbsp. Worcestershire sauce

¼ cup apple cider vinegar

¼ tsp. freshly cracked black pepper

½ tsp. chili powder

½ tsp. smoked paprika

⅛ tsp. ground cloves

kosher salt

Preheat oil in a medium-sized saucepan over medium heat. Once oil is hot, sauté diced onion over medium heat until translucent, stirring frequently, about 10 minutes. Add ginger to onion and sauté for another minute. Stir in remaining ingredients and bring to a simmer. Reduce heat to low. Simmer over low heat, stirring occasionally, for 25 minutes.

Transfer, mixture to a blender. Blend until very smooth. If sauce is too thick, thin out with 1 tablespoon water at a time until consistency of thick barbecue sauce is reached. Season to taste with kosher salt. Transfer sauce to an airtight container or jar and let sit, refrigerated, for at least 12 hours so that the flavors have time to marry. Barbecue sauce can be made up to 1 week in advance and stored chilled until ready for use.

HORSERADISH MAYONNAISE:

⅓ cup mayonnaise

1 Tbsp. prepared horseradish

1 Tbsp. coarse-grain mustard

freshly cracked black pepper, to taste

Whisk all ingredients together well in a small bowl. Store chilled until ready for use. Makes about 4 servings.

IRISH WHISKEY GANACHE:

½ cup heavy cream

6 oz. semi-sweet chocolate chips

2 oz. Irish whiskey

Place chocolate chips in a heat-proof bowl.

Heat cream over medium-high heat until simmering—but not boiling—stirring occasionally. Pour hot cream over chocolate chips and stir until chocolate has melted and ganache is smooth and silky. Add whiskey and stir until fully incorporated. Let ganache cool to room temperature. Refrigerate for about 30 minutes, stirring every 10 minutes, until ganache is the thickness of a frosting.

MACERATED STRAWBERRIES:

1 quart fresh ripe strawberries,
    hulled and quartered

2–3 Tbsp. granulated sugar,
    depending on sweetness of berries

1 Tbsp. tequila

1 Tbsp. rosewater

1 tsp. freshly squeezed lemon juice

pinch of salt

Toss strawberries with remaining ingredients in a non-reactive mixing bowl. Allow strawberries to macerate at room temperature for 1 hour, stirring occasionally. After one hour, move berries to the refrigerator and allow berries to macerate, chilled, for another 2 hours, stirring occasionally.

MANGO-BANANA SALSA:

1 slightly green banana, peeled and diced

1 mango, peeled, pit removed and diced

½–1 jalapeño, minced
    (depending on desired heat)

1 Tbsp. fresh cilantro, minced

juice from 1 lime

1 cup micro greens (optional)

kosher salt and freshly cracked black pepper

Add all ingredients to a bowl. Toss and season to taste with kosher salt and freshly cracked black pepper.

MEXICAN CORNBREAD:

Dry **ingredients:**

1 cup cornmeal

¼ cup flour

½ tsp. baking soda

½ tsp. baking powder

½ tsp. kosher salt

¼ tsp. dried oregano

½ tsp. granulated garlic

½ tsp. onion powder

½ tsp. ground cumin

½ tsp. chili powder

1 Tbsp. granulated sugar

Wet **ingredients:**

1 cup + 2 Tbsp. buttermilk

1 egg

3 Tbsp. melted butter

For **greasing the pan:**

1 Tbsp. butter, room temperature

Preheat oven to 450 degrees.

Coat a regular-sized 12-muffin tin liberally with 1 tablespoon room temperature butter.

Whisk together all dry ingredients in a large mixing bowl.

Whisk together wet ingredients in a separate bowl.

Pour wet ingredients into dry ingredients and whisk until combined. Let set for 5 minutes.

While cornbread batter is resting, place the liberally buttered muffin tin into the hot oven. Heat the muffin tin for 4 minutes at 450 degrees. The butter in the tins may brown and that's okay.

Remove hot tin from the oven. Using a ¼-cup scoop, quickly fill hot muffin tins evenly with cornbread batter. Bake at 450 degrees for 12 to 14 minutes or until a toothpick inserted into middle of the muffins comes out mostly clean. A couple of crumbs on the toothpick are okay but no batter! Remove from oven and let cook 10 minutes before removing from tin and serving. Cornbread is best eaten the same day it is made.

MINTED BLACK-EYED PEA HUMMUS:

1 cup cooked or canned black-eyed peas (if canned, rinse beans)

1 cup cooked or canned garbanzo beans (if canned, rinse beans)

¼ cup tahini

juice from ¹ or 2 lemons

¼ mint leaves

3 cloves garlic, peeled

⅓ cup water

¾ tsp. kosher salt, plus extra

⅓ cup good olive oil

Place all ingredients except oil into a blender. With blender running, drizzle in olive oil until smooth. Adjust seasoning to taste with more kosher salt. If the hummus is still too thick, thin it out with a small amount of water until

the desired consistency is reached. Chill and let flavors marry for at least 30 minutes before serving.

MUSTARD STOUT CHEESE DIP:

½ cup stout beer

1 Tbsp. butter

1 Tbsp. flour

¾ cup whole milk, at room temperature

3 Tbsp. coarse grain mustard

2½ oz. Gruyere, grated

2½ oz. white extra sharp cheddar, grated

kosher salt and freshly cracked black pepper

Reduce beer in a saucepan over medium-high heat to about ¼ cup, stirring frequently. Beer will frequently foam up while reducing, so keep a watchful eye over it. Add beer reduction to whole milk and set aside.

Melt butter in a separate saucepan over medium heat. Add flour to melted butter to make a roux. Cook roux, whisking constantly, for about 1 to 2 minutes to cook off the raw flour flavor. Do not let the roux brown at all—if necessary, remove pan from heat to slow down the cooking. While vigorously whisking, slowly

drizzle in warm beer-milk mixture until smooth and completely incorporated. Add mustard and whisk again. Cook over medium heat for 5 to 10 minutes, stirring frequently, until simmering and thickened slightly. Once thickened, remove from heat and add cheese. Stir until melted. Adjust seasonings to taste with kosher salt and freshly cracked black pepper.

ORANGE-SAGE VINAIGRETTE:

¼ cup freshly squeezed orange juice

1 Tbsp. red wine vinegar

1 Tbsp. whole grain mustard

¼ tsp. granulated garlic

¼ tsp. onion powder

½ tsp. freshly cracked black pepper

2 medium fresh sage leaves, minced

½ tsp. kosher salt

3 Tbsp. canola oil

In a mixing bowl, whisk together all ingredients *except* canola oil. While continuing to whisk vigorously, slowly add canola oil in a thin stream to form an emulsified vinaigrette. Adjust seasoning to taste with kosher salt and freshly cracked black pepper.

PINEAPPLE FILLING:

1 Tbsp. butter

1 ripe pineapple, peeled, cored and diced

½ tsp. salt

1 cup (packed) brown sugar

2 oz. rum

1 Tbsp. water

1 Tbsp. cornstarch

Melt butter in large sauté pan over medium heat. Add pineapple, salt, and brown sugar to the pan and stir. Sauté until simmering. Pour rum into pan with sautéing pineapple. Carefully light rum on fire. (There is such a small amount of rum compared to the other liquid in the pan that it won't burn for long.) Let pineapple simmer over medium to medium-low heat for about 45 minutes, stirring occasionally, until all but 1 cup of liquid from pineapples remains in the pan.

Whisk together water and cornstarch in a small bowl until cornstarch has completely dissolved. Pour cornstarch slurry into pan with simmering pineapple and stir. Simmer until liquid has thickened into almost a gel consistency, stirring occasionally, for 2 to 3 minutes. Remove from heat and let cool to at least room temperature before using as a cake filling.

PIZZA CRUST:

2 ¼ cups bread flour

1 tsp. salt

1 tsp. sugar

1 package dry active yeast

¾ cup + 2 Tbsp. warm water, about 105 degrees

2 Tbsp. olive oil

semolina flour or cornmeal, for dusting

olive oil, for greasing

Preheat oven to 500 degrees or as high as it will go.

Liberally oil a bowl and set aside.

Whisk flour and salt to a mixing bowl or the bowl of a stand mixer.

In a separate bowl, dissolve sugar and yeast in water. Stir to combine. Let yeast mixture sit for about 5 minutes until foaming and bubbly. If the yeast is not clearly active after 5 minutes, discard mixture and start again with fresh ingredients.

Add active yeast and olive oil to flour. Stir until flour pulls away from the bowl and forms a ball. If using a stand mixer, attach the dough hook and knead at medium speed for 6 minutes. If kneading by hand, turn dough out onto a lightly floured surface and knead for 10 minutes. Form kneaded dough into a ball and place in oiled bowl. Turn ball of dough around to coat with oil. Cover bowl with greased plastic wrap, greased-side down, and a kitchen towel. Place in a warm, draft-free area to rise. Let dough rise until doubled in size, about 1 hour. Punch down dough and let rise for another 30 minutes until it's doubled again. Alternately, you can punch down dough and refrigerate overnight to allow yeast to ferment longer and have a better flavor. If you choose this option, remember to let dough sit at room temperature until it doubles in size, about 1½ hours.

Divide dough in half; dough recipe will make 2 pizzas.

Grease a large sheet pan with olive oil and dust with cornmeal or semolina flour.

Dust your hands with flour and dough ball with cornmeal or semolina flour. Take one dough ball in your hands. Working from the outer ½-inch edge of dough, pinch and lightly pull dough, working around it in a circle, until you have formed the outer crust. Next, using your hands balled into fists, begin gently pulling dough out slightly and rotating, tossing it slightly into the air and rotating as you gently stretch out the dough. Keep your fists toward the outside of the dough as the center will stretch as the edges do. Continue stretching, tossing, and rotating until you have a large, thin, rounded crust. Place crust onto the prepared baking sheet.

Top as desired. Bake in a super hot oven for 10 to 12 minutes or until crust is crisp and golden on the bottom and the cheese is golden and bubbly.

POMEGRANATE HARISSA VINAIGRETTE:

1 tbsp Harissa

1/2 tsp pomegranate molasses

1 tbsp red wine vinegar

1/4 tsp kosher salt

1/8 tsp freshly cracked black pepper

3 tbsp canola oil

Combine first 5 ingredients for the vinaigrette in a mixing bowl. Whisk. While continuing to whisk vigorously, slowly drizzle in the canola oil to form an emulsified vinaigrette. Adjust seasonings to taste with kosher salt and freshly cracked black pepper.

PRESERVED LEMONS:

8–10 lemons

coarse flaked kosher salt, like Morton's

fresh squeezed lemon juice, as necessary

1 large sterilized jar

Scrub lemons very clean, removing any dirt from the rind.

Pour enough kosher salt into sterilized jar to cover the bottom.

Cut about a dime-sized slice off of both ends of the lemons to remove stem area. Stand one lemon up onto a cut end. Slice lemon as if you were going to cut it in half lengthwise, but only cut about three-fourths of the way through lemon, keeping base fully attached. Make a second cut, perpendicular to the first, so that lemon is basically quartered yet attached at the bottom. Liberally season lemon, inside and out, with about 1 tablespoon kosher salt, packing salt into the cavity of the lemon. Place lemon into prepared jar. Repeat slicing and salting process with remaining lemons, stacking lemons on top of one another and compacting them as much as you can in the jar. Once you've packed as may salted lemons as possible into the jar, top with 2 tablespoons kosher salt and add enough freshly squeezed lemon juice

so that lemons are completely submerged. Place lid tightly onto the jar.

Let lemons sit on the counter for 2 to 3 days. Flip jar upside down every 12 or so hours and let sit upside down until you flip it again so that the top lemons have an equal chance to preserve. After 2 or 3 days, transfer jar of preserved lemons to the refrigerator. Let lemons continue to preserve for about 3 more weeks before using, flipping jar upside down occasionally. Once preserved, remove pulp from lemon and rinse thoroughly before using rind in recipes. Store in refrigerator completely submerged in salted lemon juice for up to 6 months.

PRESERVED LEMON OLIVE GARNISH:

½ preserved lemon, pulp removed, rinsed, and minced

4 green olives, pitted and minced

1 Tbsp. cilantro, minced

1 pinch red pepper flakes

1 pinch freshly cracked black pepper

Place all ingredients into a small bowl. Toss to evenly distribute. Will keep in refrigerator for up to 2 days. For a longer shelf-life, wait to add cilantro until ready for use.

RASPBERRY JAM

8 oz. fresh ripe raspberries

1 cup granulated sugar

¼ tsp. salt

1 Tbsp. fresh-squeezed lemon juice

Add all ingredients to a saucepan and place over medium heat. Stir and mash the berries with a fork or potato masher to assist in the breakdown process. Once the sugar has dissolved into the juices from the berries, let the mixture come to a boil. Boil for about 3 to 4 minutes until thickened slightly into a gel. Remove from heat and let cool for about 30 minutes at room temperature then transfer to an airtight container. Place container into the fridge and chill for 24 hours before using. If refrigerated the whole time, jam will stay good for up to 1 month.

RED WINE DEMI-GLACE SAUCE:

1 bottle red wine

1 sprig rosemary

2 cloves garlic

1 tsp. whole black peppercorns

3 oz. lamb (or beef) demi-glace, store-bought or homemade

kosher salt

Simmer first 3 ingredients in a saucepan over medium-high heat, stirring occasionally until reduced to about ¾ cup liquid. Strain reduction and return to heat. Add demi-glace and stir until completely melted and incorporated. Remove from heat. Adjust seasoning to taste with kosher salt. Different brands of store-bought demi-glace have varying levels of sodium. If you use store-bought demi-glace and the sauce is too salty without adding any extra seasonings, dilute with water until palatable.

ROASTED CARROT SAUCE:

15 baby carrots

1 tsp. extra virgin olive oil

kosher salt and freshly cracked black pepper

½ cup chicken stock

¼ tsp. ground cumin

⅛ tsp. ground ginger

⅛ tsp. cayenne

small pinch ground cinnamon (about 1/16 tsp.)

small pinch ground cloves

Preheat oven to 350 degrees. Place carrots onto a baking sheet. Coat with olive oil and season with kosher salt and freshly cracked black pepper. Place carrots into preheated oven. Roast at 350 for 1 hour, tossing every 15 minutes, until caramelized on all sides.

Add carrots into a blender with remaining ingredients. Puree until very smooth. If necessary, thin sauce out with a touch more stock. It should be thick for a sauce but thinner than a puree. Adjust seasoning to taste with kosher salt and freshly cracked black pepper. For a smoother sauce, strain through a fine mesh sieve.

ROASTING CHILES AND PEPPERS:

To roast fresh chiles or peppers, toss with a small amount of oil to coat. Using tongs, hold chiles directly in the flame of a gas burner, rotating occasionally, until charred on all sides. If you don't have access to a gas burner, you can place the lightly oiled chiles/peppers on a sheet pan under a preheated broil. Broil, flipping occasionally, until charred on all sides. As soon as chiles are charred, place in a resealable plastic bag or in a bowl sealed with plastic wrap. Let chiles steam for at least 20 minutes. Once steamed, the papery exterior skin of the chiles should be easy to remove by hand. Remove skin and discard seeds and stems before using.

ROASTED GARLIC:

1 whole bulb garlic

canola or olive oil

kosher salt and freshly cracked black pepper

Preheat oven to 350 degrees.

Cut off just the tip of the pointed-end of garlic bulb to expose tips of each clove. Drizzle exposed cloves with canola oil, and then sprinkle with kosher salt and freshly cracked black pepper. Wrap completely in aluminum foil with exposed-clove side facing up inside the packet. Place foil packet into oven and roast at 350 for 1 hour. Remove from oven and let cool enough to handle. Remove cloves by squeezing base of bulb until cloves push out.

ROASTED GARLIC SMASHED RED POTATOES:

1½ lb. red skinned potatoes, quartered

4 Tbsp. butter

⅓ cup whole milk, plus extra

cloves from 1 bulb roasted garlic,
  roughly chopped

kosher salt and freshly cracked black pepper

Place quartered red potatoes in a pot and cover with 1 inch water. Liberally season water with a handful of kosher salt. Bring pot with potatoes to a boil over high heat. Boil potatoes until very tender and skin starts peeling away from the potato. To check tenderness, stab a potato quarter with a fork. Drain off all water. Place potatoes back into pot. Add butter, whole milk, and roasted garlic to potatoes. Using a potato masher, smash the potatoes, working in all of the butter, garlic, and milk until fluffy, leaving some lumps of potato. If potatoes appear dry, add 1 tablespoon milk at a time, stirring until incorporated, until potatoes are moist and fluffy. Season to taste with kosher salt and freshly cracked black pepper.

ROASTED GARLIC TURNIP PUREE:

cloves from 1 bulb of roasted garlic

1½ lb. turnips, peeled and cut in 1½-inch cubes

2 Tbsp. butter

¼ cup whole milk, plus extra, if needed

kosher salt and freshly cracked black pepper

Bring a pot of water to a boil over high heat.

Add a handful of kosher salt and allow water to return to a boil. Add turnip cubes. Boil until tender and easily pierced with a fork, about 15 minutes. Strain well.

Add cooked turnips, butter, roasted garlic, and milk to a food processor. Process until smooth. If necessary, thin with more milk. Season to taste with kosher salt and freshly cracked black pepper.

ROASTED JALAPEÑO VINAIGRETTE:

2 roasted jalapeño peppers

2 Tbsp. sherry vinegar

juice from 1 lime

1 large clove garlic, roughly chopped

2 Tbsp. cilantro

¼ tsp. freshly cracked black pepper, plus extra

¼ tsp. kosher salt, plus extra

6 Tbsp. canola oil

Place roasted jalapeños and all other ingredients for the vinaigrette *except* canola oil into a food processor or blender. Process until well pureed. With the machine running, slowly drizzle in canola oil to form an emulsified vinaigrette. Adjust seasoning levels as desired with more kosher salt and freshly cracked black pepper.

SALTED CARAMEL FROSTING:

½ cup salted caramel sauce

8 oz. cream cheese, at room temperature

2 cups powdered sugar, sifted

Beat together all ingredients until smooth and free of lumps using either a whisk, hand-beater, or stand mixer.

SAUTÉED ONIONS AND PEPPERS:

1 Tbsp. olive oil

1 red onion, peeled and sliced

1 red bell pepper, stem and seeds removed, julienned

1 orange bell pepper, stem and seeds removed, julienned

2 cloves garlic, minced

½ tsp. dried oregano

kosher salt and freshly cracked black pepper

juice from ½ a lemon

Heat olive oil in a large sauté pan and place over medium-high heat. Once pan and oil are hot (just before oil starts to smoke) add onions and peppers to the pan. Sprinkle with dried oregano, kosher salt, and freshly cracked black pepper. Sauté, stirring occasionally, for 5 minutes. Add minced garlic and sauté for another minute. Squeeze lemon juice over vegetables and stir to deglaze the pan. Remove from heat and taste. Adjust seasoning to taste with kosher salt and freshly cracked black pepper.

SESAME BRITTLE:

1 cup sesame seeds

⅔ cup sugar

½ tsp. salt

3 Tbsp. honey

1 Tbsp. water

Line a sheet pan with aluminum foil, shiny side-up.

Toast sesame seeds in a dry sauté pan over medium heat until golden, stirring frequently. Remove from heat and place onto a plate to cool.

Add sugar, salt, honey, and water to a medium-sized saucepan over medium heat. Whisk until the sugar dissolves into a thick syrup.

Once sugar has dissolved, let mixture boil until amber, carefully swishing the pan to distribute heat rather than stirring during boiling process. The sugar mixture will be *extremely* hot, so be careful from this point on. Stir toasted sesame seeds into caramel and quickly pour mixture onto the foil-lined pan. Working quickly so that the candy doesn't harden, use an off-set metal spatula to spread candy into a thin ⅛-inch layer. Let firm until completely cool, and invert brittle onto a cutting board and peel off foil. Break into shapes as desired. Store in a sealed container at room temperature for up to 3 months.

SMOKY ROASTED RED PEPPER SAUCE:

2 thick-cut slices bacon

½ yellow onion, diced

3 cloves garlic, minced

2 roasted red peppers, diced

3 sprigs fresh thyme

1 (14.5-oz) can diced tomato

¼ tsp. ground cayenne

½ tsp. smoked paprika

⅓ cup heavy cream

kosher salt and freshly cracked black pepper

Render fat from bacon in a large sauté pan

over medium heat until bacon is brown and crispy, flipping after one side has browned. Remove from pan and drain on paper towels. Drain off all but about 2 teaspoons bacon fat from pan. Return pan with remaining fat to heat and add diced onions. Sprinkle with a pinch of salt and stir. Sauté the onions over medium heat, stirring occasionally, until translucent, about 10 minutes. Add garlic and sauté for another 60 seconds, stirring occasionally so that the garlic doesn't brown. Add roasted red peppers, thyme sprigs, cayenne, and paprika. Stir and cook for another minute. Stir in tomatoes, cream, and browned bacon. Let simmer over medium heat, stirring occasionally, for 20 to 25 minutes until thickened slightly. Remove bacon and thyme sprigs and discard. Transfer contents of the pan to a blender. Blend until smooth. Season to taste with kosher salt and freshly cracked black pepper.

SPICY MANGO PEANUT SAUCE:

1 ripe mango, peeled pitted

1 Tbsp. Sambal Oelek (or less, for less heat)

1 Tbsp. creamy peanut butter

juice from 1 lime

3 Tbsp. water

¼ tsp. kosher salt, plus extra

Blend all ingredients in a blender until very smooth. Adjust seasoning to taste with kosher salt.

SPICED POMEGRANATE PISTACHIOS:

¼ tsp. hot paprika

¼ tsp. ground cumin

¼ tsp. freshly cracked black pepper

½ tsp. kosher salt

½ tsp. pomegranate molasses

½ cup shelled unsalted pistachios

Preheat oven to 350 degrees.

In a small bowl, stir together first 4 ingredients. until evenly distributed. Add pomegranate molasses. Stir to thoroughly combine. Add pistachios to pomegranate spice mixture. Using your hands, toss to coat nuts evenly. Spread seasoned pistachios onto a sheet pan in a single layer.

Roast seasoned pistachios at 350 degrees for 8 to 10 minutes, tossing halfway through, until caramelized and toasted. Remove nuts from baking sheet immediately to prevent further cooking. Let cool at least 15 minutes and then roughly chop.

SWEET POTATO FENNEL AND ANCHOVY GRATIN:

1½ cups heavy cream

2 cloves garlic, peeled and minced

6 anchovy filets, minced (or about 1 Tbsp. anchovy paste)

2 Tbsp. fennel fronds, minced

1 ½ cups + 2 Tbsp. heavy cream

3 sweet potatoes, peeled and sliced ⅛-inch thick

1 large bulb of fennel, trimmed and sliced ⅛-inch thick

kosher salt and freshly cracked black pepper

Preheat oven to 375 degrees.

Whisk together the first 4 ingredients.

Drizzle 3 tablespoons cream mixture over the bottom of an 8x8-inch square baking dish. Spread cream mixture to evenly coat the bottom of the pan. Arrange an even layer of sweet potatoes, slightly overlapping, in the bottom of the dish. Drizzle potatoes with 3 tablespoons cream mixture. Sprinkle lightly with kosher salt and freshly cracked black pepper. Scatter a few pieces of fennel over seasoned potato layer. Add another even layer of sweet potato slices, pressing down firmly on potatoes to pack down the gratin. Repeat process of drizzling with cream, seasoning with salt and pepper, scattering with fennel slices, topping with more potatoes, and compacting the gratin until all ingredients have been used, ending with a top layer of potatoes drizzled with cream. For the top layer, brush cream mixture evenly over potatoes so the whole surface area is coated with cream. Sprinkle with salt and pepper.

Bake at 375 degrees for 60 to 75 minutes or until nearly all cream has been absorbed and the top is golden brown. If the top browns faster than cream cooks away, loosely cover the dish with aluminum foil to prevent further browning. Remove from oven and let sit for 10 minutes before cutting and serving.

THAI RED CURRY BEURRE BLANC:

½ cup dry white wine

2 tsp. Thai red curry paste

1 tsp. freshly squeezed lime juice

4 Tbsp. butter, very cold, cut in 6 even pieces

Whisk together first 3 ingredients in a small saucepan over medium-high heat. Reduce white wine mixture down to a little more than 2 tablespoons liquid. Do not over-reduce.

Once liquid has reduced, reduce heat to low. Add one piece of cold butter at a time to reduction, whisking constantly after each addition until fully incorporated. If the butter is added too quickly or at too high of a temperature, the sauce will separate. Once all butter as been added, serve immediately or keep warm in a metal bowl placed over a saucepan of hot water until ready to serve.

TOASTING NUTS AND SEEDS:

To toast most nuts, preheat oven to 350 degrees. Spread nuts out in a single layer on a sheet pan. Toast at 350 degrees until golden, tossing every 3 to 4 minutes. Remove from oven and let cool to room temperature before eating or chopping. Different nuts will take different amounts of time to toast.

To toast pine nuts (pignoli), sesame seeds, or pepitas (hulled pumpkin seeds), preheat a dry sauté pan over medium heat. Once the pan is hot, add nuts or seeds. Toast in the dry pan (without oil), tossing frequently for even toasting, until golden.

VANILLA BEAN WHIPPED CREAM:

seeds scraped from ½ vanilla bean

1 cup heavy whipping cream

pinch salt

1½ Tbsp. granulated sugar

Place all ingredients into a small saucepan over medium heat. Bring to a bare simmer, stirring frequently. Remove from heat and place into the refrigerator to chill until cold—at least 2 hours.

Beat chilled, sweetened cream (either using a stand mixer with whisk attachment at medium speed or whisking vigorously by hand) until stiff peaks form. (If whipping by hand, the task will be much easier if you get the cream and the bowl very cold before whipping.)

WATERCRESS PESTO:

1 clove garlic

2 Tbsp. walnut pieces

1 cup packed watercress leaves

juice from ½ a lemon

1½ Tbsp. olive oil

¼ tsp. kosher salt

¼ tsp. freshly cracked black pepper

¼ cup freshly grated Parmigiano Reggiano

Process garlic and walnuts in a food processor until minced. Scrape down the sides of the bowl and then add remaining ingredients. Puree until all ingredients are finely chopped and form a thick paste. Adjust seasonings to taste with kosher salt and freshly cracked black pepper.

WHIPPED CREAM:

2 cups heavy whipping cream, very cold

¼ cup granulated sugar

Place whipped cream and sugar into the bowl of a stand mixer with the whisk attachment. Whip the cream at medium speed until the whipped cream holds relatively stiff peaks.

Whipped cream can also be beaten by hand in a large mixing bowl with a whisk. Whisk vigorously until the whipped cream holds stiff peaks.

WHIPPED WHITE CHOCOLATE GANACHE:

1 cup heavy whipping cream

6 oz. high-quality white chocolate chips

½ tsp. high-quality vanilla extract

pinch salt

Scald whipping cream in a small saucepan over medium heat, bringing cream almost to a boil but removing it from the heat just before it begins to boil. Stir occasionally to prevent scorching on the bottom of the pan.

While cream is heating, place remaining ingredients for ganache into a heat-safe mixing bowl.

Once cream has scalded, pour it over the white chocolate chips. Whisk slowly until chocolate has completely melted and the mixture is smooth and silky. Let ganache cool at room temperature for about 30 minutes and then cover and refrigerate for 12 hours to 2 days. It is important that the ganache gets very cold before whipping.

Using a whisk, hand-beater, or stand mixer, beat ganache mixture until very thick streaks occur and mixture is whipped and fluffy.

YOGURT-CILANTRO CHUTNEY:

½ cup plain yogurt, not non-fat

2 green onions, roughly chopped

1 cup cilantro leaves

juice from 1 lime

1 serrano chile, stem removed (use more or less depending on preferred heat)

¼ tsp. ground cumin

¼ tsp. ground fenugreek

⅛ tsp. ground coriander

1 clove garlic

1 tsp. ginger, minced

½ tsp. kosher salt, plus extra

Blend all ingredients in a blender or food processor until smooth. Adjust seasonings to taste with kosher salt and freshly cracked black pepper. Refrigerate for 30 minutes before serving so the flavors have a chance to marry.

Specialized Ingredients

Achiote Paste:

A tangy, thick, deep red paste made from the seeds of the annatto tree, garlic, citrus, salt, and spices. Achiote paste is commonly used for marinating pork, chicken, fish or other proteins. Originating from the Yucatan region of Mexico, achiote paste is also known as *recado colorado*. Available in the Hispanic foods sections of some grocery stores, gourmet markets, Mexican markets, or at http://www.mexgrocer.com.

Anaheim Chile:

A long green chile with mild heat; also known as a California green chile. Available fresh in the produce section of most grocery stores.

Ancho Chile:

The dried version of a poblano chile; heat levels vary from mild to medium. Available in most grocery stores, gourmet markets, Mexican markets, or at http://www.mexgrocer.com.

Anchovy Paste:

Made from cured anchovies and primarily used in sauces and spreads. Available in most grocery stores, gourmet markets, or at http://www.igourmet.com.

Asian Pears:

Also known as apple pears, these pears are sweet, juicy, and crisp in texture without the graininess found in European varieties. Available in the produce section of most grocery stores and Asian markets.

Baby Kiwi:

Also known as a hardy kiwi, this small green fruit can be eaten whole and tastes just like it's larger, furry cousin. Although it originated in Asia, it is commercially grown in Oregon and New Zealand. Available seasonally at markets such as Trader Joe's, Whole Foods, and other gourmet markets.

Blood Oranges:

A variety of orange with crimson colored flesh. U.S. blood oranges are grown in Texas from December to March and in California from November to May. Available seasonally in the produce section of some grocery stores, gourmet markets, or at http://www.localharvest.org/store/.

Buffalo Meat:

Also known as bison, buffalo meat tastes similar to beef but is leaner and lower in cholesterol. Buffalo meat is widely available across the U.S. in the butcher department of some grocery stores, gourmet markets, and at http://www.jhbuffalomeat.com/

Buffalo Mozzarella:

Fresh mozzarella cheese made using buffalo milk. Stored in whey and best eaten within days of being made. The flavor of buffalo mozzarella is slightly tangier than cow's milk mozzarella but is equally creamy. Available at some grocery stores, gourmet markets, cheese shops, and at http://www.markys.com

Calrose Rice:

A variety of japonica medium-grain rice that was developed in California in the early 1970s. Once cooked, the grains are soft and stick together easily, making it a perfect rice for sushi. Available in most grocery stores, gourmet markets, Asian markets, or at http://www.sushimaven.com.

Cara Cara Navel Oranges:

A variety of navel orange with rosy flesh, ranging anywhere from pinkish to deep red. Cara Cara oranges are low in acid and have a naturally sweet flavor. Available late November to January in the produce section of some grocery stores such as Trader Joe's or Whole Foods, gourmet markets, and at http://www.pearsonranch.com.

Cardamom:

A pungent and aromatic spice native to India and Southeast Asia. Sold in whole-seed pods, seeds removed from the pods, or seeds removed and ground. Available in the spice section of most grocery stores, gourmet markets, or online at http://www.penzeys.com.

Celery Root:

Also known as Celeriac, celery root is a lumpy tuber vegetable in the celery family with a thick brown outer skin, which should be peeled before using, and a cream colored flesh. Available in the produce section of most grocery stores or produce markets.

Chile de Árbol :

A spicy, bright red dried chile that is curved and narrow in shape. Available in most grocery stores, gourmet markets, Mexican markets and online at http://www.mexgrocer.com.

Chile Pequin

A very spicy, small, dried red chile commonly called a pinhead pepper, chile mosquito, chile petin, or chiltepin. Available in some grocery stores, Mexican markets, and online at http://www.mexgrocer.com.

Chipotle in Adobo:

Canned chipotle peppers (smoked jalapeños) stored in adobo sauce—a sauce made from vinegar, tomatoes, onions, garlic, spices, and other chiles. Available in most grocery stores, gourmet markets, Mexican markets, and online at http://www.mexgrocer.com.

Chorizo:

A bright red pork sausage, available both dried and fresh, and boldly seasoned with smoked chiles, peppers, and other spices. Chorizo originated from the Iberian Peninsula and is now available in three distinct styles: Spanish, Portuguese, and Mexican. In recipes in this book, fresh Mexican chorizo is typically recommended. Available in the butcher's department of most grocery stores, specialty butcher's shops, Mexican markets, and online at http://www.mexgrocer.com.

Cotija:

A hard Mexican cheese made from cow's milk used for grating or crumbling. Fresh Cotija resembles Feta cheese in flavor and texture, while aged Cotija is used more like Parmigiano-Reggiano. Available in the cheese section of most grocery stores, Mexican markets, and online at http://www.mexgrocer.com.

Crème Fraîche:

A thick, slightly soured cream product made by letting unpasteurized cream—or pasteurized cream with the addition of buttermilk or yogurt—sit at room temperature until thickened. The flavor of crème fraîche is less sour than that of sour cream and it does not "break" when acid is introduced or if added to other sauces. Crème fraîche can be found in the dairy department of some grocery stores, gourmet markets, cheese shops, and online at http://www.markys.com.

Cremini Mushrooms:

The same strain of mushroom as a portabella, harvested after 40 days of growth, whereas the portabella is harvested around 45 days. Cremini mushrooms are brown and slightly earthier than button mushrooms but still mild in flavor, making them a great all-purpose mushroom. They are available in most grocery stores, although they may be sold under the name "Baby 'Bellas."

Dandelion Greens:

The edible leaves of the common yellow dandelion family. Bitter in flavor and most tender when picked before the flowering stage. Available seasonally in your backyard, the produce section of some grocery stores, and gourmet markets.

Dried Chili Mango:

Dried mango that has been tossed with chili powder and often lime juice. Available in the dried fruit section of some grocery stores, Mexican markets, and at http://pattysnack.net.

Dried Tart Cherries:

Made from slightly sweetened dehydrated tart or sour cherries. Flavor is similar to that of dried cranberries. Available in the dried fruit section of some grocery stores, gourmet markets, and online at http://www.mi-cherries.com.

Enoki Mushrooms:

Tiny mushrooms with long slender stalks and small umbrella caps, sold in clusters still attached at the base. Commercially cultivated enoki are white in color due to the lack of sunlight during the growing process, while wild enoki are anywhere from yellow to orange-brown. Available at some grocery stores such as Whole Foods, gourmet markets, Asian markets, and online at http://www.sidwainer.com/.

Fenugreek:

A Eurasian spice that comes in the form of dried brownish yellow seeds or leaves and is an essential spice in Indian cooking and most curry dishes and curry powders. Available in the spice section of some grocery stores, gourmet markets, Middle Eastern and Indian Markets, and online at http://www.penzeys.com.

Frangelico:

A hazelnut-flavored liqueur. Available in liquor stores and online at http://www.bevmo.com.

Ginger Beer:

A non-alcoholic soda flavored predominantly with ginger root. Of the ginger beers available on the market, Stewart's brand ginger beer is the strongest and, in our opinion, best for using in mixed drinks. Stewart's ginger beer can be found in various grocery and convenient stores. While Stewart's ginger beer is not available online, you can purchase other gingers beers at http://www.bevmo.com

Grape Leaves:

Pickled leaves from grape vines sold in jars. Used for dolmas and other variations of stuffed grape leaves such as the Vietnamese dish *thit bo cuon la luop.* Available in some grocery stores, gourmet markets, Middle Eastern markets, and online at http://www.greekinternetmarket.com.

Greek Yogurt:

Plain, unflavored yogurt that has been strained for a thick consistency. Fage is a terrific brand of Greek-style yogurt and is available in the dairy department of most grocery stores, gourmet markets, and online at http://parthenonfoods.net.

Gruyère:

A nutty, hard cow's milk cheese in the Swiss family. Available in the specialty cheese section of most grocery stores, gourmet markets, at cheese shops, or online at http://www.igourmet.com.

Guajillo Chiles:

Dried medium-spicy chiles with a reddish-brown, shiny, smooth exterior and a tough, thick skin that requires a longer soaking time than other chiles. Available in some grocery stores, gourmet markets, Mexican markets, and online at http://www.mexgrocer.com.

Harissa:

A spicy North African condiment made from chiles, garlic, coriander, cumin, and caraway. Harissa is easy to make (see page 234) or can be purchased in some grocery stores, gourmet markets, and online at http://www.markys.com.

Insta Cure No. 1:

The ingredient that will give your corned beef it's typical vibrant pink color. It is a compound of sodium nitrate and salt that is used when curing and smoking meats to prevent botulism. Insta Cure No. 1 can be purchased in 8-ounce, 1l-pound, and 5-pound packages online from http://www.sausagemaker.com

Lamb Demi-Glace:

A rich, concentrated stock made from lamb bones, aromatic vegetables, and tomato paste. Time consuming but easy to make at home (see page 231) or available in high-end, or specialty gourmet stores, and at http://www.thespicehouse.com.

Lemongrass:

A tall, perennial grass with a citrus flavor that is used frequently in Southeast Asian cuisines both fresh and dried. Available fresh in the produce section or dried in the spice section of some grocery stores, gourmet markets, Asian markets, and online at http://grocerythai.com.

Linguiça:

A mildly spicy smoked pork sausage from Portugal. Available in many grocery stores, gourmet markets, butchers, and at http://foodoro.com.

Mache:

A small, mild-flavored, velvety-textured, spoon-shaped salad green. Also known as lamb's lettuce. Available in the produce section of some grocery stores such as Trader Joe's or Whole Foods, gourmet markets, or produce markets.

Manchego:

A buttery sheep's milk made in the La Mancha region of Spain, aged between 60 days and two years. Younger Manchego is consider a semi-firm cheese good for melting, while aged Manchego is a firm cheese perfect for grating. Available in the cheese section of most grocery stores, gourmet markets, cheese shops, and online at http://www.markys.com/.

Masa Harina:

Literally translated from Spanish as "dough flour," Masa Harina is a fine, powdery, instant corn flour made from corn kernels that have been treated with an alkali to loosen their outer casings. Used to make tortillas and tamales. A popular brand that I recommend is Maseca. Available in the Hispanic food section or baking section in some grocery stores, gourmet markets, Mexican markets, and at: http://www.mexgrocer.com/.

Mascarpone:

A thick, spreadable, cow's milk, triple-cream Italian cheese with a mild and slightly sweet flavor. Often used in desserts and most well-known for its use in Tiramisu. Available in the cheese or dairy section of most grocery stores, gourmet markets, cheese shops, or online at http://www.markys.com/.

Medjool Dates:

The extremely sweet fruit of the date palm tree, which is dried before eating. Often called the "king of dates" due to their large, meaty size and easy-to-remove pit. Available in the dried fruit section of some grocery stores, gourmet markets, and online at http://foodoro.com/.

Mexican Oregano:

An herb with a similar—yet slightly stronger and less sweet—flavor than standard varieties of oregano. Mexican oregano belongs to the verbena family of plants rather than the mint family. Available in the Hispanic foods section of some grocery stores, gourmet markets, Mexican markets, or online at http://www.penzeys.com.

Micro Greens:

Any variety of edible green that harvested for consumption once the plant is 1 to 2 inches high. If harvested a few days earlier, the greens are known as sprouts and if left until full grown, the greens would be varieties of lettuce and other greens. Available in select specialty produce markets, gourmet markets, and most Trader Joe's, or you can grow your own in a matter of days with seeds from http://www.burpee.com/.

Mission Figs:

Teardrop-shaped figs first grown in California with a purplish-black skin, a reddish flesh, small seeds, and an incredibly sweet flavor. Available seasonally at some grocery stores, gourmet markets, farmer's markets, or online at

http://www.localharvest.org.

New Mexico Chiles:

A medium spicy, dried reddish-brown chile pepper with an earthy flavor that is tapered in shape. Also called chile colorado. Available in the Hispanic foods section of some grocery stores, gourmet markets, Mexican markets, or online at http://www.mexgrocer.com.

Paccheri Pasta:

A large, hollow, tube-shaped pasta. Available in the pasta section of some grocery stores, gourmet markets, or at http://www.markethallfoods.com.

Panko:

Coarsely ground, light, crispy Japanese bread crumbs. Available in most grocery stores, gourmet markets, and at http://www.efooddepot.com.

Pea Shoots/Tendrils:

The tender young shoots of the sweet pea plant that are harvested once they are about 4 inches long. Available in the produce section of some grocery stores, Asian markets, and at farmer's markets.

Pepitas:

Shelled green pumpkin seeds, most often found already roasted. A popular ingredient in Mexican and other Latin American cuisines. Available in the nuts section of some grocery stores, gourmet markets, Mexican markets, and online at http://www.nutsonline.com.

Peppadew Peppers:

The brand name of a small sweet pepper with just a hint of heat that is primarily sold pickled. If your grocery store has an olive bar, try looking there first for peppadews. Available at some grocery stores, gourmet markets, or online at http://www.igourmet.com/.

Pine Nuts/Pignoli:

The high-protein, edible seeds of pine trees. Due to their high oil content, pine nuts have short shelf-lives and should be consumed quickly or stored in the refrigerator. Known as *pignoli* in Italian. Available at most grocery stores, gourmet markets or online at http://www.nutsonline.com.

Piquillo Peppers:

Small Spanish red chile with a sweet flavor similar to that of a ripe bell pepper. Most commonly sold in jars roasted whole, and then peeled and seeded. Available at some grocery stores, gourmet markets, or online at http://www.markys.com.

Poblano Chile:

Large, fresh green chiles with thick walls that make them perfect for stuffing. Spice levels vary from mild to medium, depending on the individual pepper. Available in the produce section of most grocery stores, gourmet markets, and Mexican markets.

Pomegranate Molasses:

The sweet and tart syrup made by reducing pomegranate juice. Available at some grocery stores, gourmet markets, Middle Eastern markets, and online at http://parthenonfoods.net.

Preserved Lemons:

Whole lemons preserved in salt and lemon juice, commonly found in Moroccan and other North African cuisines. Discard the pulp and rinse the rind before using. Make them yourself (see page 238) or available in specialty gourmet stores, Middle Eastern or North African markets, or online at http://www.markys.com.

Quinoa:

The nutty, flat, round-shaped seeds of the leafy plant related to beets originating in the Andes mountains of South America. Nutritionally, quinoa is considered a super-food as it is a complete protein that is high in iron, potassium, and dietary fiber. Available in the grain section of some grocery stores, gourmet markets, health food stores, and at http://www.naturalgrocers.com/.

Rose Water:

The distilled by-product of making rose oil. Used in Middle Eastern cuisines. Rose water can be easily made at home by simmering pesticide-free rose petals in water. Available in some grocery stores, gourmet markets, Middle Eastern markets, or online at http://parthenonfoods.net.

Sambal Oelek:

A bright red, thin, spicy Indonesian condiment made from ground chiles and spices. Available in the Asian section of some grocery stores, gourmet markets, Asian markets, and online at http://www.hotsauce.com.

San Marzano tomatoes:

A variety of plum tomatoes similar to a Roma tomato but with thicker walls, fewer seeds, less acid, and a stronger and sweeter tomato flavor. Available canned in some grocery stores, gourmet markets, Italian markets, and online at http://www.vineandtable.com.

Serrano Chile:

A spicy, relatively small, skinny variety of chile. Often used in Mexican and Latin American cuisine. Available in the produce section of most grocery stores, or seasonally at farmer's markets.

Sherry Vinegar:

A vinegar made from sherry wine. Available at some grocery stores, gourmet markets, or online at http://www.markys.com.

Shiitake Mushrooms

A brown, edible mushroom with a savory, slightly meaty flavor. Grown and widely eaten in Asian cuisines. Store refrigerated in a brown paper bag for a longer shelf-life. Available fresh or dried in some grocery stores, gourmet markets, Asian markets, and online at http://www.markys.com.'

Smoked Paprika:

A spice made from peppers or chiles that have been dried by smoking and ground into a powder. Available in the spice section of most grocery stores, gourmet markets, or online at: http://www.penzeys.com.

Soba Noodles:

Thin, brown, Japanese noodles made from buckwheat. Available in the Asian foods section of some grocery stores, gourmet markets, Asian markets, or online at http://www.asianfoodgrocer.com.

Sriracha:

A Thai hot sauce made from a puree of chiles, vinegar, garlic, sugar, and salt. Often referred to as "rooster sauce" due to the image of a rooster on the bottle. Available in the Asian foods section of some grocery stores, gourmet markets, Asian markets, or at: http://www.asianfoodgrocer.com.

Star Anise:

A star-shaped spice with an intense liquorice flavor. Commonly used in Southeast Asian cuisines. One of the ingredients in the classic Chinese 5-spice blend. Available in the spice section of some grocery stores, gourmet markets, or online at http://www.penzeys.com.

Sumac:

A spice with a bright, lemony flavor made from ground purplish berries of the Rhus Coriaria species of Sumac. Commonly used in Middle Eastern cuisines. Available in the spice section of some grocery stores, gourmet markets, Middle Eastern markets, or at http://www.penzeys.com.

Tahini:

A ground paste made from sesame seeds. Commonly used in Middle Eastern cuisines. Available in some grocery stores, gourmet markets, Middle Eastern markets, or online at http://parthenonfoods.net.

Thai Red Curry Paste:

A moist blend of spicy red chiles, shallots, galangal, garlic, lemongrass, coriander, lime leaves, salt, and spices used as a base for Thai red curry dishes. Available canned in the Asian foods section of some grocery stores, gourmet markets, Asian markets, and at http://importfood.com.

Truffle Oil:

An oil made with the intention of adding the essence of truffles to a dish. Most truffle oils on the market are not actually made from truffles but from a synthetic aromatic product that is found in truffles, as it is hard to actually capture their actual flavor in oil. Truffle oils can be purchased in some grocery stores, gourmet markets, or online at http://www.markys.com.

Valrhona Cocoa Powder:

A pure, intense cocoa powder made by Valrhona—a renowned French chocolate manufacturer. Available in some gourmet markets and specialty baking stores, or online at http://www.valrhona-chocolate.com.

Wasabi Powder/Paste:

A powder or paste made from ground horseradish, mustard and green dye, as real wasabi root is extremely hard grow, making it very expensive. Both wasabi paste and powders are widely available in the Asian foods section of most grocery stores, gourmet markets, and Asian markets. Imitation and real wasabi powder are both available at http://www.penzeys.com.

White Asparagus:

Regular asparagus that has been grown without sunlight. Available seasonally at some grocery stores, gourmet markets, farmer's markets, and online at http://www.tienda.com/.

Index

0 26575 53993 6